Health Psychology Consultation in the Inpatient Medical Setting

Health Psychology Consultation in the Inpatient Medical Setting

SUSAN M. LABOTT

American Psychological Association
Washington, DC

Published by
American Psychological Association
750 First Street, NE
Washington, DC 20002
www.apa.org

APA Order Department
P.O. Box 92984
Washington, DC 20090-2984
Phone: (800) 374-2721; Direct: (202) 336-5510
Fax: (202) 336-5502; TDD/TTY: (202) 336-6123
Online: http://www.apa.org/pubs/books
E-mail: order@apa.org

In the U.K., Europe, Africa, and the Middle East, copies may be ordered from
Eurospan Group
c/o Turpin Distribution
Pegasus Drive
Stratton Business Park
Biggleswade, Bedfordshire
SG18 8TQ United Kingdom
Phone: +44 (0) 1767 604972
Fax: +44 (0) 1767 601640
Online: https://www.eurospanbookstore.com/apa
E-mail: eurospan@turpin-distribution.com

Typeset in Meridien by Circle Graphics, Inc., Columbia, MD

Printer: Sheridan Books, Chelsea, MI
Cover Designer: Naylor Design, Washington, DC

Library of Congress Cataloging-in-Publication Data
Names: Labott, Susan M., author.
Title: Health psychology consultation in the inpatient medical setting / By Susan M. Labott.
Description: Washington, DC : American Psychological Association, [2019] | Includes bibliographical references and index.
Identifiers: LCCN 2018010863 (print) | LCCN 2018013516 (ebook) | ISBN 9781433829628 (ebook) | ISBN 1433829622 (ebook) | ISBN 9781433829611 (print) | ISBN 1433829614 (print)
Subjects: | MESH: Inpatients—psychology | Behavioral Medicine—methods | Interprofessional Relations | Referral and Consultation
Classification: LCC RC512 (ebook) | LCC RC512 (print) | NLM WX 158.5 | DDC 616.89—dc23
LC record available at https://lccn.loc.gov/2018010863

British Library Cataloguing-in-Publication Data
A CIP record is available from the British Library.

Printed in the United States of America
First Edition

http://dx.doi.org/10.1037/0000108-000

10 9 8 7 6 5 4 3 2 1

To Jim—you always had my six

Contents

IV

V

Acknowledgments

Thanks to the many patients who have shared their struggles and successes as they navigated their way through difficult medical and psychological problems. Thanks also to my students and colleagues for helping me collect and articulate my thoughts about this work. Finally, special thanks and love to my parents, Arlene and Robert Labott, for everything.

Health Psychology Consultation in the Inpatient Medical Setting

Introduction

Psychological practice in the inpatient medical setting is different in many ways from both outpatient clinical work and inpatient work in a psychiatric unit. Yet psychology trainees usually begin their first clinical placement in a hospital without any guidance or coursework on how to work in that setting. The same is true of established clinicians who have not specialized in health psychology. Although supervisors usually have a good grasp of the relevant issues, there is never enough time to sit with every trainee or to run a basic seminar on hospital work before the trainee begins.

This book seeks to provide basic information on clinical and professional issues operative in the inpatient medical setting for individuals who already have skills in general clinical psychology but who have little experience in a hospital. It addresses clinical questions, such as the following:

- What is delirium and how do I treat it?
- How do I treat anxiety that is directly caused by medication, rather than due to psychological concerns?

The book also addresses ethical questions, such as the following:

- What if a patient refuses to be seen?
- How do I maintain confidentiality when I am working with a large medical team?

http://dx.doi.org/10.1037/0000108-001
Health Psychology Consultation in the Inpatient Medical Setting, by S. M. Labott

It addresses professional issues, such as the following:

- How do I handle a patient's death?
- What do I do if I am evaluating a patient and another provider also wants to see the patient?

It answers basic questions regarding consultation, including the following:

- How do I understand the medical information in the patient's chart?
- What should my report look like, and where does it go?

This book provides detailed instruction on matters of significance when working in a hospital, including interpretation of the medical record, description of major psychological problems that occur in the hospital, and conducting assessment and treatment in this setting. It also provides information on attending to particular patient needs in the hospital setting, such as evaluating decisional capacity and helping them deal with end-of-life issues.

The theoretical approach of this book follows the biopsychosocial model, the current standard of practice in clinical health psychology. In this model, the biological, social, and psychological dimensions of illness are all considered when developing a conceptualization of the patient and his or her illness. The interventions described for use with medical inpatients are based largely on cognitive–behavioral, evidence-based approaches. For some of the thorny questions in this book, there is no empirical literature; these are discussed from a practical perspective based on the author's many years of clinical experience in this setting.

The book is divided into five parts. Part I focuses on the hospital setting and inpatient consultation models. Chapter 1 explains the structure of hospital units and the hierarchy of medical teams, as well as relevant hospital standards, including credentials and privileges. Differences between hospital and outpatient practice are discussed, as well as documentation and infection control procedures. Chapter 2 describes the biopsychosocial model—the foundation of inpatient health psychology consultation—as well as various types of consultations and consultation services in which a psychologist can work.

Part II addresses the nuts and bolts of performing an inpatient consultation. Chapter 3 describes background preparation before seeing the patient and includes information on understanding the referral, interpreting the medical record, and generating specific topics to be addressed in the interview with the patient. Chapter 4 describes the patient interview and includes tips on getting it started, specific content to cover, common problems in conducting inpatient interviews, and providing feedback to the patient. Chapter 5 discusses gathering collateral information, integrating data, and providing written and verbal reports to the patient's medical providers.

Part III addresses common psychological issues in the hospital setting. Chapter 6 defines and describes adjustment problems faced by hospitalized patients and describes theories of adjustment, relevant tasks and interventions to aid adjustment, and factors that can influence adjustment. Chapter 7 addresses anxiety and describes etiologies of anxiety that can occur in the hospital, such as premorbid anxiety, new anxiety due to the current medical situation, medical disorders that can present with anxiety, and anxiety symptoms caused by medications. Treatments to address anxiety are presented, including education, medication, and cognitive–behavioral interventions. Chapter 8 addresses depression and includes a description of its various etiologies, including premorbid depression, new-onset depression secondary to a medical problem, medical disorders associated with depression, and depression due to medication. Suicide in hospitalized patients is discussed, as are relevant risk factors. Interventions to address depression and depressed mood are described and include education, cognitive–behavioral strategies, social support, and psychotropic medication. Chapter 9 defines delirium, its clinical features, and its causes. Means to assess and diagnose delirium are described, together with strategies for the management of delirious patients. Chapter 10 focuses on substance use and abuse and begins with a description of referrals for substance use. The prevalence and impacts of illicit and prescription drug use are presented, as well as assessment strategies. Psychological treatments for drug and alcohol overuse are then delineated.

Part IV is focused on special issues in the hospital, that is, those occurring frequently in the hospital but less often in the outpatient setting. Chapter 11 addresses decisional capacity and describes referrals, criteria for capacity, the evaluation to determine capacity, and implications if the patient lacks decisional capacity. Chapter 12 deals with nonadherence to medical recommendations and outlines the implications of nonadherence and relevant theoretical models. Factors that influence adherence are presented, as are strategies to establish initial adherence, evaluate adherence problems, and interventions to address nonadherence. Chapter 13 is focused on pain and includes sections on assessment, factors that affect pain, and psychological interventions to decrease pain. Chapter 14 deals with end-of-life issues. It includes details about the primary concerns of dying patients, advance directives, death with dignity legislation, and steps the psychologist can take to promote a good death.

Part V focuses on ethics and professional issues. Chapter 15 discusses ethical issues that are especially relevant in the hospital, such as confidentiality, respect for other professionals, and culture and diversity issues. Chapter 16 provides guidance for training students in the hospital setting, as well as billing matters. Developing a professional identity, caring for oneself, marketing inpatient psychology services, and other professional challenges are also discussed.

My perspective on health psychology inpatient work is derived from a university-based medical center, but the information and examples are also applicable for consultants working in nonacademic hospitals. The cases and medical record samples are based on real patients and provider notes, but identifying information has been altered to protect patient privacy. Throughout the book, I have made some patients and providers male and others female to avoid the cumbersome use of "he or she."

THE INPATIENT SETTING AND CONSULTATION MODELS

I

The Hospital Milieu

1

Providing psychological services in an inpatient medical setting can be intimidating to those who have not previously worked in a hospital. The pace can be fast, the logistics of seeing patients are different from the outpatient setting, and most patients have not requested any psychological evaluation or treatment. There are also rules and norms to be followed that may be wholly unfamiliar to professionals who have worked exclusively in outpatient settings. An understanding of the structure and expectations of the hospital setting will facilitate the health psychology consultant's work and also enhance her reputation among medical colleagues. These topics are described more fully in this chapter.

Hospital Units, Medical Teams, and the Health Psychology Consultant

Most hospitals are separated into at least some specialized units. Even small hospitals may have specialized obstetrics, pediatric, and intensive care units (ICUs). The larger the hospital, the more specialized units there are likely to be, with certain floors dedicated to patients with specific medical needs, such as cardiology, general medicine, oncology, or orthopedics. Some hospitals

http://dx.doi.org/10.1037/0000108-002
Health Psychology Consultation in the Inpatient Medical Setting, by S. M. Labott

may even have specialized ICUs, for example, for cardiology, neurosurgery, or transplant. When a referral is received, the location of the patient may provide a clue to the patient's main medical issue. At times, however, floor assignment is a result of bed availability.

In teaching hospitals, patients are treated by teams of physicians. These teams are headed by the attending physician (referred to as *the attending*), who is a faculty member in the medical school and is involved in teaching, supervision, research, and patient care activities. The attending is ultimately responsible for the patient's care, although much of the actual treatment is performed by other members of the team. There is often a *fellow*, who has completed his medical residency and is now completing specialty training (such as in emergency medicine, cardiology, or pulmonary disease), usually for 2 to 3 years. The treatment team may also include one or more medical residents. Residents have finished medical school and are working on their medical residency, which is required before becoming an independent practitioner. They are sometimes referred to as *house staff* because they manage all patient care under the supervision of the attending. Residents work long hours because they are frequently on call, spending many sleepless nights in the hospital dealing with emergent medical issues. There may also be medical students on the team who are currently in medical school and have little experience in patient care. One motto of medical training is "see one, do one, teach one"; in practice, this means the individuals on the treatment team who are providing patient care will have varying levels of experience in interviewing, performing medical procedures, and negotiating the hospital system.

Members of the primary medical treatment team will see the patient each day to evaluate the patient's progress and to perform procedures. The entire team will round together once daily, visiting all of the patients for whom they are responsible. During rounds, members of the team describe the patient's status, plans are made regarding next steps in the treatment, and the attending provides supervision. If the health psychology consultant is present at the time of the primary team's rounds, it is useful to listen to the team's discussion of the patient as well as their meeting with the patient, if appropriate. This will provide the psychologist with details about the treatment issues and the team's decision-making about them, as well as an opportunity to observe interaction patterns between the patient and his medical providers. Rounds may also provide a forum for the health psychology consultant to update the team about the psychological issues and the psychological treatment plan. Although it may perhaps be anxiety provoking initially, the psychologist should be prepared to address questions from the treatment team any time they are encountered; this is a good opportunity for the health psychologist to provide relevant information and to demonstrate his usefulness to the medical team and the patient.

All members of the primary medical team rotate on and off, and not all on the same schedule; for example, the attending may be "on service" (which means he is leading a team in the hospital) for a month, whereas the fellow and residents may be on the team for several months, under the supervision of different attendings. The primary treatment team is assigned certain patients; for example, the cardiology team will see patients admitted for cardiac problems. In a large hospital, many of these patients will be located in one unit. If a patient from a cardiology unit is transferred to the ICU, the cardiology team will likely follow (i.e., continue to treat) the patient there, although the ICU medical team may take primary responsibility while the patient is in the ICU. In most cases, a health psychology consultant who is following a patient will continue to treat that patient if she moves to a different unit. An exception to this is if the new unit has other psychological services available, for example, if a cardiology patient is transferred to a psychiatry unit after she is stable medically. In that case, the health psychology consultant would ensure continuity of care, while transferring the patient to a new mental health provider located on that unit. The health psychology consultant could continue to see the patient if he has been working with the patient on a specific issue that cannot be readily managed by a provider on the new unit (e.g., if teaching specific imagery techniques for pain management, if there are no mental health providers on the new unit with expertise in this area).

Because most of the day-to-day care of the patient is provided by the fellows and residents, these are the people with whom the health psychology consultant will interact most often. They will typically order consultations, including those for health psychology, and are usually the contact person for providing feedback after the patient has been seen.

Nonacademic hospitals, including large community medical centers and small community hospitals, are staffed differently. Here, doctors who are private practitioners may see their own outpatients when they are admitted to the hospital. In these settings, the attending is the senior physician who is assigned to the case and who will "follow" (i.e., treat) the patient while she is in the hospital. In the nonacademic hospital setting, there is generally no team of fellows, residents, and medical students.

Nurses are a great source of information for the health psychology consultant. They are generally updated on the most recent changes in the patient's situation and are aware of issues that have not yet made it into the patient's medical record. Many nurses treat the same patients day after day and have spent a significant amount of time with them. They are usually good listeners and have had ample time to observe the patient. Patients often confide in their nurses, making them privy to information that others are unaware of. They may be aware of family and social dynamics from observing patients with their visitors. Nurses are on the front line for management of a patient's behavior and safety, for example, in the case of a patient who is delirious or aggressive. Not only will a nurse be able to describe the patient's behavior in detail, she may also be able to compare the patient's current status with his baseline behavior and cognition, aiding the psychologist in making the correct diagnosis. In certain units of a hospital, *nurse practitioners* may be allowed to prescribe medication and may be the main point of contact with the medical team for the psychology consultant.

Most hospital units also have a dedicated *ward clerk* who answers telephones, locates nurses and patients, pages staff, directs visitors, and handles many other tasks to keep the unit running efficiently. Ward clerks know who is responsible for what on the unit and how to find everyone; they can provide much helpful information to the health psychology consultant, especially on an unfamiliar unit or when the relevant providers are unknown.

Unless there has previously been a strong health psychology presence in the hospital, medical personnel may not have a clear idea of who a health psychology consultant is and what he has to offer to the patients and medical staff, so the health psychology consultant will need to educate others about his role. This is done by explicitly telling others what the role of the health psychologist is, as well as by demonstrating it through patient treatment and liaison with medical teams. This education sometimes involves contrasting the work of the health psychology consultant with someone whose role the medical team already understands, such as that of the psychiatrist or the social worker.

One of the best ways to educate others about the role of the health psychology consultant is to describe our work to them as we provide feedback on a particular patient. That is, providing a brief conceptualization of the patient's problem and our treatment plan can show the primary medical team how we think about patients and what we can do to help (see Exhibit 1.1).

At times, the psychologist's response to a referral question will help the members of the medical team do *their* work (e.g., in an assessment of a patient's decisional capacity). If a patient is refusing treatment, the psychologist's conclusion about the patient's decisional capacity will allow the medical team to determine what their next steps should be. In other cases, making plans to help the medical team manage a difficult patient can make the patient's treatment easier and will demonstrate ways in which the health psychology consultant can help them with the management of patient behavior. The brief script in Exhibit 1.2 demonstrates how the health psychology consultant can work with the medical team to manage a patient's behavior.

Once the medical providers understand the role of the health psychology consultant, they can be encouraged to inform patients when a health psychology consultation is being ordered so that patients are not surprised when the consultant arrives. This is best done by describing a team approach to patient care and the role of the health psychology consultant in helping patients to manage the stress of medical illness, rather than by describing the consultation in terms of mental illness.

EXHIBIT 1.1

Describing the Consulting Psychologist's Role on the Health Team

"You asked us to see Ms. X because she is crying and seems anxious. She *is* anxious—she has never really been sick before, and she is scared about what her test results will show. Also, her husband died in this hospital about 2 years ago, and being back here has stirred up a lot of emotions for her. We are teaching her ways to manage her anxiety and she is doing well with that. We are also working with her to manage her grief, and will provide outpatient grief therapy referrals if she needs that when she is ready for discharge."

EXHIBIT 1.2

Explaining How the Health Psychologist Can Help Manage a Patient's Behavior

"Ms. Y has been calling at all hours with additional questions that you have already answered for her. She is anxious, and does better when she has information, but she has a poor memory, so she does not recall what you have told her, and so she asks again and again. We are working on some organizational strategies with her and suggested that she write down her questions as well as the answers you provide. We have also encouraged her not to call you each time she has a question but to save her questions for morning rounds. We have also arranged to have the patient's daughter come each morning, so that she is present when you round. She will help the patient make notes and will also remind the patient if she forgets things that you told her. We will also plan to see the patient later each day to help her review and process the information you have given her and to teach her additional anxiety management techniques."

Credentials, Privileges, and Medical Staff Membership

Like any other provider in a hospital, a health psychology consultant should always wear appropriate medical center identification. To practice in a hospital, the health psychology consultant must be certified by the hospital as a qualified professional who provides certain defined services. *Credentialing* refers to the process in which a provider's credentials (i.e., education, licensure, and training) are reviewed by a hospital board to determine that the psychologist meets required criteria to provide psychological services. All providers in the hospital are subject to this process. Once credentialed, there is typically a review to recredential the provider every few years. This recredentialing process may involve a review of the provider's work and may include a review of reports in the medical record—both for content and timeliness—and also letters of support from colleagues.

Privileges refer to the specific services that a credentialed provider is allowed to perform in the hospital. These are requested by the provider, then approved (or not) by a review board. These privileges are typically also revisited every few years and adjusted as needed. The process is the same for other medical providers; for example, an oncologist may have privileges for ordering chemotherapy, performing biopsies, and infusing stem cells but would not be approved to do psychotherapy or neuropsychological assessment. Hospitals vary in the number of privileges available to providers and the detail with which these privileges are defined. That is, a small hospital may allow psychologists to provide inpatient psychological services, outpatient psychological services, or both. In other places, privileges for psychologists may be further differentiated into inpatient psychological services that include consultation, group therapy, pediatric treatment, or neuropsychological assessment. The psychologist requests the privileges based on his training, experience, and expected practice and then must practice within these categories of privileges until other privileges are requested and granted. See Robiner, Dixon, Miner, and Hong (2010) for a detailed discussion of privileges for psychologists who work in hospitals

Physicians in hospitals are members of the medical staff, typically pay dues to belong, and are involved in governance of the institution and their profession. Depending on the setting, psychologists may or may not be full voting members of the medical staff and may be designated as an affiliate or some other category of membership that has fewer rights and responsibilities. To the extent that psychologists can be involved in the workings of the medical staff, they can provide input on issues that will affect the practice of psychology in the hospital, consistent with American Psychological Association (2013) guidelines.

Practical Issues When Treating Medical Inpatients

Some of the practical issues to consider when consulting as part of a medical team include reframing one's professional role and relationship with patients, understanding the pace and workflow in a hospital, and quickly internalizing procedures and expectations with regard to infection and documentation.

OUTPATIENT PROVIDER VERSUS PSYCHOLOGICAL CONSULTANT

Many psychologists have experience as an independent provider in an office or clinic setting, consulting with other providers as needed. In the hospital setting, the health psychologist may perform evaluation and intervention, but in the role of a consultant, a role that is somewhat different from that of an independent provider. The consultant works with the primary medical team, but the patient belongs to them, not to the consultant. The psychological treatment should always be coordinated with the medical treatment and should not interfere with it in any way. Some patients will need intense psychological treatment, but much of that may need to be postponed until the patient is an outpatient. The priority in the hospital is the medical treatment, and although the psychological treatment can be an important part of that, it is secondary to the medical treatment. The health psychology consultant provides feedback to the primary treatment team, which in turn makes the overall decisions on the patient's care. Specifically, this means that the health psychology consultant would typically not write orders for the patient but would make recommendations to the treatment team, such as for neuropsychological testing, physical therapy, or a psychiatry evaluation that the primary treatment team can then choose to follow or not.

It is important to be accessible to the primary treatment team, so that they can contact the health psychology consultant with any questions they have about the patient's psychological care; this is especially relevant as the patient nears discharge and plans for any outpatient psychological follow-up need to be made. In the outpatient setting, returning a telephone call within 24 hours is often acceptable. In the inpatient setting, however, pages or texts need to be returned within a few minutes because the hospital setting has a faster pace than the outpatient setting, and decisions need to be made and implemented more quickly.

INPATIENTS GENERALLY DO NOT REQUEST SERVICES

Most psychologists have experience with clients who make an appointment and come to the office, seeking help with a specific presenting problem. Those clients choose to seek mental health services and are motivated to achieve some outcome that they desire. In the medical inpatient setting, this is typically not the case. Patients rarely ask to be seen for a psychological evaluation; instead, one of their medical providers deems the psychological consultation necessary and orders it. Patients may not know what a health psychology evaluation involves or feel that it is warranted, nor are they always even aware that the consultation has been requested for them. In these cases, then, the visit by the health psychology consultant is a surprise to the patient. The reason for the visit should be described to patients so that they have an idea of what to expect because many have never seen a mental health professional before. Providing a general idea of what the consultation is about will help patients adhere to the treatment plan and increase their comfort with the interview (see Chapter 4, this volume, for more detail on explaining this to patients).

SCHEDULING, WORKFLOW, AND PACE

Most inpatient work is not scheduled as an outpatient visit is, that is, with an appointment at a particular time on a specific date, although there can be exceptions. If a patient is very busy with appointments, such as on an acute rehabilitation unit where several hours of physical therapy and occupational therapy are required daily, it may be possible to informally schedule an appointment, usually with the patient's nurse, to be sure you are able to see the patient on a certain day. Flexibility is important, as other activities may still interfere. More commonly, medical professionals have a list of patients they need to see on a particular day, and they circulate around the hospital until all the work is completed. The most urgent issues need to be prioritized. One implication of this system is that several people from different services (e.g., health psychology, neurology, infectious disease) may need to see the same patient and will need to work around each other so that they can all get their work done. If a patient is newly admitted or if new medical issues have developed, there may be a host of people who need to see and evaluate the patient in a short amount of time. For example, if a patient was admitted with a fall and possible stroke, the primary service may request consultations with orthopedics, neurology, physical therapy, and health psychology all on the same day. Each of these consultants typically has 24 hours to complete the evaluation and provide recommendations to the primary medical team. All of these providers will come and go throughout the day, making it very busy for patients at times.

The system dictates that providers will need to work around each other to get all the work done. There are unwritten rules about how this works, and the individual consultants need to work this out on a case-by-case basis. The main issue that dictates which service has priority is the importance of the information to be gained from the evaluation provided by that specialty area. For example, in the preceding case, a neurological evaluation is necessary to determine whether the patient has had a stroke and what treatment is warranted. Although the health psychology evaluation will be important to the patient's overall coping and adjustment with the medical condition, in the acute phase while the diagnosis is being determined, the neurology consultation is more important. If the health psychologist is in the process of an evaluation when the neurologist arrives, a health psychologist who is a good team player will make plans to return to finish the interview later so that the neurologist can complete her evaluation in a timely manner.

Another variable that enters into this decision of whose work takes precedence is the amount of time the provider needs to complete her evaluation with the patient. The health psychology evaluation takes a lot of time, relative to many of the medical interviews. Sometimes other providers will only need to ask the patient a few basic questions to proceed with their work. If the health psychology evaluation is underway and the patient's medical resident arrives to ask the patient a few questions about his home medications (to be sure the orders for the inpatient admission are properly written), it makes sense for the health psychologist either to step aside and let the medical resident interrupt to get the information she needs or step out of the room briefly and then continue the evaluation when the resident is finished. The rules for whose visit takes priority may seem vague, but common sense will help one figure out what to do in each specific situation. Learning to negotiate this issue as a professional will be important in the long term because the health psychology consultant will meet the same people from other disciplines repeatedly in patient rooms, and building collaborative relationships will pay off over time.

The amount of time spent with a hospitalized patient is variable and depends on the work that the health psychologist needs to do with the patient. For example, an initial evaluation will take longer than a follow-up visit. It also depends on other factors in the hospital (e.g., the patient needs to go for an ultrasound). Comprehensive initial evaluations can take an hour or longer. Follow-up visits for treatment or monitoring could occur daily for 10 to 20 minutes or might only occur every few days, depending on the issues being addressed. Some patients may be followed for the duration of their hospital stay, especially those who have difficulty coping with a new diagnosis and treatment. Others may be seen only for a few visits—for example, when assessing decisional capacity, especially if nothing else needs to be addressed after the evaluation.

Because of the pace of the inpatient hospital setting, the health psychology consultant needs to be able to access information quickly, to be able to answer questions and make decisions about patient care promptly. Exhibit 1.3 is a list of resources that will enable the psychologist to function efficiently, while avoiding calls to others or trips to the library to get necessary information. Some of these resources can be carried electronically, and others will be on paper in a lab coat pocket or on a clipboard.

EXHIBIT 1.3

Resources for the Health Psychology Consultation

Mental status examination questions
List of common medical abbreviations (see Chapter 3 and Appendix A)
Telephone and pager numbers for interpreters, social work, psychiatry on call
Frequently used outpatient psychology, psychiatry, and substance abuse referrals
Consultation questions outline (see Chapter 4, Exhibit 4.1)
Psychiatric medications and standard doses
Causes of delirium
Pens and paper for notes and patient drawings
Information relevant to special settings (e.g., oncology drugs that cause psychological side effects)

DOCUMENTATION

All interactions with patients must be documented in the patient's medical record. Placing notes in the medical record informs other members of the treatment team about the work the psychologist is doing with the patient and can facilitate coordinated care. Although patient care is the main function of documentation, it is also necessary for legal and billing purposes. Medical record documentation is generally concise, while providing enough detail so that others can understand the content and relevant details.

All providers regularly make decisions about what specific content to place into the medical record. As a health psychology consultant, there are times when less detail is desirable, such as when a patient provides specific information regarding sexual abuse or marital conflicts. Health psychology inpatient notes are not separated from the rest of the record as outpatient psychology treatment notes may be, so if medical records are requested for any reason, health psychology notes are sent out along with the rest. Further, doctors, nurses, and many other providers in the hospital have access to these notes. Therefore, consideration must be given to the reporting of sensitive issues; specific and detailed information on issues such as sexuality, abuse, and other potentially sensitive issues should be avoided unless they are directly pertinent to the medical problem. For example, if a patient reports detailed information on a spouse's infidelities and how this has affected her depression and noncompliance with medical treatment, rather than providing details about the infidelity in the patient's medical record, the report could refer to "marital stressors" that played a role in the patient's emotional state and nonadherence. As Robinson and Baker (2006) noted, "One simple rule of thumb is not to write anything in the medical record that a psychologist does not want other people, including the patient, to know" (p. 266). Although medical records are confidential, there are still many people who could learn information from the psychologist's report that they do not need to know and that could negatively influence their interactions with the patient.

A psychologist might not document a lesbian relationship if the patient has adequate social support and the relationship is stable. Yet that information could be relevant if the medical team is setting up postdischarge care for the patient. Medical staff who are aware that she is in a lesbian relationship can rephrase their typical questions about her husband and his ability to help her after discharge.

There are times when explicit detail is absolutely necessary in the medical record, such as when describing a patient's risk for suicide. The cardinal rule of documentation is that "if it wasn't documented, it didn't happen." Although certainly important for the patient's care, detailed documentation of the psychologist's evaluation of suicide potential is critical if litigation occurs later.

Notes and reports from the health psychology consultant may need to follow a particular format, depending on the rules at a particular institution, and there may also be rules about the placement of psychology notes in the medical record, as well as specific information to include in those notes, such as billing codes. If there is no specific format dictated by the institution, initial evaluation reports can follow the format demonstrated in Chapter 5. Follow-up notes would be shorter and would generally focus on the specific issue for which the patient is being treated (also see examples of these notes in Chapter 5). All notes should include contact information for the health psychology consultant to facilitate communication with other providers if they have questions or input on the patient and his care.

Documentation on work done with hospitalized patients must be completed promptly or it is not useful. For example, adding a report to the medical record that describes the behavior of a delirious patient 24 hours after the evaluation may be irrelevant because the patient's presentation may be completely different by then. Many medical centers have rules on how quickly documentation needs to be finalized in the medical record. Regardless of formal documentation, verbal feedback on initial evaluations and serious issues should be promptly provided to the treatment team.

INFECTION CONTROL PROCEDURES

Standard precautions to control infection include handwashing; avoiding touch; wearing gloves when contacting secretions, blood, and fluids; and proper handling of sharps, spills, and medical equipment (World Health Organization, 2002). These procedures are to be used with every patient in the hospital, regardless of the patient's diagnosis, to prevent transmission of infection. For psychologists, because there is no expected contact with blood or bodily fluids, standard precautions require handwashing before and after seeing the patient. Proper handwashing is the single most important behavior that providers can use to protect themselves and patients from infection and involves washing hands thoroughly with soap and water or with a hand disinfectant (usually located outside of patient rooms).

Transmission-based precautions are put in place for cases in which standard precautions are not sufficient to interrupt the spread of infection. These are instituted for patients who have been diagnosed with specific infections or an infection that is suspected but as yet undiagnosed. The additional level of precaution is indicated with a sign near the patient's room. Contact precautions are a type of transmission-based precaution for patients who have infections that can be transmitted to others, such as vancomycin-resistant enterococcus (VRE), methicillin-resistant *Staphylococcus aureus* (MRSA), and *Clostridium difficile* (*C. diff*). Although it is possible that a healthy health care provider could contract one of these infections from contact with the patient, it is more likely that the provider will carry the infection to another patient who is less able to resist the infection and who will then contract it. Contact isolation procedures include wearing a gown and gloves, in addition to handwashing before and after the interaction with the patient. The gown and gloves are put on before entering the patient's room and then removed and left inside the patient's room in the garbage after the visit (so that the infection is not taken outside of the room). Even though a health psychology consultant generally has no intention of touching any blood or body fluids, and perhaps not even of touching the patient at all, these procedures must be followed for two reasons: (a) a provider never knows when a patient may become delirious, pull an IV line, vomit, bleed, or do a variety of other things that would put the provider in unexpected contact with bodily fluids; and (b) hospitals can get into serious trouble with regard to their accreditation if someone is seen not following the appropriate precautionary procedures.

Other organisms are transmitted by droplets in the air, such as influenza and pertussis, and require droplet precautions. Transmission of these organisms is most likely to occur when the patient is coughing or sneezing or during access to mucous membranes, such as during a bronchoscopy procedure. In addition to standard precautions, droplet precautions include wearing a mask as a barrier so that the provider does not inhale the droplets.

Airborne precautions are put in place for patients who have (or are suspected of having) an organism that is transmitted through the air, such as tuberculosis or measles. Organisms transmitted by air are made up of small particles (much smaller than droplets) that remain suspended in the air, and so special ventilation systems are used in the rooms of patients who have organisms that can be transmitted in this way. In addition, the provider must wear a specific type of respirator (mask), typically the N95 type. This is a more solid mask than that used for droplets, and it does not allow the organisms in the air to pass through and be inhaled.

The respirator needs to be fitted yearly for each provider (called *fit testing*), and the provider needs to know which size to use and also how to adjust it properly for maximum effectiveness. Therefore, if a health psychology consultant has not been fitted for this specific type of mask, he is not able to enter the patient's room. See Siegel, Rhinehart, Jackson, Chiarello, and the Health Care Infection Control Practices Advisory Committee (2007) for more information on transmission-based precautions.

Neutropenic precautions are for patients whose immune system is impaired, that is, they do not have sufficient neutrophils to protect themselves from infection. A low neutrophil count can occur after chemotherapy, during a stem cell transplant, and at other times. Neutropenic precautions are sometimes referred to as *reverse precautions* because the purpose is to protect the patient, rather than the provider. During the time of neutropenia, the patient can contract infections and even die from organisms that would pose no threat to a healthy person. In the case of neutropenic precautions, providers wear a gown and gloves, often a mask, and perhaps also booties over the shoes. Recall that in the case of contact isolation, the gown and gloves are left inside the patient's room, but in the case of neutropenic precautions, these are worn out into the hallway after the visit with the patient, and thrown away there, to avoid the provider leaving any potentially dangerous organisms inside the patient's room.

PRACTICAL ISSUES REGARDING INFECTION CONTROL PROCEDURES

Although many providers will shake hands with a patient when introducing themselves, hand-shaking should be avoided for infection control reasons. Some mental health providers will make a point of shaking hands, especially with certain patients (e.g., someone newly diagnosed with HIV) to indicate to the patient that they are not stigmatized. However, given the risks to patients of infections that can be transmitted by their providers, it is desirable for providers to demonstrate respect for their patients in other ways.

If the health psychology consultant has a cold or other transmittable infection, she should take additional precautions to protect patients—*all* patients, regardless of neutropenic or other precautions that are in place. This could include avoiding contact with the patient (e.g., call the patient on the telephone rather than going in to the room or have a colleague cover the patient's treatment temporarily), keeping visits as short as possible, and wearing a mask to avoid infecting the patient. Patients are appreciative when providers take any and all measures available to protect them from infection.

Following these precautions can be uncomfortable and cumbersome. Many people, when wearing a mask for more than a few minutes, become hot and feel faint. If that occurs, visits need to be kept short to avoid the provider passing out in the patient's room. Wearing gloves can make it difficult to take notes, so it is usually easiest to skip notes when in the patient's room, do a briefer interview, and make notes when back outside the room. If notes are warranted with a patient on transmission-based precautions, the clipboard and pen need to be disinfected or thrown out, and paper notes (e.g., patient drawings from a mental status examination) need to be immediately copied and thrown out. The health psychology consultant will notice that other providers will take similar precautions (e.g., a dedicated stethoscope is left in the patient's room for all providers to use with only that patient; patients use plastic silverware, cardboard trays, and paper dishes that can be thrown out rather than cleaned and used again with another patient). The general rule is that any object that goes into the room of a patient on transmission-based precautions does not come back out to be used elsewhere.

Summary and Additional Suggestions

The hospital setting is unique, and psychologists who have not worked in this setting will need to educate themselves so that they can function responsibly and effectively in the hospital milieu. The American Psychological Association (1985) has provided

EXHIBIT 1.4

Suggestions for Psychologists in the Hospital

Use plain English, not "psychologese": Be aware that your notes and reports are not being written for other mental health professionals, so avoid psychological jargon and abbreviations (e.g., SI for suicidal ideation).

Be action-oriented. Medical providers in the hospital may ask what to do; don't hesitate to tell them (e.g., discuss the treatment plan with the patient again; explain what needs to happen prior to discharge).

Be brief. Written and verbal reports need to be clear and to the point, or you will lose your audience and not be perceived as helpful to them.

Know what you are doing, and know your limits. If you don't know something, admit it.

Doctors are generally quite willing to explain a medical issue. If there is a question you can research to find the answer to, especially of a psychological nature, do it and report back. Never say you will find something out and then drop it without an answer.

Be polite, friendly, and helpful when it is appropriate. Be friendly to hospital staff members, remember their names, demonstrate that you can be helpful with the patient.

Do not feel like a second-class citizen. You have a right to be in the hospital, and your work will demonstrate to your medical colleagues that you have skills and resources that can be valuable to them and their patients.

Be flexible in how you practice. Be aware of different contexts on specialized units of the hospital (e.g., preferences for immediate call backs on patients versus reports at daily team meetings) and adjust your work appropriately.

Do not form inappropriate alliances on the treatment team. While a social worker and psychologist might tend to see things similarly, do not collude to push certain agendas.

At times it may be appropriate to offer support to a member of the treatment team, but it is not your responsibility to care for their mental health needs or to resolve conflicts between others.

Respect the hierarchy of the situation. Be aware of issues of rank and respond appropriately. Remember that you are treating the medical team's patient. You may also need to provide feedback to several members of the team independently to ensure that everyone is on the same page.

Note. Adapted from *A Hospital Practice Primer for Psychologists* (pp. 29–30), by the Committee on Professional Practice of the Board of Professional Affairs, 1985, Washington, DC: American Psychological Association. Copyright 1985 by the American Psychological Association.

a list of suggestions for psychologists who are working in a hospital setting, designed to help the psychologist establish credibility and fit in. These are listed and expanded upon in Exhibit 1.4. Colleagues and other hospital staff can also be good resources who can answer questions on credentialing, documentation, precautions, and other issues. As the health psychology consultant begins to function in the hospital, he will develop his own professional style, discussed more in Chapter 16.

Consultation Models and Content

2

The biopsychosocial model is the foundation on which all of health psychology inpatient consultation is built. Initially proposed by Engel (1977, 1980) in response to the limitations of the biomedical model, the biopsychosocial model includes psychological and social aspects of the human experience, which were not previously considered in the conceptualization of medical illness. There is currently general agreement that medical treatment is most successful when the conceptualization of a patient's illness includes biological, psychological, and social factors. Using the biopsychosocial model, a holistic conceptualization of the medical problem can be translated into a comprehensive treatment plan that is informed by all relevant factors.

Medical treatment is less successful if the biological, psychological, and social factors are not considered simultaneously. Consider Mr. S, who is a patient with diabetes mellitus and end-stage renal disease. His doctor recommends treatment with insulin and hemodialysis. However, Mr. S does not understand the relationship between these proposed interventions and his disease, so he has no motivation to deal with the inconvenience of these treatments. He also has no social support to help him understand the treatment plan, learn to self-administer insulin, and organize transportation to dialysis. As a result, he does not adhere to the treatment recommendations.

http://dx.doi.org/10.1037/0000108-003
Health Psychology Consultation in the Inpatient Medical Setting, by S. M. Labott

Although the treatment would have a good likelihood of managing his illnesses successfully, it is not utilized because of psychological and social factors that were not considered when developing the treatment plan.

Similarly, a patient with chest pain and shortness of breath (SOB) is diagnosed by an outpatient psychologist with panic disorder and treated with cognitive and behavioral interventions, but there is no improvement in symptoms. Coincidentally, the patient has an annual physical and is diagnosed with chronic lung disease, which has been responsible for the respiratory symptoms. In this case, the psychologist attended to only psychological symptoms and consequently misdiagnosed the problem. Including a consideration of the medical issues resulted in a correct diagnosis that could then be properly treated. The psychologist in this case should now reevaluate the patient because the symptoms of lung disease (SOB, chest pain) could also be associated with secondary anxiety, which might warrant additional psychological treatment in conjunction with the medical treatment.

Belar and Deardorff (2009) presented a general outline for the assessment and conceptualization of the patient's situation, based on the biopsychosocial model, shown in Table 2.1. The major domains assessed include the biological, affective, cognitive, and behavioral. Further, the patient, family, health care system, and sociocultural context are all to be included in the assessment. Finally, these authors recommended that the psychologist should assess the patient's current situation, past history, and also changes that have occurred since the illness began. Using detailed information that covers the biopsychosocial components will increase the likelihood of an accurate understanding of the patient's situation as well as successful intervention.

Melchert (2015) recently proposed a modification of the biopsychosocial model in which biological, sociocultural, and psychological factors interact over time. He argued that there are two main foundations of biopsychosocial practice: scientific evidence and ethics. Specifically, scientific evidence is the framework for conceptualization and practice and should be used to evaluate theory, rather than the traditional approach in which clinicians espouse a theory, even though there may be little or no evidence to support it. Melchert suggested that this change requires a paradigm shift to an approach that is based exclusively on scientific evidence, rather than belief. Further, biopsychosocial practice requires an understanding of ethics so that science can be appropriately applied, that is, to address the "care" aspect of health care.

Approaches to Inpatient Consultation

The two basic approaches to inpatient consultation involve a *comprehensive* evaluation or a *focused* evaluation. Both approaches ultimately address the referral question, but the process and time commitment involved in each differ. These approaches are not mutually exclusive and may be used together as the patient's treatment unfolds; for example, if a patient has repeat hospital admissions, a comprehensive evaluation at the first visit may be followed by focused evaluations at following admissions.

TABLE 2.1

Targets of Assessment

Domain of information	Patient	Environment: Family	Environment: Health care system	Environment: Sociocultural context
Biological or physical	Age, sex, race Physical appearance Symptoms, health status Physical examination Vital signs, lab data Prescribed medications Over-the-counter medications Psychophysiological data Genetic history and risks Constitutional factors, disabilities History of injury, disease, surgery, reproduction	Characteristics of the home setting Economic resources Family size Familial patterning (e.g., headache history) Other illness in family Immigration status	Characteristics of the treatment setting Characteristics of medical procedures Availability of prosthetic aids Accessibility of health care Gender and cultural disparities in care	Social services Financial resources Social networks Occupational setting Health hazards Exposure to violence, terrorism, war Global factors (e.g., political, economic)
Affective	Mood Affect Feelings about illness, treatment, health care, providers, self, family, job, social network History of affective disturbance	Members' feelings about patient, illness, and treatment	Providers' feelings about patient, illness, and treatment	Sentiment of culture regarding patient, illness, and treatment

(continues)

TABLE 2.1 (*Continued*)

Targets of Assessment

Domain of information	Patient	Environment: Family	Environment: Health care system	Environment: Sociocultural context
Cognitive	Cognitive style Thought content Intelligence Education Knowledge about disease Health beliefs Attitudes and expectations regarding illness, treatment, health care, and providers Perceived meaning of illness Philosophy of life Spiritual/religious beliefs	Knowledge about illness and treatment Attitudes/expectations about patient, illness	Providers' knowledge Providers' attitudes toward patient, illness, and treatment	Current state of knowledge Cultural/religious attitudes toward patient and illness
Behavioral	Activity level/exercise Interactions with family friends, providers, and coworkers Health habits Health care utilization/history of treatments Substance abuse Adherence Ability to control physical symptoms	Participation in patient care/caregiving roles Reinforcement contingencies for health and illness Family interactions, interpersonal violence Primary language	Providers' skills in education and training patients Reinforcement contingencies for health and illness Providers' linguistic and cultural competence	Employment policies Laws regulating health care practice, disability, provision of care, health habits, accessibility Customs in symptom-reporting and help-seeking

Note. From *Clinical Health Psychology in Medical Settings: A Practitioner's Guidebook* (2nd ed., pp. 51–53), by C. D. Belar and W. W. Deardorff, 2009, Washington DC: American Psychological Association. Copyright 2009 by the American Psychological Association.

COMPREHENSIVE EVALUATION

A comprehensive psychological evaluation is the most common approach to inpatient consultation and includes a thorough evaluation that addresses the major aspects of a biopsychosocial evaluation. This evaluation includes information on social history, substance use, medical and psychiatric history and current issues, and mental status, including a brief cognitive screening. Chapter 4 contains more detail on the specific information to be captured in each of these areas.

Using a comprehensive evaluation makes it unlikely that the consultant will miss something of importance, and it also provides a good general description of the patient and her history that will be useful for ongoing treatment. However, this evaluation can take a significant amount of time, often an hour or longer. Sample 2.1 provides an example of a comprehensive consultation done on a patient who was newly diagnosed with cancer and due to be discharged later the same day.

Although the comprehensive evaluation can provide a wealth of relevant information about a patient, there are times in which the hospital milieu or the patient's condition will not allow for a long evaluation. In those cases, the consultant can perform a shorter evaluation that is more specifically focused on the referral question, including additional questions from the longer evaluation as warranted.

FOCUSED EVALUATION

A specific and focused evaluation will target information that is relevant to the referral question exclusively and will not involve a thorough evaluation of the patient's symptoms and functioning. For example, if the referral question is about depression, the consultant would do an evaluation sufficient to answer that question and would go no further (unless clues about other problems were elicited during the focused evaluation). The problem facing the consultant is to gather sufficient information to address the referral question, with the concern being that a focused and specific evaluation of a particular aspect of the individual's experience might result in the consultant missing some important issue that was not queried.

The focused evaluation is most useful in certain specific circumstances, for example, if there is a need for a consultation and intervention for a specific adjustment issue in a patient who has not demonstrated any significant psychopathology or cognitive problems. However, a focused consultation could result in the psychologist responding to the wrong issue. Although some referral questions are on target, others do not address the appropriate issue, and that issue can be missed if the consultant simply addresses the question that is asked. For example, a referral is received regarding anxiety, and the psychologist interviews the patient using a focused approach, then calls back the report to the resident physician, concluding that the patient is not experiencing significant anxiety. At the time the verbal feedback is given, the referring physician notes additional concerns about depression because the patient had a past suicide attempt, of which the health psychology consultant was unaware. The depression and past suicide attempt would likely have been discussed in the context of a comprehensive evaluation, but if it did not come up in the focused evaluation, she will need to further evaluate the patient.

Sample 2.2 provides a focused evaluation for the same cancer patient described in the thorough consultation in Sample 2.1. The purpose of the consultation was to determine whether the patient needed any outpatient follow-up to help her deal with the cancer diagnosis and poor prognosis, even though there was no clear evidence of adjustment problems.

Note that Samples 2.1 and 2.2 describe the same patient, but the quantity of information obtained from the patient in the two evaluations is quite different. The comprehensive evaluation is generally more useful because it provides more information than the focused evaluation and lessens the likelihood that important information will be missed; it is definitely the most appropriate evaluation to use when training students.

Structure of Inpatient Consultation Services

There are several frameworks in which a psychologist can work when providing services to medical inpatients. Traditionally, inpatient psychiatric services are provided in hospitals by a consultation-liaison (CL) psychiatry service. Psychiatrists and residents who staff a CL service are available around the clock, usually in conjunction with emergency department personnel, and manage any and all consultations and psychiatric issues. The services provided include consultation, evaluations for psychotropic medication management, and patient behavior management (e.g., orders for restraints or sitters). The focus is on consultation and emergency management, with little ongoing follow-up with patients or use of psychological (nonpharmacological) interventions. As physicians have discovered the utility of psychological services to help inpatients cope with medical matters, there has been pressure to expand the services offered by CL psychiatry. One answer to this problem has been to expand the CL psychiatry service to a multidisciplinary team in which various members provide specialized services. The multidisciplinary team might consist of psychiatrists and psychiatry residents to address the traditional psychiatric issues, nurses to deal with problems of pain and conflicts between staff and patients, and psychologists to provide psychological therapy and to teach patients skills such as relaxation, imagery, and biofeedback. All members of the team have specialized skills, yet there is significant overlap in the work they do.

A second framework is that of an independent psychology (typically health psychology) consultation service, run and staffed by only psychologists. Psychology consultation services were developed by psychologists to address the psychological needs of medical inpatients that were not met by traditional psychiatric CL treatment. An independent health psychology service will typically provide both consultation and intervention services. The health psychology consultation service may be small, staffed by only a psychologist or two, or it may be a larger team consisting of psychology postdoctoral fellows, interns, and externs.

Psychologists who work in an outpatient medical specialty clinic (e.g., with neurology or pulmonary) may be enlisted to see patients from that specific outpatient practice when they are admitted to the hospital. Finally, psychologists in private practice may develop a relationship with a hospital and see inpatients on occasion, providing evaluation, intervention, or both.

In all cases, psychologists must have proper credentials and privileges to provide services in the institution (see Chapter 1, this volume). One important distinction among these frameworks is their relationship with the providers of psychiatric services. If the psychologist is part of a multidisciplinary team in the CL model, the relationship with psychiatry is built in, and requesting a psychiatrist to see a patient for medication management is usually relatively easy. In the other models, psychologists must develop relationships with the psychiatry service in the institution, so that those services can be obtained for a patient when warranted, keeping in mind that a referral to another service generally requires a formal order from the patient's primary medical team. Another advantage of the CL model is that mental health providers from various specialties can collaborate more easily on the treatment of a patient and can also learn from each other. One disadvantage is that because psychiatrists are in charge of this multidisciplinary service, medication management often takes precedence over psychological, nonpharmacological, interventions. The independent health psychology consultation service can avoid this problem and easily maintain a focus on the biopsychosocial issues that affect the patient. The independent psychology service is also more likely to provide ongoing inpatient follow-up of the patient throughout the inpatient admission, consistent with the focus on intervention and therapy, rather than consultation only.

Sample 2.1
Report From Comprehensive Consultation

Referral. Patient referred by Dr. D for evaluation of adjustment issues following new abdominal CA (*cancer*) diagnosis and poor prognosis.

Medical and substance use. Patient had abdominal surgery last week, plans to discharge to home today. She also has HTN (*hypertension*), well controlled with medication. Patient does not smoke tobacco, drinks alcohol minimally and rarely; no leisure drugs.

Social. She is a 34 y/o Caucasian woman, married with 2 children, ages 7 and 9. She completed college and works as a coordinator of programs for medical continuing education.

Psych history. Patient denies any previous history of psych treatment, including inpatient and outpatient treatment and psychotropic medication. She does report one brief period of mild depression after her first child was born. This lasted about 5 weeks, did not interfere with her functioning, and resolved on its own.

Psych symptoms. Patient reports mild sleep disturbance over the past few weeks, in anticipation of surgery, and then while processing her prognosis, but she denies sleep problems generally. She describes her mood today as "overwhelmed" although she denies symptoms of anxiety, panic, irritability, or depressed mood. She also denies hopelessness, helplessness, decreased interest, suicidal ideation. She does report some decreased energy since surgery. Patient also denies any strange experiences, including hallucinations.

Mental status. On mental status exam, she is alert and oriented × 3. Registration intact, short-term memory mildly impaired (2/3). Judgment, abstract thinking, long-term memory, attention/calculation all intact. Thinking is linear and goal-directed. Speech normal in rate, prosody, and tone.

Intervention. Discussed with patient any needs for psychological follow-up after discharge. She currently reports that she has good support and that she needs some time to get home and process the information about her medical situation and to determine future plans for treatment. Pt is eager to get back home with her kids and has plans to explain (with her husband) her situation in general terms so that they have awareness appropriate to their developmental level.

Also discussed the adjustment process and the variety of strong emotions the patient may experience, as well as coping strategies she can use to help her deal with them. Patient reports being good at relaxing with books, music, and hot baths when she has needed to relax in the past. She also reports taking advantage of her social supports and finding ways to distract herself when necessary. She has a good record of seeking information from her treatment team to help her make the best medical decisions she can.

Pt was informed about outpatient health psychology services available to her if she wishes to take advantage of them in the future, and she was provided with contact information for that (xxx–xxxx).

Summary: Patient with mild episode postpartum depression about 9 years ago, otherwise no history of significant psych issues or treatment. She is facing a new CA diagnosis with poor prognosis. Pt is currently coping well, and has good social support. She is aware of coping strategies she can use. She also has contact information for outpatient health psychology services, and was encouraged to contact us for follow-up as needed.

Thanks for the consult; please call with questions. Discussed with Dr. D.

S. Smith, PhD, pager 2223.

Sample 2.2
Report From a Focused Evaluation

Patient referred by Dr. D. She had abdominal surgery yesterday; new diagnosis CA and poor prognosis.

Patient was seen with husband before discharge home. She denies past psych history. She reports feeling sad and overwhelmed and is eager to get home to see her young children. She has a plan to tell them about her medical problems, and she reports very good social support from family and friends. Patient reports some mild sleep disruption past few weeks, denies significant anxiety or depressed mood. She reports needing some time to collect her thoughts and denies psychological needs at present. No gross mental status changes noted.

Discussed the adjustment process, and emotions Pt can expect to experience. Discussed coping strategies, including social support, seeking information, distraction, and relaxation. Provided patient with contact information for outpatient health psychology services (xxx–xxxx) and encouraged her to call if we could be of service after discharge. She appears to be coping well at present.

Thanks; please call with questions. Discussed with Dr. D.

S. Smith, PhD, pager xxxx.

THE INPATIENT EVALUATION

II

Preparing for the Consultation 3

This chapter describes typical referral questions for a health psychology consultation. Reviewing the medical record is discussed at length, sample reports from the medical record are interpreted, and information regarding laboratory tests and medical procedures is provided. The chapter concludes with a summary of issues to consider before seeing the patient. Much of the advice and descriptive information provided in the chapters in Part II are based on clinical experience, with literature cited for specific points that are research-based.

Understanding the Referral

Medical teams refer patients for health psychology evaluations for a variety of reasons. Typically, the medical team's goals for the psychological consultation involve (a) aiding the patient in coping with limitations or dealing with a diagnosis or treatment, (b) providing a psychiatric diagnosis and treatment recommendations, or (c) helping the medical team to manage the patient's behavior. Common reasons for referral for psychological consultation include

- a new diagnosis of cancer;
- refusal of a lifesaving amputation;

http://dx.doi.org/10.1037/0000108-004
Health Psychology Consultation in the Inpatient Medical Setting, by S. M. Labott

- overuse of pain medications;
- patient is listless and uncooperative with treatment;
- anxiety about surgery;
- recent stroke, trouble coping with limitations;
- long hospitalization, and patient appears depressed;
- history of schizophrenia; and
- a terminal diagnosis.

These referrals are fairly specific and provide a basic idea of the referring physician's concerns. The consultant can evaluate the patient while attending to the question the referring physician or team has raised.

However, not all referrals are as clear as those just listed. For example, it is not uncommon to receive referrals to address "mood and coping" without any specific information about the patient's situation (although this can often be determined by reviewing the patient's medical record). Further, medical professionals without expertise in mental health will vary in their understanding of patients' psychological needs and may not have the terminology to adequately describe the behavior or the ability to diagnose what they see. In that context, the referral question may be vague or may not reflect the actual problem. If it is unclear what information the medical team is requesting, it is best to contact them to get more information; in a brief phone call, the referral source can describe what motivated the request for a psychological consultation. Descriptions of the patient's behavior (e.g., patient threw a tray at the nurse, will not wake up when we try to examine him, does not seem to understand the medical condition, cries continually) can be helpful in directing the consultant's evaluation.

Table 3.1 provides data on 2 months of consecutive consults from the Health Psychology Inpatient Consultation Service at the University of Illinois at Chicago in 2013. These data reflect a total of 114 referrals. Common referral issues are listed on the left, followed by the percentage of consults that listed this topic as the referral question. Note that questions about mood, depression, and coping were the most common referral questions. The right column shows the percentage of the consulta-

TABLE 3.1

Consult Referral Questions and Outcomes

	Referral (%)	Outcome (%)
Mood	46	4
Depression	16	25
Coping	14	27
Anxiety/panic	7	10
Cognition/delirium	4	17
Stress, social issues	4	4
Addiction; adherence	2	2
Pain	2	4

tions that resulted in a "diagnosis" of each of the topics on the left. It is important to note that the initial reason for the consultation (Referral column) did not necessarily reflect the consultant's primary conclusion after the consultation was completed (Outcome column). For example, referral questions about mood accounted for almost half of the referrals received, but only 4% of the consultations were thought to be primarily about mood problems after the consultation was completed. Most striking, perhaps, was that only 4% of the referral questions were about cognitive changes or delirium, but 17% of the patients were diagnosed with cognitive problems as their primary issue at the conclusion of the consultation.

One reason for a lack of consistency between referral questions and outcomes is due to comorbidity. That is, many individuals have more than one problem (i.e., hospitalized patients experiencing symptoms of anxiety may also be experiencing symptoms of depression). Often symptoms of both disorders occur in patients who are overwhelmed with medical procedures or a new diagnosis. Similarly, patients may be having difficulty coping with pain and may also be experiencing cognitive changes associated with pain medication. Certainly there is confusion regarding overlapping terms and definitions; for example, if a patient appears to have depressed mood, would that be a referral for mood or depression?

Coping is a common referral for an inpatient psychological consultation and can refer to a wide variety of issues. In the medical context, coping may refer to the patient's struggle to deal with a difficult medical situation, such as acute leukemia or chronic respiratory problems. It may also refer to behavioral problems or poorly managed psychological symptoms that affect the patient's ability to cope with the hospital admission and medical diagnosis. It is the job of the psychologist to provide the correct conceptualization of the problem (and a psychiatric diagnosis, if warranted) so that the appropriate treatment may be instituted.

Although "coping" may be unclear as a reason for a referral, the term *coping* in many ways captures the essence of the intervention provided by a health psychology consultant. Regardless of the specific problem experienced by the patient, the consultant's task is to help the patient cope with his hospital experience. If the patient's experience involves anxiety, cognitive changes, or family conflicts, the purpose of the psychological intervention is to help the patient manage whatever social, psychological, cognitive, or medical issues he is facing. (Interventions to address the referrals listed in Table 3.1 are described in later chapters.)

Reviewing the Medical Record

The medical record contains a wealth of information that can guide the consultant's evaluation. For example, if the referral question is about depression, the medical record may contain information about the patient's mental health history or current medications that can focus the consultant's interview questions. Sometimes it is not feasible to read the entire medical chart, especially for a patient who has multiple medical problems and many hospital admissions or physician visits over years. In this case, the psychological consultant can start with the medical record notes that are most likely to be relevant to the current evaluation. Although the psychologist might not review each note in a chart, a patient is entitled to work with a psychologist who has done her homework and is aware of the patient's history and current medical concerns.

Initially, most psychology consultants are not familiar with the interpretation of notes in the medical record, due to minimal experience with medical terminology and abbreviations. It will be important to have access to resources that describe the clinical issues associated with a specific medical diagnosis, its typical course, and relevant treatments. Although the psychological consultant is not responsible for explaining the implications of the patient's disease to him, knowledge of the basic realities associated with the disease lends credibility to the consultant's work (both with physicians and patients) and facilitates rapport. If the psychologist does not have an adequate understanding of the disease, she can't put the patient's experience into the proper context. (Although the health psychology consultant will often ask the patient why she is in the hospital, this is done to assess the patient's understanding, not because the consultant doesn't know.) Several good Internet resources provide information on medical diagnoses in layperson's terms; these include WebMD (https://www.webmd.com), the Cleveland Clinic (https://my.clevelandclinic.org/health), and the Mayo Clinic (https://www.mayoclinic.org) websites. Many books also provide this information. A list of common medical abbreviations is in Appendix A; similar lists can be found in Belar and Deardorff (2009) and on many websites. Most hospitals provide comprehensive lists of abbreviations approved for use in the medical center; be aware that there can be some variability from one hospital to another.

Exhibit 3.1 is a list of the most relevant aspects of the medical record for the psychological consultant to review before seeing the patient. The current admission (*admit*) note is critical because it provides a description of the patient's active medical issues upon admission to the hospital. Second in importance are any reports that relate to the patient's mental health history, if there are any. Reports from other consultants and providers may also be relevant, depending on the referral question, for example, if there is a question about cognitive changes, a recent or past evaluation from Neurology is useful. Current inpatient progress notes will provide specific information on the

EXHIBIT 3.1

Aspects of the Medical Record to Review

- Admission note
- Reports of any mental health treatment
- Consultations from other specialists
- Recent inpatient progress notes
- Discharge summaries
- Medications
- As needed:
  - Laboratory test results
  - Procedure notes
  - Vital signs

patient's current medical status, and past discharge summaries from either psychiatric or medical inpatient admissions can provide good descriptions of the patient's medical or psychological history and problems. Any notes may contain data regarding how the patient interacts with medical professionals and may demonstrate problems in those relationships. In many cases it is important to review other parts of the medical record to gain information on medications, laboratory results, and medical procedures. Each of these sections of the medical record is described more fully in what follows.

Each of the samples of medical record notes in this chapter is abstracted from actual patient medical record notes, but with identifying information changed or deleted to protect patients' privacy. Note that they are not all written in the same format. Medications are often referred to with generic names, but brand names may also be used. Abbreviations are used heavily, and it is generally acceptable to write using phrases rather than complete sentences provided that the content is clear (e.g., "Pt married, with 3 kids").

The goal of the chart review is to discover a host of background information about the patient to inform the interview. The psychological consultant may not choose to share all of that information with the patient but will always use it to tailor the interview to get the most information about the relevant issues as quickly as possible. Especially if there are concerns about the patient's honesty or ability to report accurately, the interviewer can choose questions to target specific and accurate information. For example, in a patient with a history of documented drug use, if the patient says he does not use drugs, the consultant can then question more specifically to resolve the inconsistency. Similarly, results of a recent toxicology screen from the medical record would be useful when seeing a patient with possible substance abuse problems. The consultant may not choose to share toxicology screening results with the patient, unless the patient continues to insist that he does not use drugs.

The patient's medical record is an extremely valuable source of information, but the consultant must not assume that everything found in the medical record is correct: Important information in the medical record needs to be verified. It is common for people to make mistakes in medical notes, and once a mistake is made—especially in electronic medical records—the information may be copied into the notes of others and repeated over and over. Therefore, even if information is found repeatedly in the patient's medical record, this does not mean that it is accurate or that more than one provider has obtained that information.

CURRENT ADMISSION NOTE (ADMIT NOTE)

The inpatient admit note is typically written by the resident or attending physician soon after she evaluates the patient once he has arrived in the hospital room. This note provides important information, such as details on the patient's current symptoms that warranted the admission to the hospital, medical diagnoses to be considered or ruled out, an overview of the patient's past medical history, and information on substance use and prescription medications. This note should provide a good picture of the patient's current medical situation.

The admit note may also provide additional information that is especially relevant to a psychologist, such as observations of the patient's behavior that may suggest specific psychological or cognitive issues. For example, notes may contain details regarding the patient's presentation, for example, the patient was irritable and demanding, confused, or somnolent. These observations are especially important because the behaviors demonstrated during that evaluation may no longer be present when the patient is seen by the health psychology consultant but may be relevant to the patient's current situation or diagnosis. For example, consider an elderly patient who was admitted with fever and delirium and who was combative on admission. If the psychologist is asked to see the patient a few days later, the cause of the patient's fever was likely treated, and the patient may be calm and presenting with only a few or no cognitive changes at all. Knowing how the patient looked a few days earlier helps the psychological consultant to conceptualize the patient's situation and plan for appropriate intervention.

Admit notes may also contain information about psychiatric history or current emotional symptoms. Certainly information on psychiatric history and current symptoms will be evaluated by the psychologist, but these notes can provide valuable data on history and on psychological symptoms and behavior witnessed by others that can be evaluated further in the psychological consultation. For example, the admit note could mention that the patient has a history of posttraumatic stress disorder or that the patient was paranoid when admitted.

The admit note may also provide some insight into nonadherence. Many patients are admitted to the hospital because they have not followed the recommended treatment for a medical problem. Nonadherence could involve not taking medications as directed, not following up to get prescribed testing to provide further diagnostic information on a cancer that has been discovered, or a range of other possibilities.

See the sample admit note in Sample 3.1. Comments in italics are not part of the original note but are placed in the sample to help with the interpretation of the note. Ideas the psychologist should consider while reviewing the materials are also presented in italics in the context of the note itself.

From the admit note in Sample 3.1, the psychological consultant gets a picture of a patient with likely cardiac problems and complaints of chronic leg pain. She has been diagnosed with schizophrenia and takes several psychotropic medications, although current psychiatric status is not mentioned. The patient lives in an assisted living facility, has memory problems, and is unable to describe her pain and symptoms well, all suggesting impairment of cognition or functioning generally. This admit note, then, provides a significant amount of detail that can help the health psychology consultant to develop hypotheses about the patient's current psychological status.

NOTES FROM MENTAL HEALTH PROVIDERS

Any and all current and past notes in the medical record from psychologists, psychiatrists, social workers, and other mental health providers should be reviewed. Many patients in the inpatient medical setting have had no past psychological or psychiatric treatment, so there will be nothing to review. However, if a patient has detailed information on inpatient or outpatient psychological treatment, this will provide additional data to aid in the development of a current conceptualization of the patient's situation and will also help to plan intervention. Sample 3.2 is an evaluation for a kidney transplant, performed by a social worker. (Italics again interpret abbreviations and indicate issues for the psychological consultant to consider in planning the psychological evaluation.)

On the basis of the sample note in Sample 3.2, the patient had no formal psychiatric history at the time of the evaluation. Cognition appeared WNL (*within normal limits*), although mental status was not formally tested. The patient apparently had some depression associated with her medical condition but was not interested in seeing Psychology. The referral to Psychology was made anyway. The consultant reviewing this information should determine whether the patient was ever seen by Psychology after this evaluation by the social worker and, if so, the outcome of that.

INPATIENT PROGRESS NOTES

Any patient in the hospital has a daily note written by a member of their primary medical team (see Sample 3.3 for an example). This note will be more focused on the immediate medical issue than an admit note and will address the medical symptoms and changes in the patient's medical status that have occurred each day. Inpatient progress notes contain specific information that may be of concern to the patient as well as plans for care, including information on tests and procedures that have been or will be performed. Progress notes become more important as the time between the admission and the consultation grows because medical issues will unfold and change as time goes on. Reading these daily notes can provide a good understanding of the course of the illness during the patient's admission, which is important because the course of the illness may influence emotional reactions the patient is experiencing.

CONSULTANT REPORTS

All consultant reports (both outpatient and inpatient) are valuable because they are typically comprehensive evaluations that provide additional data on the current problem; for example, if the current referral is about drug use, the health psychology consultant could look for past evaluations from an addiction or pain service. Some consultants' reports include a wealth of data relevant to a psychological conceptualization of the patient, especially those written by neurologists and psychiatrists. These are likely to contain psychological and cognitive data that can provide much information to help the psychologist develop hypotheses about current psychological problems. If the referral question is about cognition, a neurologist's evaluation of the patient, even if not recent, will provide data that can contribute to an understanding of the patient's current situation. See the sample neurology consult report in Sample 3.4.

DISCHARGE SUMMARY

Discharge summaries are similar to admit notes in that they contain a wealth of background information. The discharge summary will often include pre–post data on the medical problem, so the course of the medical issue can be tracked. The note shown in Sample 3.5 is a discharge summary following a psychiatric admission. This one is especially helpful for a psychological consultant because it contains a great deal of information regarding the patient's psychiatric history.

MEDICATIONS

The patient's medications are listed in many notes in the chart, as well as perhaps in a separate section that tracks medications and adjustments in them throughout the hospital admission. As discussed in later chapters, many medications can result in psychological symptoms, such as anxiety-like symptoms, depressed mood, or cognitive changes, and reviewing the medications can provide hypotheses regarding the etiology of current symptoms. In addition, a review of the patient's medications can provide information as to the specific medical issues the patient is dealing with, as well as their severity and chronicity. Many psychological diagnoses may be understated or missed completely in the medical notes (especially if the chief complaint is not psychological in nature), but all outpatient medications should be listed in the patient's medical record, so the psychological consultant can determine some basic information about the patient's psychological status from this list. For example, if Paxil (paroxetine), Zoloft (sertraline), or Prozac (fluoxetine) is listed in the patient's medication list, the psychologist would consider that the patient may have a diagnosis of depression, even if that is not stated clearly in other notes.

LABORATORY TEST RESULTS

When working in the inpatient medical setting, a working knowledge of common laboratory tests and their meanings will help to inform the psychologist about the patient's medical situation. For example, a patient who has had a stem cell transplant may be eagerly awaiting discharge but will not be allowed to leave the hospital until the white blood cell (WBC) count is at an appropriate level to protect him from infection outside of the hospital. In this case, the patient may follow his blood "counts" daily, and this will be a topic of conversation as it relates to his emotional state. Anxiety is common in a situation like this because the patient is at risk for infection until levels of certain blood components have recovered and will have a significantly worse prognosis if they do not recover. The consultant's intervention may be focused on anxiety management, and an understanding of the laboratory results and the typical course of recovery will inform the psychological treatment. Likewise, when seeing a patient to address a substance abuse issue, an understanding of toxicology results is imperative.

Knowledge of laboratory results can also be used if the medical team requests help in seeking the etiology of acute cognitive changes. As discussed in Chapter 9, delirium involves acute cognitive changes and often psychotic symptoms that are caused by a medical problem. There are many etiologies for delirium, and the medical team may seek help from the health psychology consultant in the search for issues that could be causing the symptoms. Infections and electrolyte imbalances are reflected in laboratory results and demonstrate only a few of the medical causes of delirium (Kalish, Gillham, & Unwin, 2014).

Finally, in many cases a psychological consultant is called on to help a patient understand her medical situation and make decisions about treatment. Typically the medical team would give the patient information about the medical diagnosis and treatment options as well as the pros and cons of each. The psychologist can follow up with the patient afterward, to help her process the information and make decisions about treatment. A good understanding of the medical situation, including laboratory results, can inform the discussion with the patient. At times, the psychologist may need to ask the medical team for additional information to help the patient understand the relevant medical issues if the material is unclear.

Medical centers typically have a laboratory manual that describes the laboratory tests that can be ordered, normative values, the meaning of test results, and sample collection procedures. For the health psychology consultant, the most relevant piece of information is the interpretation of the test values. If a consultant works exclusively with one medical specialty, that psychologist will learn a host of very specific information about lab results in that specialty area. For consultants who do more general work with a variety of specialty areas, a working knowledge of some of the more common lab tests and their meanings is warranted. It is rare for the psychologist to need the specific value for the lab result; most often a general idea of the value being high or low is sufficient. (One exception would be the patient mentioned earlier who is monitoring his WBC counts daily.) See Appendix B for a description of some common laboratory tests and their meanings. There are also some good books that can be used as additional resources, such as Fischbach and Dunning (2015) and Pagana and Pagana (2014).

In most medical records, a patient's lab results are listed alongside the normative values, and values that are not within the normal range are indicated as being low or high, so it is easy to see which lab values are out of range. Table 3.2 shows a sample of part of a complete blood count (CBC) report. Note here that the samples were

TABLE 3.2

Example of Complete Blood Cell Count Results

Date	2/14/15	2/14/15
Time	0430	1350
WBC	H 12.4	H 11.8
RBC	4.3	4.4
HGB	13.0	13.2
HCT	40.0	39.4
RDW	14.0	14.6
PLT	L 46	L 48

Note. HCT = hematocrit; HGB = hemoglobin; PLT = platelet; RBC = red blood cell; RDW = red cell distribution width; WBC = white blood cell.

collected and tested at two times on the same day (i.e., at 4:30 a.m. and 1:50 p.m.). High and low values are indicated with H and L next to the values here, although in electronic medical records, nonnormative values are often indicated in color. Normative values may differ slightly from institution to institution. In Table 3.2, it can be seen that the patient has a high WBC count, likely indicating an infection, and also low platelets (PLT), indicating poor blood clotting and perhaps a bleeding risk.

In medical notes, physicians may put lab values into a diagram, such as the one shown in Figure 3.1 (Spaulding & Silverblatt, 1993). On the diagram, the abbreviations for each lab value indicate where in the diagram the value of that specific lab result is located, for example, the patient's sodium level is located on the top left corner of the first grid, and the platelet result is located on the far right of the second grid. See the Inpatient Progress Note (Sample 3.3) for an example of these diagrams used in medical notes to convey lab results. Note that in the electronic medical record, the diagrams are not as clear as those in Figure 3.1.

PROCEDURE NOTES

As with laboratory results, the health psychology consultant would not be involved with medical procedures or with the interpretation of those reports, but there are situations in which some basic understanding of the procedures is relevant. Many people fear bone marrow biopsies because they can be associated with pain and are performed repeatedly in patients with leukemia. A general understanding of this procedure and the potential pain and emotional consequences can enable the psychologist to help the patient to cope with this procedure more effectively. Similarly, some patients are afraid of needles or of enclosed spaces, making certain medical procedures particularly frightening for them.

Frequently it is not the procedure itself but the possibility of bad results that creates anxiety in patients. Patients are afraid they will be given bad news that will have significant implications for either their quality or quantity of life. In these cases, the focus is not on the procedure itself; instead, it is on the potential implications of the results. It is helpful, for example, for the consultant to understand enough about

FIGURE 3.1

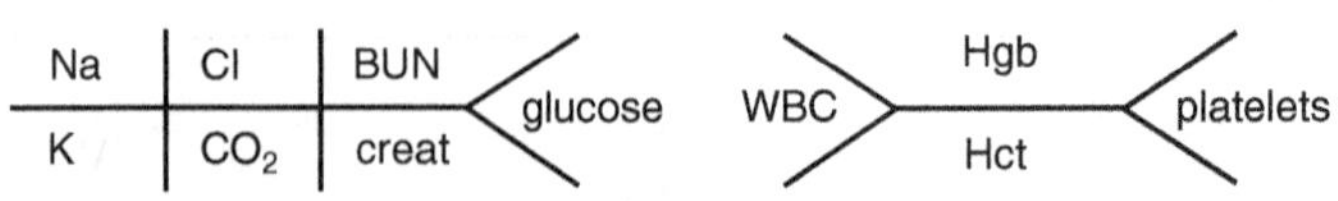

Sample diagram showing lab values. BUN = blood urea nitrogen; Cl = chloride; CO_2 = carbon dioxide; Creat = creatinine; Hct = hematocrit; Hgb = hemoglobin; K = potassium; Na = sodium; WBC = white blood cell. From "Using Grids to Document Laboratory Results" by A. Spaulding and F. J. Silverblatt, 1993, *Annals of Internal Medicine, 119*, p. 863. Copyright 1993 by the American College of Physicians. Reprinted with permission.

the procedure to assess its purpose and implications (e.g., the procedure has been performed to determine whether the cancer has metastasized).

VITAL SIGNS

"Vitals" include respiration rate, heart rate (pulse), body temperature, and blood pressure. The values for the vitals may be found in a physician's note (see the sample of Inpatient Progress Note in Sample 3.3) or in nursing notes. Vital signs are good indicators of gross physical functioning. Although these offer few data to inform specifics of the health psychology consultant's evaluation, they do provide valuable information on the patient's physiological functioning that can help the consultant to understand the patient's overall medical situation. Normal values for vitals can differ slightly from one institution to another. Exhibit 3.2 shows normal values for vital signs provided by Medline Plus (n.d.).

What to Think About Before Seeing the Patient

Once the medical record has been thoroughly reviewed, the consultant can integrate all the relevant information and prepare to interview the patient. Table 3.3 contains the list of some possible referral questions from the beginning of this chapter, followed by issues that the consultant should be considering when reviewing the chart and preparing to evaluate the patient. In each case, it will be important for the consultant to know something about the specific medical diagnosis. When learning to perform inpatient consultations, it is important to research each new diagnosis; although it is not the job of the psychologist to explain aspects of the medical diagnosis and treatment to the patient, it is important that the consultant have a general idea of what the diagnosis entails, as well as its typical course and treatment. It will also be important to keep in mind that each patient is unique, and there are always new medical treatments that may not be listed in the resource materials that the psychologist has reviewed.

The information from the medical record provides a context for the evaluation: It will help the health psychology consultant understand the patient's current medical issues, will be useful in conceptualizing the patient's current situation, and also assists

EXHIBIT 3.2

Normal Values for Vital Signs

Blood pressure: 90/60–120/80 mm/Hg
Respiration rate: 12–18 breaths per minute
Pulse/heart rate: 60–100 beats per minute
Temperature: 97.8–99.1°F (36.5–37.2°C)

Note. Data from Medline Plus (n.d.).

TABLE 3.3

Referral Questions and Issues to Consider for Evaluation

Referral question	Issues to consider
New diagnosis of cancer	Prognosis? What will treatment involve? How is the patient's social support?
Terminal diagnosis	Any physical or cognitive limitations? Estimated time left? Family situation?
Patient refusing amputation or other procedure	Does patient understand implications? Any cognitive problems? Relevant beliefs?
Overuse of pain medications	Is pain controlled? Substance abuse problem? Does the patient understand proper dosing?
Patient listless or uncooperative	Depression? Delirium? Personality?
Anxiety about surgery	Does patient have specific concerns? Medical questions? Needs anxiety management?
Recent stroke, trouble coping with limitations	What are the limitations? If cognitive, is patient able to cope effectively? Other barriers to effective coping?
Long hospitalization, appears depressed	Depression? Boredom? Giving up?
History of schizophrenia	Is patient medicated properly this admission? Does patient have outpatient follow-up in place?

in developing an appropriate plan for intervention. Knowledge about the relevant medical issues also lends credibility to the consultant's interactions with both the patient and the medical team.

For example, consider a referral for coping and stress in the patient with multiple sclerosis (MS) admitted with exacerbation of MS symptoms (see the Neurology Consult in Sample 3.4). After considering coping issues generally, details regarding the course of MS and its treatment, and a review of the patient's medical record, the psychology consultant will likely be considering the following issues:

- This is not a new diagnosis of MS, but has the patient adjusted to having MS and its implications?
- MS is associated with major depression and also with cognitive changes. What is the patient's status regarding these issues, especially given that her neurology note indicated that she is on psychotropic medications and has history of depression?
- What do we know about her past psychiatric history?
- The patient is unwilling to take steroids to manage the exacerbation. Does she understand the advantages and disadvantages of the steroid treatment? She does understand that steroids can be associated with weight gain. Is this a realistic concern in her case, or a reflection of vanity or an eating disorder?

In summary, the psychologist needs to understand the referral question and can review medical record notes, laboratory results, and other materials to generate hypotheses that may guide the consultant's evaluation to the most relevant topics for this particular patient. However, the historical data from the medical record should not result in the exclusion of basic questions from the psychological evaluation, which could result in important information being missed. These medical record data should be used as a guide for the consultation, with the consultant rechecking important aspects of the history with the patient and then evaluating the current status of relevant issues in depth.

Sample 3.1 Admission Note

CC: "Chest and leg pain" *(Patient's chief complaint [CC], in her own words, is "chest and leg pain")*

HPI (*history of present illness*): 42 y/o obese female smoker w/pmhx (*past medical history)* of untreated HTN *(hypertension)*, asthma, and schizophrenia presents to ED *(emergency department)* for 2 distinct chief complaints: 1. Chest pain × 2 weeks, 2. LLE *(left lower extremity—left leg)* pain × 2 months. Although a poor historian *(why is she a poor historian?)*, pt *(patient)* describes a 2-week hx *(history)* of exertional L *(left)*-sided parasternal chest pain of a "tight" and "burning" quality that is aggravated by physical activity (walking, lifting objects) and relieved after 2–3 minutes of rest. Endorses an occasional concurrent numbness in all digits of her L hand, although this seems to be more chronic than the chest pain. Pain does not radiate to shoulder or up the neck. Pt also endorses concurrent dyspnea *(shortness of breath)* and cough, which she was experiencing at the time of our encounter. Cough is productive but color not noted. No hemoptysis *(coughing up blood)*. Pt claims to have also experienced vomiting 2×/week for the past month, usually during episodes of chest pain. Chest pain had resolved at time of encounter. Regarding her atraumatic LLE pain, pt states that for the past 2 months, she has had difficulty ambulating around her assisted living facility *(Why is 42-year-old patient in an assisted living facility? Suggests significant impairment of some sort.)* due to persistent pain that begins in the knee and radiates up L thigh and down the anterior shin. Pt does have a documented hx of lumbar radiculopathy *(pinched nerve)*; it is unclear if sciatica is playing a role in her pain due to her difficulty articulating the pain's quality. She notes occasionally her whole leg will "lock," and she will be unable to move it, although the writer was unable to elicit in which joint (hip or knee) she experiences this locking sensation. Takes no medication for CP *(chest pain)* or LLE pain.

Schizophrenia is not the presenting issue but will almost certainly be relevant. Patient is a poor historian, so getting accurate information during an interview may be difficult.

PMedHx *(past medical history)*:

1. HTN *(hypertension)*
2. Obesity
3. Asthma

4. Schizophrenia
5. Seizure disorder
6. Hypothyroidism
7. Nephrolithiasis *(kidney stones)*
8. Latent syphilis

Multiple medical problems—schizophrenia noted again. Thyroid issues can cause psychological symptoms; syphilis can result in cognitive problems but does not seem to be a major issue currently.

<u>Meds:</u>

Paroxetine 30 mg QD *(daily)*
Risperidone 2 mg BID *(twice daily)*
Trazodone 100 mg QPM *(daily at bedtime)*

These meds suggest depression, psychosis, and sleep problems. Does patient get her psychotropic meds from a PCP (primary care physician), or does she have her own psychiatrist, either here or outside this hospital?

<u>SocHx: *(social history)*</u>

1. Smoker (2 cig/day recently, although former 1PPD *(pack per day)* smoker × >10 years)
2. "occasional EtOH" *(occasional alcohol use, in the patient's own words)*
3. Previous Utox *(urine toxicology)* +cocaine, though denies use

Not clear what "occasional alcohol" use means to the patient. She had a previous urine test that was positive for cocaine, wonder how long ago that was, and she denies use.

ROS *(Review of systems)*

Gen *(general)*: no fevers, chills, unintentional weight loss, changes in sleep or appetite
HEENT *(head, eyes, ears, nose, throat)*: no headache, blurry vision, change in hearing, nasal congestion, or sore throat
CV *(cardiovascular)*: As in HPI (*history of present illness)*
Resp *(respiratory)*: As in HPI
GI: + N/V *(nausea/vomiting)*, no heartburn, difficulty swallowing, abdominal pain, constipation, or diarrhea
GU *(genitourinary)*: + dull suprapubic pain with urination, "I was told I have blood in my urine"
Ext: no muscle weakness, joint pain, joint swelling, or extremity edema
Skin: no rashes, bruising, or ulcers
Psych: + schizophrenia; "I forget things"
Neuro: + headache, no dizziness, gait/balance disturbances, numbness, tingling, or weakness
Endocrine: no heat or cold intolerance, excessive sweating, or excessive thirst

Besides schizophrenia, patient is also reporting forgetfulness and headache.

Physical Exam:

Gen: AO×4 (*alert and oriented to person, place, time, event*)
Skin: warm, dry, no rashes
HEENT *(head, eyes, ears, nose, throat*): head atraumatic, PERRL *(pupils equal, round, reactive to light)*, EOMI *(extraocular movements intact)*, sclera anicteric *(not jaundiced)*, no sinus tenderness, no nasal mucosa inflammation, oral mucosa moist, no lesions in mouth
CV *(cardiovascular)*: RRR *(regular rate and rhythm)*, normal S1 and S2, no MRG *(murmurs, rubs, and gallops)* appreciated. NT *(not tested)* costal margins.
Resp: CTAB *(clear to auscultation bilaterally)*
Abd: BS *(bowel sounds)* present, soft, nontender, no rebound tenderness or guarding
Neck: supple, normal ROM (*range of movement)*, no enlarged lymph nodes, no masses
Vascular: no edema, good peripheral pulses, no carotid bruits *(vascular murmur)*
Neuro: AO×4, CN *(cranial nerves)* II–XII intact, 5/5 strength in UE *(upper extremity)* and RLE (*right lower extremity)*. Pt *(patient*) unable to tolerate exam of LLE *(left lower extremity)*.
Psych: disheveled, dysphoric, poor insight
Ext: LLE diffusely tender, popliteal fossa and ant tib plateau. Effusion difficult to appreciate due to habitus *(body build)*. Guarding during exam; ROM *(range of motion)* unable to be elicited. No erythema *(skin redness)*. Neurovascularly intact.

Dysphoric, disheveled, poor insight—helpful behavioral observations for use by the psychologist.

Assessment and Plan: 42-year-old female w/history HTN, obesity, hx smoking, paranoid schizophrenia presenting with L-sided chest tightness for the last 2 weeks that occurs with exertion, associated with dyspnea on exertion. Initial ECG *(electrocardiogram)* and cardiac enzymes negative. Patient admitted for full ACS *(acute chest syndrome)* r/o *(rule out)*. Pain likely from stable angina. Patient also presenting with LLE pain, which has been assessed in outpatient setting w/recommendations for PT *(physical therapy)*.

Stable Angina

- Follow cardiac with second and third set of cardiac enzymes and ECGs at 6 hour intervals for full ACS r/o
- Obtaining Urine drug screen in setting of recent cocaine positive test
- Will start metoprolol 12.5 mg Q BID *(two times daily)* AM
- Will start aspirin 81 mg QAM
- Nitro sublingual prn *(as needed)* for chest pain

Left Lower Extremity Pain

- Will provide pain control with Norco 5 Q6H *(every 6 hours)* prn pain
- XR *(x-ray)* b/l *(bilateral)* knees

Schizophrenia

- Continue outpatient psych medication: Trazodone, Paroxetine, Risperdal

FEN (fluids, electrolytes, nutrition)

- Follow daily Chem 7 *(set of lab tests)*
- Replete electrolytes prn
- NPO *(nothing by mouth)* during ACS r/o

PPx (prophylaxis):

- Heparin Sq *(subcutaneous)*

Code status: Full

Sample 3.2
Note From Social Worker

CLINIC NOTE
DATE OF SERVICE: 08/xx/2016
DATE OF BIRTH: Pt is 58 y/o Hispanic woman
PSYCHOSOCIAL ASSESSMENT FOR SOLID ORGAN TRANSPLANT:
PHONE NUMBER: xxx–xxxx is the patient's home. Patient does not have a cell phone.
PRESENT FOR INTERVIEW: Patient only.
ORGAN TYPE: Kidney.
ETIOLOGY OF ORGAN FAILURE: Diabetes diagnosed 39 years ago.

SOCIAL HISTORY: The patient states that her mother has passed. Her father is living and is healthy. She has three children. One is biological. The other two are her niece and nephew, whom she has raised.

The patient has 4 siblings, and all have diabetes as well. The patient states that she lives with her son and nephew, ages 22 and 18 years, and they are both healthy. Patient's marital status is single. Pt's niece will likely be the primary support person for her after surgery. The patient does not drive, but she does have transportation available to her. She reports having no mobility impairments. She ambulates independently with no devices.

She reports no hearing or visual deficits and is independent with ADLs *(activities of daily living)*. She has one flight of stairs to enter her home.

EDUCATIONAL HISTORY: The patient states that the highest level of education she completed is GED.

OCCUPATIONAL AND FINANCIAL HISTORY: The patient states that she last worked in 2008. She had been working in a shelter for several years but stopped when the job moved. She reports no significant financial concerns at this time. Insurance is Medicaid. The patient states that she is not a veteran.

SUBSTANCE ABUSE: The patient reports that she last smoked cigarettes 15 years ago. She states that she has about two alcoholic beverages a month. The patient reports no use or history of illicit drugs. She states that she is on Vicodin currently for gout and reports appropriate use of this med.

EMOTIONAL AND PSYCHIATRIC HISTORY: The patient admitted to some depression because of her illness. She states that she has never been under the care of a mental health professional. She reports having no inpatient psychiatric stays, and she states that she has never taken any medication for any mental health concerns. The patient denies suicidal thoughts, homicidal thoughts, hallucinations, symptoms of mania, and delusions. The patient states that she would not like to see a psychologist to learn ways to cope with her depression and her illness.

MENTAL STATUS: The patient was well groomed and clean; her behavior was cooperative. Her speech was normal rate and tone. Her mood was congruent. Her affect was normal. Her thought process was linear. Her thought content was free from paranoia. Patient appeared to have good insight and good judgment. The patient appeared alert and oriented ×3 throughout this interview. The patient's memory was sufficient for this interview. The patient appeared to have good concentration and a good fund of knowledge. The patient was fluent in English.

MEDICAL HISTORY AND COMPLIANCE: The patient states that she started hemodialysis in October of 2014 and that she has never missed dialysis. The patient states that she never forgets to take her medications and she never forgets doctor's appointments.

POWER-OF-ATTORNEY FOR HEALTH CARE: She does not have a power of attorney for health care at this time, and she is not interested in obtaining one.

ASSESSMENT AND RISK STRATIFICATION: It is the impression of this social worker that the patient is a reasonable risk for kidney transplantation at this time. The patient appears to have a good knowledge of her present illness. She appears to have adequate insurance coverage for transplant and posttransplant needs. The patient appears to have a stable financial situation. She appears to have no substance abuse history. She appears to have a good support system from her niece and other family members. The patient appears to have an appropriate discharge plan, and she appears to be mentally stable, although she does endorse some depression. Social worker will make referral for a psychologist, but patient's listing candidacy should not be dependent on this.

Sample 3.3 Inpatient Progress Note

Subjective

Pt seen and examined this morning, no acute events were reported overnight. He denies nausea/vomiting and has not had any bowel movements. He denies LE *(lower extremity)* pain. He started on oral Keflex approx 2 days ago. Thinks overall cellulitis is improving, less red and painful. No chest pain, SOB *(shortness of breath)*, chills/fevers.

Objective

Vitals (Past 5 vitals in past 24 hours):

Date	Temp (°F/°C)	BP	Pulse	RR (*respiration rate*)
09/17 04:25	98.1/36.7	121/74	87	20
09/16 23:55	98.2/36.8	104/64	87	20
09/16 22:48	98.6/37.0	133/88	94	20
09/16 14:26	97.5/36.4	129/68	110	22

24 Hour Max Temp: 37.0C at 09/16 22:48

Physical Exam:

General: Pt lying in bed comfortably, cooperative, NAD *(no acute distress)*
HEENT *(head, eyes, ears, nose, throat)*: no scleral icterus *(jaundice)*
Heart: RRR *(regular rate and rhythm)*, normal S1S2, no murmurs
Lungs: CTAB *(clear to auscultation bilaterally)*, symmetric chest movement, no wheezes/crackles/rhonchi
Abdomen: soft, nontender, nondistended, no organomegaly, no guarding, bowel sounds present
Extremities: erythema, warmth and mild induration in lower extremities has remained below the marked border, nontender, no drainage, no areas of fluctuance, slightly improved from yesterday

Active Scheduled Medications:

cefazolin 2 Gm, INJECTION, IVPB *(intravenous piggyback)*, Q8HR
clotrimazole 1% topical 1 appl, CREAM, TOPICAL, BID, Routine, Apply to feet and toenails
esomeprazole, 40 mg, INJECTION, IVPB, Q24HR
hydrochlorothiazide 25 mg, TABLET, PO *(by mouth)*, DAILY, Routine
lisinopril 10 mg, TABLET, PO, DAILY

Active PRN Medications:

acetaminophen 650 mg, TABLET, PO, Q6H PRN, For pain
morphine injection 4 mg, INJECTION, IV PUSH, Q4H PRN, For pain
ondansetron 4 mg, INJECTION, IV PUSH, Q4H PRN, For nausea and/or vomiting: Anticipatory

Active IV Fluids and Medications:

NaCl 0.9% 1,000 mL 1,000 mL/hr, 1,000 mL per Bag

Laboratory Studies

MOST RECENT RESULTS: 09/16 18:27

(see Figure 3.1 for an explanation of the following diagrams)

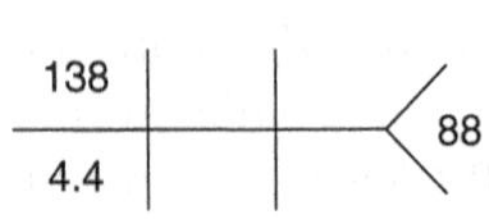

Ca	9.1
Mg	2.0
Phos	4.7

7.3 〉 12.7 / 39.2 〈 152   PT 16.7
INR 1.3

Documented Diagnostic Problem List:

Essential hypertension
Onychomycosis *(fungal infection of nail)*
Hyperpigmentation of skin
Tinea pedis *(dermatological foot infection)*
Body mass index 40+—severely obese
Steatosis of liver
Obstructive sleep apnea syndrome
Vitamin D deficiency

Allergies: NKA *(no known allergies)*
Code Status: Full Code

Assessment and Plan

32-year-old man w PMHx *(past medical history)* HTN *(hypertension)*, morbid obesity, fatty liver, LE *(lower extremity)* cellulitis L >R presenting w coffee-ground emesis *(vomiting)* and black stools × 1 day as well as lower extremity cellulitis.

#) coffee-ground emesis, melena *(blood in feces)*: Possibly due to upper GI *(gastrointestinal)* bleed, uncertain of etiology, pt denies recent NSAID *(nonsteroidal antiinflammatory drug)* use. Pt has a hx of fatty liver and etoh abuse, last drink was 2 weeks ago. Differential includes PUD *(peptic ulcer disease)*, gastritis.
- Hb *(hemoglobin)* 12.7→11.3
- continue esomeprazole 40 mg IV q24h *(every 24 hours)*
- Zofran for N/V *(nausea/vomiting)*
- tele monitoring
- will monitor vitals
- GI on consult, appreciate recommendations, will perform EGD *(esophagogastroduodenoscopy)* today, NPO *(nothing by mouth)* for now

#) LE cellulitis L>R: Improving. Likely inoculation due to tinea pedis.
- outline of cellulitis marked on pt's leg at OSH *(outside hospital)*, no increase in erythema over demarkation
- will switch IV *(intravenous)* cefalexin to PO *(by mouth)*
- morphine 4 mg q4h PRN *(as needed)* for pain
- treating tinea pedis with clotrimazole cream

#) HTN—controlled
- cont HCTZ *(hydrochlorothiazide)*, lisinopril

#) onychomycosis
- cont topical antifungal
- pt w elevated liver enzymes, not candidate for oral antifungals at this time

#) morbid obesity, BMI *(body mass index)* 64.6
- pt currently seeing nutrition, has already lost 26 lb
- will make appt w surg for poss gastric sleeve when has accomplished more wt loss

#) FEN *(fluids, electrolytes, nutrition)*
- NPO since midnight
- IVF *(intravenous fluids)*

#) Prophylaxis
- NO HEPARIN, encourage ambulation

This patient was admitted with pain, vomiting blood, black stools, possibly due to a GI bleed. The patient has a history of alcohol abuse. No psychological or cognitive symptoms noted in this progress note.

Sample 3.4 Neurology Consultation Report

Reason for Consultation: Multiple Sclerosis
Consult Requested by ED *(emergency department)*
Age: 50
Gender: F
Handedness: R

History: Pt is a 50 yo F with a pmhx *(past medical history)* of MS *(multiple sclerosis)*, presenting to the ED after a fall with resultant fracture of her occipital bone with resultant SAH *(subarachnoid hemorrhage)*. Pt reports that she has had increased frequency of falls over the past 3 weeks. Pt reports that she has been compliant with her medications. She reports that she has been more unsteady on her feet. She feels that she is has been having a flare for the past 2 weeks. She reports that she is not interested in starting steroids at this time due to concern for her gaining weight.

Pt reports that she fell at work today and hit her head. She denies loss of consciousness. She was brought to the ED and was found to have a SAH and an occipital bone fracture.

Consultant should determine what the patient's weight is to evaluate the concern about gaining weight with steroids.

<u>Neurological Review of Symptoms:</u>

Bladder symptoms: Negative
Bowel symptoms: Negative
Pain: Negative
Numbness or tingling: Negative
Confusion: Negative
Memory loss: Negative

Speech disorder: Negative
Convulsions: Negative
Blackouts or syncope: Negative
Weakness: Negative
Muscle twitching or cramping: Negative
Headaches: Negative
Vertigo or dizziness: Negative
Tinnitus: Negative
Hearing loss: Negative
Imbalance or falling: Negative
Blurred vision: Negative
Visual loss: Negative
Double vision: Negative
Difficulty with gait or walking: Negative

General Review of Symptoms:

ENT: Negative
Eye: Negative
Cardiovascular: Negative
Gastrointestinal: Negative
Hematological/lymphatic: Negative
Respiratory: Negative
Allergic/immunological: Negative
Dermatologic/breast: Negative
Musculoskeletal: Negative
Genitourinary: Negative
Endocrine: Negative
Psychiatric: Negative
Constitutional: Negative

Note that psychiatric symptoms are negative at the time of the consult.

Medication List

Active Medications

Ordered

acetaminophen: 1,000 mg, 2 tab, PO, Q6HR, PRN: Pain.
acetaminophen-hydrocodone: 1 tab, PO, Q4H, PRN: Pain.
baclofen: 20 mg, 2 tab, PO, BID.
dalfampridine: 10 mg, PO, BID.
docusate: 100 mg, 1 cap, PO, Q12H.
famotidine: 20 mg, 1 tab, PO, Q12H.
heparin: 5,000 units, 0.5 mL, SC, Q12H.
ibuprofen: 600 mg, 1 tab, PO, QID, 40 tab, PRN: for pain.
interferon beta-1a: 44 mcg, SC, Q M & W & F, 36 kit.

interferon beta-1a: 44 mcg, SC, Q M & W & F, 90 Days.
levetiracetam: 500 mg, 1 tab, PO, Q12H.
lorazepam: 0.5 mg, PO, PRN
lorazepam: 1 mg, 1 tab, PO, QHS, 90 Days, PRN: Sleep.
methylprednisolone: 128 mg, PO, DAILY, 30 tab.
methylprednisolone: 1,000 mg, IVPB, DAILY.
morphine: 2 mg, 1 mL, IV PUSH, Q4H, PRN: Pain.
olanzapine: 5 mg, 1 tab, PO, QHS.
omeprazole: 20 mg, 1 tab, PO, DAILY, 90 tab.
oxybutynin: 15 mg, PO, TID.
paroxetine: 50 mg, 2 tab, PO, DAILY, 180 tab.
sulfamethoxazole-trimethoprim: 1 tab, PO, BID.

Note psychotropic medications (lorazepam, olanzapine, paroxetine), but no psychiatric symptoms noted earlier in ROS.

Allergies: nkda
Illnesses: MS, depression, HLD (*hyperlipidemia)*
Note history of depression reported by the neurologist.
Tobacco: denies
Alcohol: denies
Other drug use: denies
Education: some college
Occupation: secretary
Family history: noncontributory
Objective
Vital signs

Vitals (Past 5 vitals in past 24 hours):

Date	Temp (°F/°C)	BP	Pulse	RR	SaO2 (*oxygen saturation*)
03/27 23:02		109/51	74	21	94 (room air)
03/27 22:00	98.1/36.7	119/59	74	16	93 (room air)
03/27 21:00		138/68	71	21	94 (room air)
03/27 20:00	99.0/37.2	109/54	75	22	97 (room air)
03/27 18:45	98.1/36.7	133/63	75	19	95 (room air)

	Height (cm)	Weight (kg)	BMI
03/27 20:00	170	96.5	33.39

Note that BMI = 33 as related to concerns about weight noted by the patient: BMI >30 is designated as obesity.

General Appearance: Well-nourished
Carotids: No bruits heard
Heart: No murmurs
Peripheral pulses: Normal

Ophthalmologic Exam
Optic disk: Normal
Retinal: Normal
Retinal arteries: Normal

Mental Status
LOC *(level of consciousness)*: Alert
Attention: Normal
Orientation: Oriented to person, time, and place
Memory: Normal
Language: Normal
Fund of Knowledge: Normal

Several aspects of mental status were either tested or observed to be normal.

Visual-Spatial ability: Normal
Cranial Nerves
II (visual fields): Full
II (visual acuity): Normal OU *(both eyes)*
II (Fundi): Normal OU
III, IV, VI (EOMS *[extraocular movements]*): R INO *[internuclear ophthalmoplegia]*, upbeat nystagmus at up gaze
V (sensation, mastication): Normal
VII (facial strength): Normal
VIII (hearing): Normal
IX, X (swallowing, phonation): Normal
XI (shoulder shrug): Normal
XII (tongue protrusion): Normal
Gait and station: deferred—pt in c-collar
Tandem gait: deferred—pt in c-collar

Motor Strength	Right	Left
Deltoids	5	5
Triceps	5	5
Biceps	5	5
Grip	5	5
Hip flexors	5	5
Knee flexors	5	5
Knee extensor	5	5
Foot plantar flexors	4	4
Foot dorsi flexors	4	4
Muscle tone	Normal	Normal
Sensory		
Pinprick	Normal	Normal
Vibration	Normal	Normal
Biceps	2+	2+

Triceps	2+	2+
Knee	2+	2+
Ankle	2+	2+
Babinski sign	Absent	Absent
Finger jerks	Absent	Absent
Jaw jerk	Absent	Absent
Coordination		
Finger-to-nose	Normal	Normal
RAM (*rapid alternating movements*)	Normal	Normal
Heel-along-shin	Normal	Normal

Medical Decision-Making:

Assessment: 50 y/o female with MS, presenting to the ED after fall and subsequent fracture of the occipital bone and SAH. Concern that the pt is having flare of her MS symptoms as she has had prior symptoms of falls in previous flares. Pt does not want to start on steroids for acute exacerbation. Given that steroids do not alter the course of the disease, aside from shortening a flare, it is reasonable that the pt could follow up as an outpatient with her primary neurologist. However pt would warrant rule out of a pseudo exacerbation *(a flare of MS symptoms caused by an event other than new neurological damage as in a true exacerbation; not a pretend event or a psychological issue)*. At this time would check a UA *(urinalysis)* and urine culture, chest x-ray. Continue pt on rebiff and ampyra. Would also order an MRI *(magnetic brain imaging scan)* brain with contrast to examine progression of disease.

Attending: I have examined the patient with the Neuro team and reviewed the pertinent findings. I agree with the above assessment and plan. Suggested course of iv steroids, pt/ot *(physical therapy/occupational therapy)* possible rehab after cleared by NS *(neurosurgery)*. Hopefully, she will reconsider. (*Initial note was written by the resident physician; this is the attending physician's agreement and summary attestation.)*

Patient with apparent significant psychological history of depression and on three psychotropic meds. She is refusing treatment with steroids for presumed MS exacerbation.

Sample 3.5 Psychiatry Discharge Summary

ADMIT DATE: xx/xx/xxxx
DISCHARGE DATE: xx/xx/2013
Note date of admission; how long ago was this admission to inpatient psychiatry?
ATTENDING: Dr. P
ADMISSION DIAGNOSIS:
impulse control d/o *(disorder)*; depressive disorder—unspecified; intellectual disability: mild.

HISTORY OF PRESENT ILLNESS:

Patient is 30 y/o female with intellectual disability and unclear psychiatric history, with multiple admissions at outside hospital for management of aggressive behavior. Pt was brought to the ER by her caretaker (currently in process of getting guardianship) because of aggressive behavior (both verbal and physical), hypersexuality, suicidal ideation and inability to take care of her needs. In the past 2 days, the patient became very angry for no specific reason, and she has been grabbing knife, throwing microwave, yelling at people, at times she would take her clothes off, walked naked in front of people, also make sexually inappropriate gestures. Pt also expressed suicidal ideation with plan to cut herself with the knife. Patient has a history of 1 suicidal attempt when she tried to cut herself with a knife. Pt lives with 5 y/o daughter, her husband (intellectually disabled), and a caretaker. DCFS *(Department of Children and Family Services)* is involved. Caretaker is Ms. S, who is in the process of obtaining guardianship over patient and her family. She reported history of multiple hospitalizations, with limited success in managing pt's behavior issues. After last admission at OSH *(outside hospital)* she was discharged on Sertraline (Zoloft) 100 mg QHS *(at bedtime)* and Depakote (divalproex sodium) ER 500 QHS; her psychiatrist is Dr. R.

Per collateral (caretaker): Patient has been acting out more frequently over the past couple months, getting angry or tearful, yelling, grabbing knife in kitchen. She was most recently hospitalized around 1 month ago, at which time Depakote was added to her regimen (was taking only Zoloft previously). Caretaker does not believe this is helping. She believes patient is acting out more because patient may be thinking about experience 2 years ago when patient was molested by an uncle. Caretaker reports patient is welcome back home and is interested in opportunities available for pt to engage in more structured daytime activities.

Note that the patient's husband also has an intellectual disability and they have a 5-year-old child. DCFS is already involved, raising concerns about abuse and neglect. Is this too much for the caretaker to handle?

MENTAL EXAMINATION:

on admission:

Gen: short caucasian woman appearing somewhat younger than stated age with short hair, smiling and inappropriately laughing throughout interview, avoidant eye contact, cooperative. good grooming/hygiene.

Speech: somewhat dysarthric *(imperfect articulation)*

Mood: "depressed"

Affect: at times inappropriate/mood-incongruent, smiling/laughing when talking about depression, somewhat anxious, stable

TP *(thought process)*: concrete, linear/goal directed

TC *(thought content)*: denies current SI *(suicidal ideation)*/HI *(homicidal ideation)*, no AVH *(auditory or visual hallucinations)*

I/J *(insight/judgment)*: limited

on discharge:

Gen: childlike—smiling and giggling throughout interview, fair eye contact, cooperative. good grooming/hygiene.
Speech: somewhat dysarthric
Mood: "good"
Affect: smiling/laughing during interview, pleasant, stable
TP: concrete, linear/goal directed
TC: denies current SI/HI, no AVH
I/J: limited

HOSPITAL COURSE:

Patient was admitted to psych unit under formal voluntary conditions, was oriented to the unit and placed on safety checks for self-harm, elopement and aggressive behavior. She was seen initially by the treatment team to be very pleasant, smiling/laughing at times inappropriately throughout interview even when speaking of feeling depressed. She admitted she had been feeling suicidal and "aggravation" at home, sleeping "4–6 hours" a night. She reported feeling "a little sad once in a while" and angry more recently, although she did not wish to speak about what has bothered her and stated there were no changes at home. Patient was restarted on her outpatient medications of Zoloft 100 mg qhs and Depakote 500 mg qhs. *(Had she been off meds, and if so, for how long?)* Depakote level on admission was 63 *(low normal)*. Due to mood instability and more aggressive behavior at home, in addition to her endorsing somewhat poor sleep, her Depakote was increased to 750 mg po qhs. Patient did not display any self-injurious, aggressive, or violent behavior while on the unit. She maintained good hygiene, was calm/pleasant, and appeared to enjoy engaging in groups. She reported she no longer felt suicidal or angry, identifying her medications and groups as helping her. The treatment team believed group activities would be beneficial to her on discharge; outside agency was therefore contacted by SW *(social work)* to assist with arranging group programming for after discharge. She had no somatic complaints besides mild occasional headache in occipital/frontal areas that she states are usually relieved with Excedrin at home. She agreed to follow-up with her primary physician for further management of headaches. Patient's caretaker was contacted and made aware of plans, to which she agreed. The patient was seen to be psychiatrically stable for discharge to her caretaker's home. She voiced improved mood, sleep, and denied any suicidal/homicidal ideation on discharge.

DISCHARGE INSTRUCTIONS:

1) ACTIVITY: no restriction
2) FOLLOW-UP:
   Psychiatry—Family Services with Dr. R on 2/24 at 2:30 p.m.
3) MEDICATIONS:
   Depakote 750 mg po qhs
   Zoloft 100 mg po qhs
   MVI (*multivitamin*) daily

folic acid 1 mg daily
pt to also take Excedrin tab for headaches at home (reports relief of headaches with this medication)

4) DIET: regular
5) DISCHARGE DISPOSITION: to caretaker's home

CONDITION UPON DISCHARGE: stable

This patient has had several psychiatric admissions in the past. The note indicates issues with aggression, depression, anxiety, suicidal ideation, and behavioral problems. Intellectual disability is likely also a critical part of the picture. Psychology consultant would want to determine how the patient has been behaviorally and psychologically since this discharge summary was written.

Interviewing the Patient 4

Typically, most of the consultant's data about the patient come directly from the interview with the patient herself. This chapter discusses introductions to the patient with attention to concerns that they may have about participating in mental health interviews. The content of the biopsychosocial interview is presented next, as well as strategies to manage problems that can occur during patient interviews. The importance of providing feedback to patients and methods to do so are also presented.

Getting Started

When entering the room, the health psychology consultant should always introduce himself to the patient. This introduction should include the psychologist's name, the department or service he is from, and the reason for seeing the patient. This introduction can be more or less formal, depending on the patient and the atmosphere the psychologist is trying to develop. Less formal and more friendly (yet professionally appropriate) interactions are most conducive to gaining the patient's willingness to proceed with the evaluation.

Many physicians and nurses refer to the patient by his or her first name, ostensibly because it is more warm and familiar. However, it is also less

http://dx.doi.org/10.1037/0000108-005
Health Psychology Consultation in the Inpatient Medical Setting, by S. M. Labott

respectful than referring to the patient with the appropriate title (Mr., Mrs., Ms., Dr., etc.), at least until the relationship is stronger. If the psychologist expects the patient to refer to her with the proper title, then it would seem appropriate that we offer the same respect to them.

Many physicians will also shake hands with the patient, at least at the initial introduction. However, nosocomial infections (those acquired in the hospital) are "the most frequent adverse event in health-care delivery worldwide" (World Health Organization, n.d.) and are often transmitted to the patient from the hands of their medical providers (E. Larson, 1988). Handwashing should be performed before and after each contact with each patient, but this does not completely obviate all risk, and so handshakes should be avoided. (See Chapter 1, this volume, for more detail on infection control procedures in the hospital.)

Most patients have not requested psychological services, and they may be unaware that a health psychology consultation has been ordered for them, so the psychologist will need to explain the purpose of the visit. The explanation should be low key; for example, the consultant could describe herself as a member of the patient's treatment team who is here to see how the patient is managing the stress associated with the hospitalization. The reason for the visit can be explained in fairly vague terms, especially if the specific reason for the consultation may decrease the patient's level of trust before the interview even gets started. For example, consider the case of a patient whose medical problems are escalating because he is drinking too much alcohol. Consider these two introductions: "Good morning, I am Dr. S from the Health Psychology Service. I'm here to talk to you today about your alcohol use" versus "Hi, Mr. J. I'm Brenda Smith from the Health Psychology Service. I'm here because often people have some trouble coping with their medical problems, so I want to talk with you about how you're doing with that and see if there is anything we can do to help." The second introduction is more general, can be used with almost any specific referral question, and is unlikely to put the patient on the defensive.

A patient may ask specifically who ordered the evaluation and the reason for it; then it is appropriate to answer those questions for them. Often, however, it is acceptable to say, "Your doctors asked me to come by to talk with you and see if there is anything we can do to help out." (The formal written report, however, should explicitly state the name of the referring physician as well as the specific reason for the consultation. For example, "Mrs. S was referred by Dr. J for evaluation of acute cognitive changes" or "Mr. B was referred by Dr. W with concerns about adjustment to new diagnosis of cancer and help coping.")

Most people, even though they are not feeling well, have good social skills and will respond appropriately to a well-meaning consultant who is trying to gather information to aid the patient's overall treatment in the hospital. Some, however, will be less welcoming. Less psychologically sophisticated people, those outside the mainstream culture, and those who have had bad experiences with mental health professionals in the past may be uncomfortable with the health psychology consultant. Some people worry that they will be labeled as a "crazy" psychiatric patient and that this will stigmatize them or affect their medical care in a negative way (i.e., their providers may think their symptoms are psychiatric in nature and so will not provide appropriate medical treatment). Over time, the consultant will learn to pick up cues of patient discomfort, hesitation, or suspicion quickly when approaching the patient. Addressing any issues or questions to improve the patient's comfort with the evaluation will improve the patient's experience and will also result in better information being generated.

The goal is generally to interview patients alone, and typically any visitors or family members who are present should be asked to leave (also see Chapter 15 regarding privacy issues). Often they can be asked to get a cup of coffee and come back in a bit, but sometimes visitors have traveled a long way and may have only a short time to visit. In this case, the consultant should agree to come back later in the day, if possible. Often the benefits of supportive family and friends are as useful as the psychological treatment we plan to provide. There are times when it is appropriate to include a family member, in cases in which the patient has difficulty participating in the interview (i.e., is somnolent or impaired cognitively) or to provide emotional support for a patient, especially if they are frightened or delirious. If, as a result of a family member being present, the consultant feels the information gathered was tainted, that should be addressed after the visitor leaves.

When beginning the interview, it is good practice to let the patient know you will be asking a wide variety of questions to get to know him or her. If the patient appears comfortable with this, the health psychology consultant can pull a chair next to the bed and begin the interview. If the patient is in a chair next to the bed, they may offer the consultant a seat on their bed, but sitting there is not appropriate (due to issues of infection as well as intimacy). The consultant will often stand throughout the interview, sometimes because this is the best way to maintain eye contact with the patient if she is propped in the bed in such a way that she cannot see the consultant if he is seated in a chair next to the bed. In other cases, patients have difficulty staying awake, so if the consultant can lean over them and speak more loudly, it is more likely to help them to remain attentive.

Inpatient consultants typically need to take notes on the interview and will need to do so while maintaining eye contact and rapport. It is not uncommon for a consultant to interview several patients before sitting down to write reports. For example, if three women in their 60s were interviewed in one morning, it may be difficult to keep the details of their histories and lives straight without good notes to aid the process.

When performing an inpatient interview, there is a balance to be achieved between rapport-building and data collection that is different from that in the outpatient setting. Outpatient intake interviews are often the beginning of a therapeutic relationship, and practitioners are likely to forgo some data initially to allow clients more time to talk freely, in an effort to increase rapport. Although rapport is also important in the inpatient setting, the main goal of the inpatient consultation is to collect relevant data to conceptualize the current problem—and quickly. Therefore, inpatient evaluations need to remain more focused on data collection, and consultants will direct the conversation more in the inpatient setting than they would in the outpatient setting.

Data to Collect in the Patient Interview

The interview with the inpatient is typically a comprehensive biopsychosocial interview that is not significantly different from a traditional psychological intake interview, i.e., it includes an evaluation of the individual's social situation, psychological treatment history, and current status, substance use, and mental status. One key difference is that in the inpatient setting, there is additional attention paid to medical issues because all of the other data obtained will be considered in that context. It is important to understand the reason for the patient's current hospital admission, chronic medical issues and medications, and her coping with these issues. Further, the information regarding psychological symptoms is understood in relation to the medical issues; for example, the patient may be experiencing symptoms of anxiety and depression as a result of a new medical diagnosis, she may receive little social support from family as she struggles with chronic medical problems and associated treatments, or she is overusing medications or substances in an attempt to escape from the stress of the medical problem. In addition, the health psychology consultant will want to remain vigilant for any additional issues have been raised that warrant further assessment or discussion. The specific areas to cover in the inpatient psychological consultation interview are described in detail in the following subsections.

As with any psychological interview, the health psychology consultant will generally want to use good interviewing skills with open-ended questions. At times, however, more direct questioning will be necessary to obtain specific information in a brief time period. It is easiest for the consultant to cover the items in a consistent order, because it will then be more difficult to forget something. However, if the patient has something he wants to discuss, it is best to start with that. Otherwise, start with a general discussion of how he is doing, and then complete any sections of the evaluation that have not yet been covered. It is often best to leave formal mental status testing to later in the interview because it feels to the patients like a test and is therefore more threatening. There are exceptions: If a patient is uncooperative and seems likely to refuse a complete evaluation, it is best to ask the most relevant items right away (e.g., suicidal ideation, mental status, psychosis) in case the interview does not get completed. Exhibit 4.1 contains a list of the most relevant items that the health psychology consultant will want to cover during the interview; the consultant can write notes next to each item as the interview progresses (this is especially helpful for trainees). Some of the historic data can also be abstracted from the patient's medical record before the interview and then checked for accuracy with the patient.

MEDICAL HISTORY AND CURRENT ISSUES

The consultant will have reviewed the medical record and should have a good idea of what the patient's medical issues are and then can begin the interview by asking the patient to provide information about her current medical situation. Some patients will complain that you should have read their chart so they don't have to go over it all again; that complaint can typically be managed by explaining that you have read their

EXHIBIT 4.1

Inpatient Consultation Content

Pt name:
Age:
MR # (*medical record number*):
Room #:
Gender:
Referral source/pager:
Date and reason for admission:

Referral question

Medical history and current issues:
- Medical problems
- Meds
- Pain
- Coping with medical issues

Social situation:
- Marital status/children/living situation
- Education
- Employment
- Social support
- *Substance use:*
  - Current use/history of problems/past tx (*treatment*)
  - Tobacco
  - ETOH
  - Drugs

Psychiatric history:
- Previous psych tx—inpt and outpt (*inpatient and outpatient*)
- Psych meds
- Family psych hx
- Suicide attempts/self-harm

Current psychological status:
- Mood/depression
- Sleep/appetite
- Guilt/worthlessness
- Interest
- Energy
- Hopelessness/helplessness
- SI (*suicidal ideation*)
- Irritability
- Anxiety
- Worry
- Panic
- Manic sx (*symptoms*)
- Paranoia
- Hallucinations

(*continues*)

EXHIBIT 4.1 (*Continued*)

Inpatient Consultation Content

Mental status:
- Subjective memory concerns
- Orientation
- Registration
- Attention/calc (*calculation*)
- LTM (*long-term memory*)
- Abstract thinking
- Judgment
- STM (*short-term memory*)
- Observations

Special issues to discuss/assess (e.g., nonadherence, end of life, decisional capacity, pain control)

Referral question answered?

Note. For abbreviations that are unclear, here and in other chapters throughout the book, consult Appendix A. Thanks to past students who developed several iterations of this interview guide.

chart but that you want to hear a little bit about their situation directly from them. A discussion of the current medical issue is warranted as part of the consultation, but often the remainder of the medical history can be obtained from the medical record. For example, if the patient is dealing with a new diagnosis of Crohn's disease, the fact that he has been on medication for high cholesterol for a few years is not as relevant. In that case, the written report could reflect which aspects of the patient's history the patient reported, and which were obtained from chart review.

It is important for the health psychology consultant to know what medications patients are taking, but patients should not be expected to report on all of the medications they are taking in the hospital. There are frequent changes in medications and doses, and many patients will not be aware of some medications they have been prescribed. Most relevant for the psychology consultation are medications that can have psychological effects (such as mood and cognitive changes), and the consultant will know this information from the chart review. In addition, outpatient psychotropic medications are relevant (even if the patient is not taking them in the hospital) because they provide information on the patient's psychological history and premorbid level of functioning. Patients should be asked to confirm outpatient psychotropic medications that are listed in their chart because medical providers are often less attentive to these and changes may not be recorded, and many times patients have discontinued psychotropic medications on their own.

Adherence is also an important component of a patient's adjustment to her medical situation. If no problems with adherence have been noted, the psychology consultant could simply ask if the patient ever has problems following the doctor's recommendations or attending medical appointments. If so, then a more thorough evaluation of adherence to specific medication recommendations, diet, exercise, and special treatments (such as outpatient chemotherapy or hemodialysis) is warranted. If patients are having difficulty with adherence, reasons for that will also need to be assessed. (More information on nonadherence is in Chapter 12.)

SOCIAL SITUATION

As with any psychological evaluation, it is important to obtain information on the person's education, employment, and family. In the inpatient setting, these topics often do not need to be described in great detail, but the basic information will provide a good idea of the patient's place in life. Social support is typically relevant because it can be a great resource as patients work to navigate the medical setting. Social support is often sorely lacking when patients are struggling to manage.

SUBSTANCE USE

Information should be obtained on a patient's current and past use of tobacco, alcohol, and street drugs. Unless there are specific concerns about use or abuse or patterns of substance use that would be expected to cause problems for the patient (either socially or with their medical problems), only basic information is necessary. If there are specific concerns regarding substance use or abuse, then a more thorough assessment should be done, to include a description of substance use patterns over time as well as substance use treatment and its effectiveness. (See Chapter 10 for more information on a detailed and thorough evaluation of substance use patterns.) Certainly if patients are dealing with a medical issue that necessitates total abstinence—for example, if the patient is a candidate for liver transplantation—that should be discussed clearly and in a straightforward manner.

PSYCHOLOGICAL AND PSYCHIATRIC HISTORY

To understand the patient's situation, it will be important to know about previous inpatient and outpatient mental health treatment by psychologists, psychiatrists, and other mental health providers, as well as psychotropic medication use, whether prescribed by a psychiatrist or a primary care doctor, and family history of psychological problems. It is also useful to ask patients about a history of emotional problems, even if they have no history of psychological or psychiatric treatment, as well as a history of trauma. Note that in an initial inpatient evaluation of this type, the collection of information on the details and specifics of the trauma should be avoided. Although this could be a focus of ongoing treatment on an outpatient basis later, requests for personal and difficult information like this make people uncomfortable, especially those who have not requested an evaluation in the first place. Further, trauma experience detail is less likely to be necessary information for the current purposes.

CURRENT PSYCHOLOGICAL STATUS

Patients should be evaluated for current depression, anxiety, worry, panic, adjustment problems, mania, paranoia, and hallucinations. In many cases, the psychological terms will need to be defined for them. Alternately, the questions can be asked without using the psychological terms at all; for example, rather than asking if a patient is experiencing paranoia, the health psychology consultant could ask the patient if he feels safe. If symptoms are present, one may assess specific criteria to develop a *Diagnostic and Statistical Manual of Mental Disorders* (fifth edition; American Psychiatric Association, 2013) diagnosis, although this may not be necessary. In the inpatient setting, the specific symptoms and their intensity are more important than the formal clinical diagnosis (although the diagnosis may be needed for billing purposes; see Chapter 16). It will be important to delineate emotional symptoms that are a result of the current medical situation, such as anxiety about a new diagnosis of leukemia or due to a new medication, versus those that predate the current situation (e.g., a history of dysthymia).

MENTAL STATUS OBSERVATION AND ASSESSMENT

Mental status assessment here includes both formal mental status screening and also behavioral observations. Psychologists, in general, are good at making and documenting behavioral observations, due to their experience with this aspect of evaluation in the outpatient setting. In the inpatient medical setting, most patients are sitting calmly in bed, so behavior other than that is remarkable. Agitation, irritability, somnolence, poor eye contact, and other less common behaviors are all noteworthy. Although most patients are wearing hospital gowns, some are neat, and others are disheveled. Some people in the hospital apply complete makeup, while others have apparently not combed their hair in days. Other, more atypical behaviors may also be observed (e.g., the patient is unwilling to interrupt a telephone conversation to be evaluated, is engaged in a heated argument with his wife, or the consultant is unable to wake the patient to complete the evaluation). The latter would also warrant notification of the patient's nurse.

Additional aspects of mental status can also be observed while interviewing the patient, such as mood, thought process and content, and affect expression (as reported in a typical psychiatric interview). These may also provide data that aids the health psychology consultant in his understanding and conceptualization of the patient's situation.

The psychologist's observations of the patient may also be useful medically. For example, one elderly female patient had undergone a round of chemotherapy as part of treatment for an acute leukemia. She had been doing well, although the process had been physically and emotionally difficult for her. She had not demonstrated any cognitive changes or significant psychological symptoms. Yet, at a routine follow-up visit, the health psychologist found her to be almost completely nonverbal and appearing fearful. The patient was not able to communicate well with nods or other signals. A mental status examination could not be obtained, but the observations of her behavior clearly indicated a change. The health psychologist quickly located the patient's nurse and described what she had seen; the nurse then went to evaluate the patient herself and acknowledged that the patient's presentation was different today than previously. She contacted the patient's physician, who ordered tests to assess for problems that could be the cause of these changes. Within a few hours, it had been determined that the patient had a slow brain hemorrhage, and treatment was begun. In this case, the health psychology consultant did not know exactly what the cause of the problem was when she initially saw the patient, but she noticed that the patient's presentation was very different from her baseline. That observation was sufficient to prompt immediate diagnostic testing and medical intervention.

Formal mental status testing is also an important part of the inpatient evaluation. Psychologists with outpatient experience may be inclined to skip formal mental status testing because in the outpatient setting there is little variability in performance as most clients are cognitively intact. However, in the inpatient setting, formal cognitive screening is critical because changes in cognition occur commonly, and they may not be exposed in any other way.

Even for patients who appear to have no cognitive problems and for whom none are noted in the medical record, a brief mental status screening is warranted. It is not uncommon for patients to demonstrate mental status changes on a screening exam that were not known about previously. At times, these may reflect a poor night's sleep or some other issue that is not of significance. Other times, however, a small change on a mental status exam may be the first sign of a bigger, significant medical problem. Many medical issues can present with subtle cognitive changes while the specific signs and symptoms of the medical disorder are still subclinical; the finding of a cognitive change on the mental status exam may be the first indication that the patient has some significant medical problem that is yet undetected. For example, it is not uncommon to complete an entire interview with a patient and observe no cognitive deficits. Then, during mental status screening, the patient says the year is 1962. Even if the rest of the cognitive screener is negative for problems, this response is significant. On the basis of the screener itself, it may not be clear what exactly this response reflects, but it is a red flag to the consultant that there is some problem that needs to be noted and assessed further.

The most commonly used scale to screen for cognitive problems in the inpatient medical setting is the Mini-Mental Status Examination (MMSE; Folstein, Folstein, & McHugh, 1975). This is a cognitive screener that takes only a few minutes and provides data on orientation, registration, attention, short-term memory, language, and other aspects of cognition. The evaluator also rates the patient's level of consciousness. The MMSE has been widely used in both clinical and research settings; norms (Bravo & Hébert, 1997) and cutoff scores for dementia (Boustani et al., 2003) have been published. For the inpatient evaluation, it may be helpful to formally score the examination (which is simple to do) because the score can be monitored over time, and a score on the MMSE is often meaningful to psychiatrists and neurologists who may also be monitoring the patient's cognitive status.

The Modified Mini-Mental State (3MS) Examination (Teng & Chui, 1987) is a modified version of the MMSE. It contains some improvements over the original MMSE (e.g., more graded scoring; more items for some aspects of cognition, such as orientation and memory; and items to measure additional domains, such as similarities), but it is less commonly used in the inpatient setting.

The score on the cognitive screener is often less important than a description of the patient's responses, followed by a general impression of how the patient is doing cognitively, and the implications of this for the patient's medical treatment. Many psychology consultants will choose to use the MMSE, adding a few additional items to measure long-term memory, abstract thinking, and judgment to provide a more thorough description of the patient's cognitive functioning. Later, once the clinician has a good knowledge of what responses are typical in a specific population, he may shorten the exam to collect just the data needed for a particular purpose (although that can't be scored properly). If a consultant needs additional information on a specific area, such as fund of information, proverb interpretation, or disorientation, additional items to assess specific aspects of cognition can be added to the standard screener. Strub and Black (2000) provided a good resource with sample items to assess a wide variety of cognitive deficits.

Other professionals may have performed mental status testing previously, and this information can provide comparison data for the health psychology consultant's current examination but should not replace it. Do not be fooled by inpatient notes that say "A & O × 3" (alert and oriented to person, place, and time) without any concrete data because this may only mean that no gross deficits were noted but no formal orientation questions were asked. It is not uncommon for this to be recorded in the patient's medical record if the patient responded with "good morning, doctor" when the physician entered the room.

When patients are experiencing acute mental status changes, their cognitive functioning can fluctuate dramatically (see Chapter 9 on delirium), and then orientation, memory, and other aspects of cognition should be assessed repeatedly over time to track changes. In these cases, changes in specific aspects of cognition will change over time, and it is important to track the patient's progress back to baseline as the cause of the delirium is resolved. This fluctuation in the patient's mental status will also account for the differences in performance seen by two clinicians who assess the same patient at different times on the same day.

The mental status evaluation can provide critical information about the patient's cognitive functioning, but it is only screening. For a thorough understanding of the patient's cognitive functioning, complete neuropsychological testing should be performed. Yet there are factors in the inpatient environment (e.g., time constraints, patient fatigue) that may make a full neuropsychological exam difficult. In many inpatient cases, the mental status screening will provide sufficient data to address the acute issue, with more comprehensive neuropsychological testing scheduled for a later date in the outpatient setting, if it is still warranted after the acute phase has passed.

Some psychologists would also include a brief literacy screener to flag patients who are functionally illiterate. The Single Item Literacy Screener (SILS; Morris, MacLean, Chew, & Littenberg, 2006) can be used for this purpose. The SILS asks, "How often do you need to have someone help you when you read instructions, pamphlets, or other written material from your doctor or pharmacy?" Patients are asked to respond using a scale from 1 (*never*) to 5 (*always*). Responses of "sometimes," "often," and "always" indicate potential literacy problems. The SILS is useful as a brief screener that can be expanded on if more detail on a patient's literacy is warranted.

Health literacy may also be included as a standard part of an interview because as many as 90 million Americans have low health literacy (Institute of Medicine Committee on Health Literacy [IOM], 2004) that can affect their ability to manage their medical conditions. Patients with low health literacy may have difficulty communicating their concerns to their providers, and they face additional challenges in understanding and processing information about their health and treatment options as well as the risks and benefits of potential treatments. Low literacy is associated with a higher likelihood of hospitalization and poorer health outcomes (Dewalt, Berkman, Sheridan, Lohr, & Pignone, 2004); it is correlated with poorer education, non-White ethnicity, and older age (Paasche-Orlow, Parker, Gazmararian, Nielsen-Bohlman, & Rudd, 2005). See the IOM's (2004) extensive review of health literacy and related issues, as well as recommendations to improve low literacy.

The assessment of health literacy can be brief and can quickly reveal potential problems in understanding that can then be remedied with additional education. Although communication about health matters should be clear and understanding of important medical details should be assessed with all patients, specific data on low health literacy can provide additional motivation for providers to attend to this issue.

Several measures have been used to assess health literacy. The Rapid Estimate of Adult Literacy in Medicine—Short Form (Arozullah et al., 2007) takes only 2 to 3 minutes to administer. Patients are presented with a list of seven medical words (e.g., *antibiotics, jaundice*) and asked to read each word out loud. The score is the number of words pronounced correctly; higher scores are reflective of a higher reading grade level and better health literacy. This scale has been used frequently in research but is also useful clinically. For patients who speak Spanish, the Short Assessment of Health Literacy for Spanish Adults (Lee, Bender, Ruiz, & Cho, 2006) is a reliable and valid measure of health literacy.

Common Problems With Inpatient Interviews

It can be difficult to interview sick people in a busy hospital setting. Specific challenges that can interfere with an evaluation include patients who are uncooperative, who have complaints about their treatment, and who have problems communicating. Each of these is discussed in this section.

UNCOOPERATIVE PATIENTS

Many patients are hesitant to talk to a psychologist, but most will comply and become more comfortable as the interaction progresses. On occasion, a patient will flatly refuse an interview, sometimes even before the consultant can introduce himself to the patient. It is easy to attribute this to negative personality traits, although in the inpatient medical setting, it is more likely to be due to pain, fear, or delirium. Certainly patients have the right to refuse any and all medical treatment, including a health psychology consultation. However, patients do not have the right to refuse if their ability to make decisions is impaired. If the referral question is about decisional capacity, the patient's rights are not clear until the evaluation is completed. A patient who refuses the consultation places the consultant in a difficult position because the referring medical team is requesting specific information to aid their treatment of the patient that the consultant cannot provide without seeing the patient. As a consequence, it makes most sense to try to get the evaluation done without interfering with the patient's rights or upsetting him and then to make determinations about the patient's decisional capacity for future contacts (see Chapter 11 for more on decisional capacity).

There is an art to obtaining compliance in these situations that the health psychology consultant will learn over time. Keeping the interaction low key and minimizing the time commitment can help to gain patient agreement. Sometimes patients will agree to an interview at a time later in the day if they are not feeling up to it when the consultant first arrives. Other times patients will agree to a few minutes of an interview to address the most pressing issues, with the rest of the interview to be completed at another time. If it is clear that the patient is thinking of refusing, the consultant should try to make this appear like a quick visit (i.e., don't pull out a pad and pen, remain standing) and assess the most critical issues first.

COMPLAINTS

Often patients have complaints about their care in the hospital. Some complaints may be due to a poor understanding of the treatment or communication problems, and these can be cleared up relatively easily. For example, a patient may be angry at his nurse because she won't bring him water, not understanding that he is to be NPO (nothing by mouth) for a medical procedure later that day. An explanation of the procedure, why it is important to his treatment planning, and the rationale for being NPO will typically resolve the issue.

A second scenario occurs when patients have unreasonable expectations or are scared and very needy as a result. The neediness will usually subside (at least temporarily) if the psychologist spends time with the patient, discussing her concerns and ways to cope with them. Unreasonable expectations can also be addressed with education (e.g., a patient complains that he hasn't seen his regular doctor in 2 days, so he feels that he is not getting any care). Educating him about the workings of the hospital (e.g., in a teaching hospital, the resident physician that he has seen is discussing his care with the primary physician) may help to decrease the patient's concerns. Patients who have little contact with the medical system often do not understand that they see several physicians in a day, several of whom may be in training and acting as surrogates for their primary physician. An understanding of the process will likely resolve a complaint like this, especially when the patient is made aware that he does have access to his primary physician and can specifically request a visit when he needs to.

Even after all the miscommunications are resolved, there are times that patients have legitimate complaints about their treatment. One major category of complaint has to do with poor communication among the various medical providers, especially in large teaching hospitals. A patient may complain that his primary medical team told him this morning that he is healing nicely and could be discharged home today to follow-up in the outpatient clinic at the end of the week. An hour later, however, another consultant comes by and says there is one last test they want to run, and that would mean he has to stay here at least 1 more day. Especially if the patient has been in the hospital for a while, he is eager for discharge, and he may also need to make arrangements for someone to take off work to pick him up and get him settled at home. Unfortunately, the various professionals who are caring for a patient are sometimes not working effectively as a team, and the only way to resolve this issue is to get them to communicate with each other and to arrive at a decision about the patient's discharge so that the patient can plan accordingly.

Patients may also have complaints about nurses and how they are treated by them. Many of these complaints result from a situation in which nurses are overworked and may not spend the time with a patient that he (as well as the nurse) would prefer. Patients are often understanding of this issue, as long as they are confident that the nurse will be available for them when they need something. At other times, however, nurses take too long to respond to a patient's legitimate request for help. In these cases, patients can be encouraged to allow a reasonable amount of time for the nurse to respond. If she does not, they should be encouraged to press the call button again.

The health psychology consultant will generally be interested in hearing patient concerns, whatever they might be. Listening goes a long way to decreasing the anger or fear that patients feel in these situations. Yet while the psychologist will want to listen and empathize with the patient and her concerns, she must also be careful not to incite the patient further, to avoid appearing like she is bad-mouthing other members of the treatment team, or to make excuses for them. It is best to listen to the complaint, asking a few questions to gain an understanding of what the likely problem is, while empathizing with the patient's feelings about it, and then decide how best to manage it. On occasion, there is a patient who becomes more and more upset as the complaint is discussed (rather than calming down). In this situation, the consultant would do well to make the discussion brief to avoid stirring up the patient's anger or negative emotions and then move the discussion to a more positive topic.

Management of the complaint may be something the psychologist can help the patient to accomplish, or perhaps the psychologist can advocate for the patient with the relevant party. Exhibit 4.2 contains a list of strategies that can be used to manage patient complaints. When advocating for the patient, tact is necessary to avoid making the relevant staff member feel criticized and defensive, which will not help manage the issue. It is also important to avoid making the patient appear to be difficult and unreasonable. When advocating for the patient with medical providers, it is useful to acknowledge that they are busy, and then inform them about the patient's specific concerns, asking for their help to address the problem.

EXHIBIT 4.2

Methods to Handle Patient Complaints

Educate the patient to clear up misunderstandings.

Encourage the patient to discuss the issue further with the relevant staff member, and role play with the patient how to do so appropriately.

Advocate for the patient by raising a question or concern with the relevant physician or nurse.

Teach the patient appropriate ways to address concerns or ways to manage his or her own emotional reactions.

Provide contact information for the hospital department or staff person who handles formal patient complaints.

INTERVIEWING PATIENTS WITH COMMUNICATION PROBLEMS

Health psychology consultants commonly need to interview patients who are unable to communicate easily or at all. Patients who are on ventilators, for example, are unable to speak unless they have had a tracheotomy, and even then it may be difficult to understand them. Some of these patients are able to write, and they can do so on a clipboard. Because they are lying in bed, their writing may be poor, but an interview can sometimes be conducted by asking questions and letting them write their responses. Unfortunately, people on ventilators also often have IVs and monitors on their hands and arms, or they are not physically or cognitively able to write, making this a poor option. Patients can sometimes be presented with a list of the letters of the alphabet (available on a laminated board in some hospitals, or the consultant can write the alphabet on a pad of paper) and can point to letters to spell responses to interview questions. However, this method can be time-intensive, and patients may be too tired to complete an entire interview.

If patients are cognitively able, communication can also be achieved with head nods (for yes–no) or some other signal (one finger for yes, two fingers for no). If this strategy is used, the consultant will need to test the patient first with a few simple questions to be sure he understands the system (e.g., Is your name Brian? Are you 47 years old? Is my name Dr. S?). Once it is clear that the patient understands the system, the consultant can proceed with the interview but will need to remember to ask all yes–no questions. The entire interview, even much of the mental status assessment (asking questions such as: Is this 1984? 2012? Are we in a grocery store? A hospital?), can be done this way fairly well. Although a process like this can provide much of the necessary information, it will result in little understanding of the specifics of the patient's experience. Perhaps more detailed information can be obtained from family in these cases.

Each of these methods of communication will be time-consuming and can be frustrating for the patient, so it is best to keep the interview as short as possible. In these situations, it is often most important to assess patients' current psychological situation (anxiety, depression, fear, pain) and cognitive functioning; information about other aspects of their life can wait until later. It is important to empathize with the patient that they are in a difficult and frustrating situation. Intervention with these patients most often is done by providing patients with education about their situation, along with suggestions of how they can cope. Many times, the patient will be able to communicate more effectively later (e.g., when her lung infection improves and she can breathe on her own), then further assessment can be done, and the patient can be more involved in the intervention.

Wrapping Up the Interview and Providing Feedback

When learning to do inpatient consultation, there is an overwhelming amount of information to digest and integrate, and it is tempting to say goodbye and walk away when all the interview questions have been answered. Yet patients who are often exhausted and uncomfortable have given a significant amount of their time and energy to the interview, even though they often don't know its purpose or anticipate much (if any) benefit from it. The health psychology consultant should get in the habit of providing something to patients at the end of the interview to give them something of benefit. This might take the form of a summary of what was discussed to let the patient know she has been heard and understood by the psychologist and that her time has not been wasted. It is also always a good strategy to ask the patient to correct any information that is incorrect. Spending a few minutes to provide a patient with feedback is typically part of this process. The consultant can explain her impressions in lay terms and then describe any recommendations for treatment. The feedback provided to the patient may be similar in content to that provided to the referral source, but it should be presented in simpler terms and with more time spent discussing the intervention and how this will help the patient. It should be made clear to the patient that his experience is understandable given the situation he is facing; psychiatric terminology and pathological labels should be avoided. The consultant should present the conceptualization of the problem as a normal reaction that warrants coping, rather than a psychiatric problem that warrants psychiatric treatment.

A consultant may say,

> So, Mr. J, you seem to be managing your illness well, except that sometimes you get worried and anxious about what the future holds. So I think we should talk some more about ways to calm yourself at these times and decrease your worry. Does that make sense? Let's come up with a few ideas right now to help you to distract yourself from your worries while you are in the hospital, and I will also show you a quick way to control your breathing and help you to relax when you get anxious. Then I'll come back in a day or so to see how that's working, and we can discuss other plans to help you manage this.

The consultant will then discuss the distraction plans and show the patient how to do diaphragmatic breathing. Leaving the patient with useful tools that he can use to cope promotes a more positive feeling about the interview and the consultant. Patients also experience a greater sense of efficacy and control over their medical situation and their emotional reactions. The feedback and brief intervention also provide patients with a benefit for doing the interview and ensure that the patient will get at least some minimal treatment (especially if the patient is discharged before the consultant returns to provide additional intervention).

Note also that in the preceding example, the consultant made plans to continue to follow up with the patient. Most health psychology consultation work involves seeing patients every day or every few days to provide brief interventions to help them manage and cope with the issues they are facing. This is in contrast to much consultation psychiatry work, which includes little ongoing therapy.

Assuming the interview has gone smoothly (as most do), it is appropriate to let the patient know you will be back in a day or so to follow up and see how things are going and to provide additional intervention or education as needed. It works best to present this as a brief visit because it will most likely be so and because that will be acceptable to most patients. As demonstrated in the foregoing example, there are two important aspects to scheduling the follow-up visit: (a) keep the timing of your follow-up visit a bit vague ("tomorrow or the next day") so that you aren't in the position of disappointing a patient if the consultation service gets busy and you don't return as promptly as expected, and (b) let the patient know you will be returning but don't directly ask their permission to do so. Patients will refuse if they want to, and the consultant will need to respect that, although it can also be discussed further before the final decision is made. Asking for permission to follow up is tempting the patient to say he is OK and it isn't necessary, and then the consultant is in a position of having to convince the patient otherwise or not to return to provide an intervention that is warranted.

Finally, provide the patient with a card or a way to contact the consultant if he needs to do so before the next visit. It is rare that patients will feel a need to make the contact before a follow-up visit, but this gives them a reminder of who interviewed them and why. If discharge plans change quickly, the patient could be discharged before the consultant's next visit. Most inpatients do not follow up with the health psychology consultant after discharge, but they will at least have the psychologist's contact information if they have additional questions or problems or if they want to schedule outpatient treatment.

Wrapping Up the Consultation 5

After the patient interview, the psychologist must obtain any additional information that is necessary to complete the evaluation, and then all sources of data need to be integrated into a cohesive report. Written and verbal reports, as well as follow-up notes for ongoing evaluation or intervention, are discussed in this chapter.

Gathering Additional Information

Gathering additional information beyond the medical record review and the interview with the patient often helps to clarify the patient's history and current problems and can provide additional direction regarding the appropriate intervention. In many cases, it is helpful to obtain collateral information from nursing staff or family and friends, or additional information through a consultation from another specialty area.

COLLATERAL INFORMATION

It is always relevant to talk to the patient's nurse, and often most helpful to do so before the interview. Nurses typically have a significant amount of information on a patient's cognition and behavior. They will likely be aware

http://dx.doi.org/10.1037/0000108-006
Health Psychology Consultation in the Inpatient Medical Setting, by S. M. Labott

if the patient is somnolent, confused, or irritable. They may also have observed the patient over time, and can describe changes in behavior and cognition that will help the health psychology consultant understand the relevant issues. Patients will also often describe their concerns to their nurses, and this information can prompt specific questions during the interview with the patient. Nurses have often also observed the patient's interactions with family and will have noted any problems there.

If the patient is unable to provide accurate information on her current state and history, it will be important to involve family or friends in the initial evaluation to obtain sufficient data on the patient's history and current functioning, as well as current psychological symptoms. Their input is less relevant if the patient is able and willing to provide accurate information. However, if a patient is delirious or sedated, she may be unable to remain awake to participate in the evaluation, or she may be confused about aspects of her history. In these cases, the consultant can interview a family member—generally outside the patient's room if the family member is visiting—or can call the family member and do this over the telephone. The psychologist will need to explain who she is and the purpose of the interview, and then collect any relevant information that the family member is able to provide. If calling a family member by phone, clarify the purpose of the call early on, as family members often jump to the conclusion that something bad has happened to the patient if they get a phone call from the hospital. See Exhibit 5.1 for suggested questions to ask family members. A complete evaluation can be done by proxy with a close family member if needed (e.g., if the patient is completely nonresponsive), although in most cases the family members will only need to fill in some missing information.

Collateral information is also useful when patients are unwilling to provide the data requested. This occurs most often in the area of substance use and abuse. The patient's use of drugs and alcohol may be relevant to the treatment of his medical problem, as well as to associated psychological issues. Family members will likely be more objective in their reports of a patient's drug use than the patient would be, but depending on the relationship, a family member may not be privy to aspects of the patient's drug use or other behavior.

EXHIBIT 5.1

Sample Questions for Interviews With Family Members

How do you think he is doing emotionally while in the hospital? What have you noticed?

Have you noticed that your brother has been confused at all recently? What specifically have you noticed? Can you provide an example?

Does he have any history of problems with his memory? If so, what? Has a doctor ever given him a diagnosis for memory problems?

How about emotional problems—any depression? Anxiety or nerves?

Has he ever had psychiatric treatment? Currently? (If so, obtain details on provider, contact information, and medications.)

Does your family member use drugs? Alcohol? How much? Any history of problems in this area?

Family members can also often provide good data on the patient's behavior or cognition over time. If the family member has lived with the patient or visited frequently while in the hospital, he can report changes in the patient's behavior or cognition. Although most family members do not have a medical or psychological background and will not automatically understand what the psychologist is looking for, good questioning can elicit the information if the family member has been attentive and has information to share. Be aware that family members may misunderstand aspects of the patient's life or may be unaware of some important issues in the patient's life, so it is best to confirm the information provided with the patient when he is able.

CONSULTATIONS FROM OTHER SPECIALTIES

The input of other providers may be necessary, either to help with diagnosis of the current problem or as part of the intervention. In most hospital settings, the health psychology consultant would not formally order a consultation from another service but would describe why it is warranted to the primary medical team members, who would then make the formal consultation request. The psychologist might then want to contact the new consultant to provide additional information to facilitate his evaluation.

The psychologist's evaluation might have uncovered issues that would warrant a consultation from a psychiatrist. This could occur if the patient describes significant psychiatric symptoms that might warrant the use of psychotropic medication or if the patient already has outpatient psychiatric treatment in place but needs orders for current outpatient psychotropic medications to continue while he is in the hospital. Nonpsychiatric physicians may order the psychotropic medications, especially if the patient is stable on an outpatient regimen; the psychiatry consult may be warranted to determine if there are any new medical contraindications for the outpatient medications or to adjust doses to fit the current situation. Other specialty areas of psychiatry may also be useful to help with diagnostic issues and treatment planning, for example, a consultation with neuropsychiatry may be useful in a patient who presents a complicated mix of affective and cognitive issues.

A neuropsychological evaluation may be helpful for a patient with cognitive problems, depending on the history and the current situation. This might be especially useful if the patient appears to have a stable dementia that seems to affect her functioning and has never been thoroughly evaluated. If the patient has acute cognitive changes that are new at this admission, these can be assessed with a brief screener and would likely not warrant a complete neuropsychological battery during this inpatient admission (because it would tire the patient and will need to be redone later to assess the patient's baseline cognitive functioning when the acute issue has cleared). Often the full neuropsychological battery is ordered as an outpatient evaluation to be completed when the patient is back at her cognitive baseline.

Medical social workers are often consulted to provide help regarding the patient's disposition. They are aware of resources that are available and can help patients access them. Social workers can help with insurance questions; outpatient health care resources;

discharge planning, including transportation to outpatient medical appointments; disability applications; and other social issues. Their role may differ from one institution to the next; in some places, they may engage patients in counseling, and the psychologist will need to work with them to avoid overlap and confusion in the services being provided.

Integrating Data

Initially, integrating the large amounts of data from the medical record, patient interview, and collateral information may take some time, but it is accomplished more quickly with practice. The consultant needs to consider all the information provided and decide what is relevant for the written and verbal reports as well as the recommendations that should be made.

DISCREPANCIES IN THE MEDICAL RECORD

There will often be discrepancies in the information obtained from the various sources of data (e.g., medical record, patient, nurse, family); some of these discrepancies are important to resolve, and others are not. Consider a patient who reports a depressive episode and tells the emergency department nurse that it occurred 10 years ago, but then later tells the psychologist it was 15 years ago. The important point is that the patient had the depressive episode sometime in the remote past, rather than specifically when it occurred. The health psychology consultant will want to gather information on the symptoms and treatment that occurred at that time, other episodes and details surrounding those, and current functioning. The discrepancy about the timing of the previous episode is fairly irrelevant in terms of the psychiatric history (unless there are concerns about the patient's memory that would require more evaluation). In another case, the patient denies any use of drugs or alcohol, but the medical record notes a toxicology screen that was positive for opiates and marijuana at an admission 4 months earlier. In this case, especially if the drug use has implications for the medical issue, the psychologist would want to clarify the information. The health psychology consultant should double check the toxicology result in the medical record and then seek other relevant information—for example, does the patient have a history of drug use? Did she appear high at the previous admission? Are there notes from an addiction consultant or comments regarding substance use in notes from other providers? Perhaps additional information should also be obtained from the family to clarify the issue. The consultant might also interview the patient again to try to understand the discrepancy, for example, did the patient understand the questions about substance use? Has she stopped using substances recently? Is she not being honest about substance use?

IRRELEVANT OR SENSATIONAL INFORMATION

The consultant likely obtained information on a variety of topics during the interview with the patient that can be helpful in developing a conceptualization of this patient and her life, but every bit of that information does not need to be written into the formal consultation report. What qualifies as relevant information, however, will vary from patient to patient. For example, in most health psychology consultation evaluations, the fact that a patient does or does not have adequate social support is likely relevant, although it doesn't generally matter who provides the social support (e.g., a heterosexual or a homosexual partner; if they are married or not). However, if the patient has become unable to make his own decisions and will need a surrogate decision-maker to make decisions on his behalf, the relationship information may be relevant because some states do not allow anyone other than a family member or a spouse to act as a surrogate for a patient who lacks decisional capacity. This would cause problems for the patient in a same-sex, unmarried relationship.

Patients may describe dramatic events during the interview, but sensational details do not need to be included in the report. One patient vividly described the shooting of a woman and her two young children in the patient's neighborhood before her admission; the horrific details are not relevant to the consultation report (although they could be relevant if the patient begins therapy for posttraumatic stress disorder later) and can be described as "a recent shooting in the patient's neighborhood that has been traumatic for her."

Similarly, one patient had recently realized that her husband was cheating on her and described their conflicts and sexual problems in great detail to the consultant. The patient's husband visited her frequently and was known and liked by nursing staff. The details of his affair and their sexual issues were not directly relevant to the patient's medical treatment, yet the stress associated with their relationship was, so it was referred to in the consultation report as "marital issues that create significant stress for the patient" without additional detail. It was not important that other members of the medical team have knowledge of the details of their relationship problems.

DATA ACCURACY

It is tempting for psychologists to extrapolate and to expand on what the patient has actually said during the interview, but this can introduce error. For example, if the patient was asked about suicidal ideation and said that he did not experience it, the consultant should say something like this in the report: "Patient denies suicidal ideation." Although it is unlikely that the patient has a plan or intent if there is no ideation, it is not accurate to say, "Patient denies suicidal ideation, plan, or intent" because the patient was not asked about plan and intent during the interview. This level of concreteness may seem excessive, but it keeps the report data-based and forces the psychologist to avoid assumptions that could be incorrect. Approaching the evaluation in this way forces the consultant to ask the patient about everything that she wants to write about in the report. An exception to this could occur if the psychologist wants to present data found in the medical record, but then it should be cited as such. If the consultation report is ever part of a court case, information obtained directly from the patient will be more useful than assumptions the consultant has made.

Although electronic medical records are helpful at collecting and transmitting patient data, one of the major problems with them is that they enable providers to copy information from their own notes or those of others into future notes, making it easy to repeat a mistake if one has been made. Consider the case of a consultant who misremembered what a patient said when asked about past psychiatric history. The patient had no past psychiatric history, but the consultant confused her with another patient and wrote that she had an episode of depression in high school. When the patient next saw her primary care provider (PCP), he saw this and added "depression" to the patient's history of medical problems. Each year depression was recopied into the PCP's note, so that 5 years later, depression had been listed in the patient's chart six times. At the next inpatient medical admission, all providers, including the health psychology consultant, assumed that the patient had a history of depression. Through discussion with the patient, however, it was revealed that this was a mistake that had simply been copied into the patient's chart year after year. When a mistake like this is uncovered, the health psychology consultant should clearly note the mistake in the medical record, provide an explanation, and also a clear description of the correct information.

A similar scenario occurs when psychologists copy information from someone else's note into a psychological consultation report. This is most tempting if the patient has many medical problems, and it is easier to copy someone else's description than to describe them all oneself. While the psychologist will generally want some medical background and a reason for the current hospital admission in the consultation report, the medical team should know the entire medical history well, so this does not need to be described in great detail. The following information was copied from a medical resident's note into the psychology consultant's report: "Pt with hx of atypical Crohn's consisting of an eosinophilic panarteritis and fibrosis variant, RA/arthritis 2/2 Crohn's, migraines, GERD, presents to the ED with a 2-day history of N/V, right sided abdominal pain, and unable to take p/o." For purposes of the health psychology evaluation, a simpler statement would be: "Pt with MMP (multiple medical problems), admitted for N/V and abdominal pain." In this case, the additional detail is not relevant for the health psychology consultation report, but it is not incorrect as long as the psychological consultant is certain that the information is accurate and she understands the meaning of the medical details that are included. There is no way of controlling for a mistake in the description of the medical issues if the health psychology consultant simply copies someone else's information into her report. Further, it is not good practice to write something in a psychological report that the health psychology consultant doesn't understand and can't explain if she is asked about it. This is poor patient care and could significantly decrease the psychologist's credibility if the content of the evaluation was questioned in court.

Written Consultation Report

If the consultant does a thorough biopsychosocial evaluation, there is a multitude of information that can be written into the formal report. However, reports for medical records need to be more concise than those written in assessment settings or in graduate school, and they need to have clear conclusions and/or recommendations that communicate the most relevant issues for those who do not review the entire report.

EXHIBIT 5.2

Sections for Written Consultation Report

- Referral
- Medical
- Social
- Substance use
- Psychological history
- Current psychological status
- Mental status
- Special issues (optional)
- Summary (optional)
- Impressions and/or recommendations

It is helpful to write the report using headings that will help others to locate specific information. The headings used should correspond to the content areas covered in the interview. This format will need to be adjusted in some situations; for example, if the patient has no previous psychiatric history, that section can be combined with the current psychological status section; if the patient has been evaluated previously, sections that are less relevant can be skipped and the reader referred to a previous evaluation. See Exhibit 5.2 for a list of recommended section headings that can be used to organize a comprehensive health psychology consultation. It is less important to follow this particular outline specifically than it is to clearly present the information in a way that is user-friendly to the other providers who will read the report.

REFERRAL

This brief section at the beginning of the report is likely to include basic demographics (e.g., age, race), the name of the attending physician who has referred the patient, and the reason for the referral. Other atypical aspects of the evaluation might also be included here; this might include whether a family member was present during the interview, the interview was done using an interpreter, or the patient responded by writing rather than verbally, for example. If only a brief description of medical issues is warranted, that may also be included here. It will also be important to note whether any of the data in the report were obtained from a source other than the patient.

MEDICAL

This section might include details on the patient's medical history but is more likely to have a brief description of chronic medical issues and a statement about why the patient is currently in the hospital. Medications may be listed but are often not required in the inpatient evaluation report because they are listed in other places in the medical record. Psychotropic medications should always be listed here, along with doses if known, as well as outpatient prescriber information (e.g., psychiatrist or internist), with mention of psychiatric diagnoses if known. The frequency of use of prn (as needed) psychotropic medications should also be included here. Problems with medication and medical appointments and other aspects of adherence might also be included in this section of the written report.

SOCIAL

Most relevant here is information on the patient's social situation (marriage, children), living situation, and employment. Social support might also be included.

SUBSTANCE USE

Patient's current use of tobacco, alcohol, and recreational drugs should be described here. In addition, any history of substance use problems or treatment should be described.

PSYCHIATRIC HISTORY

For patients without a formal psychiatric history, a statement similar to the following is usually sufficient: "Patient with no previous inpatient or outpatient psych tx, no psych meds, no family hx" (assuming that the consultant asked the patient about all of these potential treatments and the patient denied them). For those patients with a significant psychiatric history, inpatient psychiatry admissions, suicidal ideation/self-harm, and any psychological or psychiatric treatment with therapists and psychiatrists should be described. More detail is required if the problems are more severe and the treatments more current. For a patient with an extensive remote history for which details are less useful currently, the treatment detail could be summarized: "Pt with 4 suicide attempts and 5 inpatient psych admissions, most recent 10 yrs ago." The implication is that the patient is more psychologically stable currently, and the details of that are described in the next section.

CURRENT PSYCHOLOGICAL STATUS

This section should describe the patient's experience of the psychological symptoms asked about in the interview (e.g., mood, sleep, appetite, guilt, worthlessness, hopelessness, suicidal ideation, anxiety, worry, panic, adjustment problems, mania, paranoia, hallucinations). Details are very relevant here. For example, if a patient reports panic attacks, the report should describe their frequency, as well as the specific symptoms experienced (e.g., shortness of breath, chest pain), the duration of the episodes, and any methods the patient uses to cope with the symptoms. There is some overlap between this section and the preceding psychiatric history section; at times it is most useful to combine these sections in the report.

MENTAL STATUS

Most important clinically is a description of the specific cognitive deficits demonstrated by the patient, including specific data. Consider the following excerpt from an inpatient health psychology evaluation report: "Patient was alert and oriented × 3 (not time). Registration, attention, language were all intact. Both short- (2/3) and long-term (2/3) memory were mildly impaired." This provides a clear description of what the patient was asked, as well as how she did on the exam, and provides useful information for other providers. Providing specific data can also help other providers (as well as the psychologist) track changes in cognition over time. If health literacy or any other brief cognitive or neuropsychological tests were given during the consultation, results from those should also be included here.

Behavioral observations are also important. However, noting that a patient was sitting in the hospital bed wearing a hospital gown is somewhat irrelevant because that is the case for most patients evaluated in the hospital. Unexpected behaviors, such as agitation, somnolence, rapid speech, and confusion, are more relevant.

SPECIAL ISSUES

This is an optional section that may be added to the standard report to address the referral question, and the heading should reflect that (e.g., Nonadherence, Decisional Capacity). In other cases, new issues that warrant attention during this admission may have been uncovered in the course of the interview, and these could be described here.

SUMMARY

This is an optional section that is used to summarize the content of the entire evaluation in one brief paragraph. The purpose is to provide a concise version of the main points of the report, which is especially useful if the report is long. This section may be skipped, especially in a straightforward evaluation, or the summary may be integrated into the Impressions or Recommendations section instead.

IMPRESSIONS

This section describes the consultant's thoughts about the patient and her issues and is solidly based on the interview data. This is not a place for hypotheses about the patient's personality dynamics or behavior unless those are well grounded in data. Often the Impressions and Recommendations sections are combined because the specific recommendations are generally closely related to the Impressions—in fact they often follow directly from them.

RECOMMENDATIONS

One important aspect of the health psychology consultation is that the consultant will provide impressions regarding what the relevant issues are for this patient, as well as recommendations for how to address them. These recommendations typically include a description of what the psychologist plans to do in terms of inpatient follow-up, outpatient referral suggestions, or recommendations for additional consultation from other specialty areas (if warranted).

The recommendations section of the written consultation report should address activities that the health psychology consultant is asking the medical team to address. For example, the psychologist may want the primary medical team to provide more education to the patient to improve the patient's understanding of a proposed treatment. Additional consultation or testing may be recommended, and the primary medical team will need to place those orders so they will need to know what is being requested and why it is relevant to the patient's treatment.

As part of the recommendations, the health psychology consultant will also need to generally explain his plans for the patient so that the primary treatment team is aware of what is being done by way of psychological intervention with the patient this admission. The psychologist will often plan to see the patient on an ongoing basis during the admission to provide treatment to address anxiety or depression or monitor mental status or coping. All recommendations should be appropriate to the hospital setting, that is, they should be brief interventions that can be implemented with short visits to achieve clear goals. Longer term issues should be addressed in the outpatient setting, and the health psychology consultant can provide referrals for that.

A referral for outpatient treatment may also be warranted if the patient has a history of significant psychiatric problems that will need to be monitored and treated on an ongoing basis with therapy or medication, or both. An outpatient referral may also be useful if the patient is to be discharged soon and there will be no time for health psychology intervention in the hospital. Further, some patients have premorbid psychiatric or social issues that would benefit from longer term therapy. Although these issues might be addressed briefly in the inpatient setting, especially if they are relevant to the current medical and psychological situation, some patients will need longer term outpatient treatment to fully treat the problem.

There are many good reasons to provide a recommendation for additional outpatient psychological or psychiatric treatment, but the health psychology consultant will want to avoid suggesting outpatient follow-up as a matter of course for all patients. Many medical inpatients would not have needs for psychological intervention if they had not developed a significant medical problem, and most will not need psychiatric or psychological outpatient follow-up. All patients, however, could be given contact information for the psychological consultant, who could then provide any assistance regarding referrals if ongoing treatment becomes relevant for the patient at a later date. It is not uncommon for a former inpatient to contact the health psychology consultant several years after the consultation in the hospital to request help with a new problem that has developed.

For some consultations, there may be no specific recommendations, and the health psychology consultant can state that clearly in the report. That is, many patients are coping well and have no significant psychiatric history or current emotional difficulties. These patients will not need inpatient or outpatient follow-up but should be provided with the appropriate contact information that they can use if new issues arise.

Exhibit 5.3 provides tips for the written consultation report, and Samples 5.1, 5.2, and 5.3 contain example consultation reports. Note that these reports vary in terms of the level of medical detail provided, as well as the report format. All, however, contain the basic information from the interview with the patient and provide appropriate impressions and recommendations. Note that the case described in Sample 5.2 contains a summary at the end of the report and that the case described in Sample 5.3

EXHIBIT 5.3

Consultation Report Writing Tips

Be clear and concise; use headings.
Avoid copying information from someone else's report in the medical record into your own report.
Be sure you understand and can explain everything in your report.
Don't extrapolate and assume information about issues you haven't asked the patient about.
Avoid hypotheses, and stick to what the patient reported.
If the evaluation is not finished for some reason, say so, and indicate that you will return to finish it later.
Pay special attention to the impressions and recommendations at the end of the report, so that they convey the most important issues and the plan for the patient's treatment this admission.
If the report contains data from sources other than the patient, cite them (e.g., per medical record, per patient's wife).

involved some psychological intervention even before the interview was started; this is often necessary in the inpatient setting.

Verbal Consultation Reports

In most medical contexts, the evaluation results and recommendations are provided to the referral source verbally as well as through the written report in the medical record. Typically the referral source is paged or called, and the consultant provides a brief summary of the evaluation and findings by phone. A verbal report could also occur in the nurses' station or in a quiet corner of the hospital hallway. It should never occur in an elevator, the cafeteria, or anywhere else that others could overhear and the patient's confidentiality could be breached. Some physicians have preferences about when these reports are delivered (e.g., before morning rounds, never from 6 to 10 a.m. because they are in surgery), and it is good to accommodate those preferences when appropriate.

The verbal report must be brief and should occur within several hours of the time the patient was seen. Never assume that other providers will review the written reports. Although many do, if there is information on the inpatient that the health psychology consultant wants to convey to the referral source, this should be done verbally. The report should generally contain a statement about the patient's psychological status, his or her cognitive status, and the response to the referral question. This summary should include a statement about what the health psychology consultant plans to do for follow-up with this patient (e.g., provide referrals, see patient during admission to teach anxiety management) as well as recommendations for what the medical team can do (e.g., provide more information to the patient about the disease, consult psychiatry to evaluate for antidepressants). Brevity is critical, and medical providers will ask questions and engage in a longer discussion of the issues if they choose. Sample 5.4 shows example verbal reports that might correspond to the written reports for the same cases described in Samples 5.1 through 5.3.

Follow-Up Notes

Recommendations from the initial consultation will determine specific interventions that the psychologist will begin with the patient. Each time the patient is seen, a note in the medical record will need to be written. As with consultation reports, the specific format of the follow-up note may be dictated by the institution and may also need to include specific information relevant for billing. The content of all notes will need to reflect the interactions with the patient, as well as the service being billed for. In general, follow-up notes are brief and provide a summary of any ongoing evaluation of cognition or mood, the psychologist's interventions, and the patient's response to them. Sample 5.5 shows two examples of follow-up notes that could have been written as follow-up for Ms. E's and Ms. R's cases, respectively. Note also that each indicates the psychologist's plans for ongoing treatment.

Sample 5.1
Consultation Report for Ms. E

Referral: Ms. E is a 75 y/o Hispanic woman with multiple medical problems admitted with leg pain. Health psychology consult requested by Dr. I for potential depression. Pt seen with the aid of a Spanish interpreter.

Pt's daughter contributed to portions of the pt's history.

Social Hx: The pt lives in a home with her daughter. Pt has six additional children. She reported a close-knit and supportive family network. She denied any formal education. Pt and daughter reported that she is completely illiterate in both English and Spanish. Daughter manages all of pt's affairs. Pt reported that before the onset of her leg pain earlier this week, she was completely mobile. Pt's daughter reported that she accompanies the pt on all outings outside of the house.

Substance Use: Pt denied any use of alcohol, tobacco, or illicit drugs.

Psychiatric Hx/Status: Pt denied any history of psychiatric treatment including hospitalizations, psychotherapy, or use of medications. She denied any current or past significant depression, anxiety, panic attacks, mania, or psychosis. With regard to current symptoms, the pt denied all symptoms of depression. Affect was bright and euthymic throughout the eval, laughing and joking with daughter and examiner. Pt reported that she did experience some depressed mood for less than 24 hours a few days ago related to leg pain and difficulty coping with intensity of the pain. Pt's daughter denied any signs of depression at home, reported that mother was at baseline mood during the eval. Pt denied any symptoms of hopelessness or inappropriate guilt. She denied current suicidal ideation, intent, or plan.

Mental Status: Pt alert and oriented to person and grossly to place, "Los Angeles" denied knowledge of state. Disoriented to season, month, and year. Denied knowledge of birth date or the birth dates of any of her children. On cognitive exam, basic reasoning ability was intact. Basic abstraction abilities were impaired. Attention/concentration was intact on a basic test of counting from five to one backward. Recall of three items after a brief delay was 1/3, improved to 2/3 with cues. Pt was able to name three common objects and name 3 types of coins. In contrast to impaired cognitive testing, thought processes during interview appeared linear and goal-directed. Thought content was appropriate throughout eval. Speech was normal in rate, prosody, and tone.

Impressions/Recommendations: Ms. E is a 75 y/o Hispanic woman with multiple medical problems admitted with c/o leg pain.

With regard to depression, the pt denied any current symptoms of depression or past history of depressive episodes. Pt noted a less than 24-hour period of depressed mood attributed to difficulty coping with current leg pain over the past week. Pt with bright and euthymic affect throughout eval. Also, pt's daughter denies any mood changes in her mother at home.

Pt with deficits on cognitive exam in several basic areas, e.g., basic orientation, memory, and abstraction. Pt and daughter attribute this to poor education. Daughter reports that pt's cognition is at baseline. Thought processes were linear and goal-directed. However, deficits on cognitive testing are significant. Pt's lack of recall of her own birth date is striking and appears to be due to more than just illiteracy. We will follow to monitor mood and cognition. Will continue to monitor mental status and continue to evaluate pt's current level of functioning.

Thank you for the consult request. Please page with any questions.

Rebecca S, PhD, #6283
Health Psychology Fellow

Sample 5.2
Consultation Report for Ms. R

Ms. R is an 82 y.o. Caucasian female who was admitted on 9/xx/16 for a robotic resection of a pancreatic mass. She has a pmh of recurrent pancreatitis, hypothyroidism, and OA (*osteoarthritis*). Health Psychology consult was requested by Dr. S to evaluate mood and coping following the suicide of pt's grandson last week.

Ms. R is widowed (husband died 10 years ago) and lives alone. She has 5 living children (her 6th child died at age 4) and 6 grandchildren. She completed 1 year of business college. She was a stay-at-home mother while her children were young and currently works 2 days a week doing clerical work for a dentist. She has worked at this job for approximately 20 years. She reported that she has frequent contact with friends and family and that she has multiple sources of social and emotional support. She reported that she has not smoked since her husband passed 10 years ago. She reported that she does not currently drink alcohol and that she previously only drank socially (1–2 drinks several times per week). She denied current/past illicit drug use.

Ms. R denied history of inpatient or outpatient psychiatric treatment. She has never taken any psychiatric medications. She endorsed current depressed mood that she attributed to the recent death of her grandson. She reported that she has been coping with this news by speaking with family/friends and distracting herself by watching TV and listening to music. She stated that she understands it will take some time for her mood to return to normal but that she knows it eventually will. She reported that her sleep has been good since beginning to take sleeping meds several days ago. Her appetite has been good overall during her hospital stay, but it has been poor since receiving the news about her grandson. She denied current/past symptoms of anxiety/worry, anhedonia, mania, worthlessness/guilt, helplessness/hopelessness, paranoia, and aud/vis hallucinations. She reported that she has had several panic attacks in the past, the most recent occurring during an MRI (*magnetic resonance imaging*) approximately 3 years ago. She denied current/past suicidal/homicidal ideation, intent, or plan.

Ms. R was alert. Her mood appeared somewhat dysphoric, although she smiled several times during the evaluation. Her thinking was goal-oriented, and her thought content was unremarkable. She was grossly oriented to time and place, although she did not know the exact date; she knew the day of the week, month, and year. The follow domains were intact: attention, concentration, registration, short-term and long-term recall, and abstract thinking. Her judgment was mildly impaired on exam, although it improved with a follow-up question.

SUMMARY AND IMPRESSIONS

Ms. R is an 82 y.o. Caucasian female who was admitted for a robotic resection of a pancreatic mass. She has a pmh of recurrent pancreatitis, hypothyroidism, and OA. Her grandson committed suicide last week. Ms. R is currently experiencing grief-related depressed mood. Overall, she appears to be coping well with her grandson's death and reported that talking with friends and family has helped her cope. We discussed the typical course of adjustment to a significant loss. Pt has experienced losses before and understands.

Thank you for this consult request. We will continue to follow while the pt is in-house to monitor mood and aid with emotional coping. Please page with questions, pager xxxx.

d/w (*discussed with*) medical team.
Samuel G, PhD

Sample 5.3
Consultation Report for Mrs. X

Referral: Pt referred by Dr. M for health psych eval to assess coping. Pt, Mrs. X, is a 69 y/o woman with multiple medical problems, e.g., DJD (*degenerative joint disease*), DM (*diabetes mellitus*), HTN (*hypertension*). She had L TKA (*left total knee arthroplasty*) last week, is admitted to acute rehab unit to address deconditioning.

On approach, pt reported there was a mix-up in her pain meds when she transferred from one unit to another, so she was quite uncomfortable (although nurse had just given her the meds; they had not yet taken effect). We discussed adjunctive pain management strategies, such as relaxation, breathing, and distraction. Pt was able to relax noticeably and breathe deeply and slowly.

Social: Pt is widowed and lives with a son and his wife, and their 3 teenagers, reports this arrangement works fine. She also has 1 other son and 2 daughters who live locally. Pt reports good family support. She is also very active in her church. She reported this is her time of life to do what she wants, and she is happy with her situation generally. She is retired now but worked managing a coffee shop in the past. She completed some community college.

Substance Use: She denies use of tobacco, ETOH, and drugs.

Psych hx and current status: Pt denies any previous psych tx, saw a psychiatrist once for a required eval when going for a promotion in a job. She denies any emotional problems in her past, with one exception. She notes that she became depressed when her husband was sick and she was overwhelmed with caretaking responsibilities before his death, about 8 yrs ago. No suicidal ideation, and she continued to function OK, although she feels she was not herself as she was unmotivated.

Pt currently denies depression, anxiety, psychotic sx. She notes being disappointed after R TKA last December, when she realized she needed to have the 2nd knee done fairly soon. However, she didn't allow this to interfere with her church activities, although she often did little after returning home at the end of the day.

Mental status: Pt notes she has forgotten names throughout her life but denies other subjective cognitive problems. On mental status exam, she was alert and oriented × 3 (not date). Registration, attention, judgment were intact. Short-term memory mildly impaired (2/3); long-term memory mildly impaired also (2/3; past presidents). Thinking is concrete.

Impressions: Pt admitted to rehab unit with L TKA. She has participated in rehab before, is motivated, and understands she will need to work hard to regain her functioning. Pain was a problem today, but pt was feeling better by the end of the interview. She has good social support and is active in her church and with other activities. One depressive episode in the past when her husband was dying, but no other major psych problems. She seems to be coping well with her current situation. We will not plan to follow; please reconsult if new issues arise.

Thanks.
Kristin Carter, PhD
pager: xxxx

Sample 5.4
Verbal Reports

Ms. E

This is Rebecca Smith from the psychology consult service. You referred Ms. E to us this morning, and I saw her earlier today. She has no previous psych history, and she denies feeling depressed currently. She does acknowledge a brief episode of depressed mood that was associated with leg pain a few days ago, but her mood has been good before and since that. She does seem to have some cognitive problems, especially with memory and orientation. Pt is illiterate, but these cognitive deficits do not seem to be due to that. We will follow her this admission to monitor her mood and cognition. Thanks; my report will be in (*the medical record*) shortly.

Ms. R

We saw your patient Ms. R this morning. She has no psych history, but she does report feeling sad about her grandson's recent death. She seems to be experiencing a normal episode of grief and she has good family support to help her manage this. We will follow her this admission, to monitor her mood and to aid with her adjustment to the loss of her grandson. Thanks.

Mrs. X

We saw your patient Mrs. X this morning in rehab. Initially she was having a difficult time with pain, but she was responsive to suggestions for additional pain management strategies to help her while she was waiting for her meds to work. Patient reports a prior episode of depression when she was caring for her sick husband several years ago, otherwise no significant psych history or symptoms. She demonstrates some mild changes in memory. She understands what rehab involves and is motivated; she seems to be coping well. We will not plan to follow; but please reconsult if something changes. Thanks.

Sample 5.5
Follow-Up Notes

Ms. E

Pt referred with concerns about depression, with altered mental status at initial eval; seen with interpreter. Pt today is alert and oriented × 3. Mood is good. Attention, judgment, short- and long-term memory all intact and improved from initial evaluation yesterday. No new psychological issues. Will continue to monitor cognition, mood, and coping.

Ms. R

Pt seen for health psych f/u (*follow-up*) to address grief re: grandson's recent death. Pt today reports she has had several visitors, and they helped to lift her spirits. She also reports improved appetite and less pain. Discussed activities she could use in the hospital to continue to improve mood and also expectations for the grief process. Will continue to follow.

PSYCHOLOGICAL ISSUES IN THE INPATIENT SETTING

III

Adjustment to Medical Illness

6

Adjustment is a process in which patients learn to live with and successfully manage medical problems and associated changes and limitations. The term *adjustment* is often also used to refer to a state that a patient achieves and maintains or the extent to which a patient has been successful at integrating the new medical changes into her life in an adaptive manner. This chapter describes common challenges that medical inpatients face, as well as theories of the adjustment process. Tasks associated with successful adjustment and clinical interventions to achieve them are described, as are factors that influence adjustment.

Changes in Medical Status

In the hospital setting, almost every patient is dealing with a new medical issue or a change in a medical problem that involves limitations and negative effects on the patient's life. These may include physical limitations (e.g., the inability to walk, perform activities of daily living [ADLs], or engage in sports or hobbies), inconvenient or embarrassing symptoms (e.g., using colostomy, frequent diarrhea), changes in appearance (e.g., weight increase or decrease, hair loss), or cognitive deficits (e.g., problems with memory or alertness).

http://dx.doi.org/10.1037/0000108-007
Health Psychology Consultation in the Inpatient Medical Setting, by S. M. Labott

EXHIBIT 6.1

Mr. R—New CVA (cerebrovascular accident; stroke)

Pt is a 55 y/o man who works as an auto mechanic. He is married for 36 years and is the father of four children, ages 18–35 y/o. Past medical history is significant only for hypercholesterolemia, for which he takes a statin. Yesterday at work he complained of a bad headache, then fell and was taken to the ER by his coworkers. Today he wakes in the hospital and is told that he suffered a stroke. He has slurred speech and weakness on one side. He is unable to walk, and he is incontinent. He also evidences some memory problems. Mr. R is tired and his thinking is slow, but he is very aware of his significant physical impairments.

Patients may need to learn to deal with new and permanent physical or cognitive limitations, impairments that fluctuate, or those that will worsen over time. Adjusting to a new medical issue may take patients a significant amount of time and generally continues long past the inpatient admission during which the new medical problem or changes were diagnosed.

Many challenges in the hospital begin with the patient being informed of a new medical diagnosis. Exhibits 6.1 and 6.2 are two descriptions of patients surprised by a new diagnosis and associated limitations that will have dramatic impacts on their lives.

While a new diagnosis may be the most difficult for patients to accept, even patients who have had a good adjustment to chronic illnesses may be admitted to the hospital with a progression of the illness that results in new impacts on their lives. Consider a patient who has learned to manage a chronic lung disease but has developed new or worsening symptoms as the disease progresses and now needs to be worked up for a lung transplant. Similarly, a patient who successfully managed the diagnosis and treatment of breast cancer and who has been disease-free for 3 years is now admitted to the hospital and learns that the cancer has recurred and that she needs to undergo treatment again. These chronic medical issues require ongoing accommodations in the patient's life as the illness progresses.

It is common for patients to experience an initial adjustment period when faced with a new diagnosis or a change in medical status, followed by a series of additional

EXHIBIT 6.2

Ms. T—New Leukemia

Pt is a 32 y/o woman who works part-time doing clerical work in an office. She is married for 10 years and has two children, ages 5 and 8. She has been complaining of fatigue for the past few months but didn't think much of it because she is busy with her family and work and often didn't get enough sleep. She recently developed some unexplained bruising and became short of breath a few times, so she scheduled an appointment with her PCP and saw him today for a checkup. Blood tests were run, and the patient was told she may have acute leukemia. She was sent directly to the hospital to confirm the diagnosis and to begin chemotherapy. She is aware this is a serious disease, although she knows little about it.

adjustments over time, unless the medical problem resolves. The patient's adaptation to these changes in medical status can be influenced by the severity of the changes the patient is facing, the absolute number of changes, and the permanence of the associated impairments or limitations. The key issue is that the patient is facing a change from his baseline physical, cognitive, or functional status.

The new medical challenges that patients face can be placed on a continuum from those that are life-changing to those that have lesser impacts on the patient's day-to-day activities. Mr. R, whose case is described in Exhibit 6.1, experienced a major change in his medical status (the CVA) that happened very quickly and resulted in significant physical and cognitive impairments. Alternately, some changes occur more slowly over time, as in the case of a patient who has slow but progressive changes in physical and cognitive functioning due to multiple sclerosis (MS). For Ms. T, described in Exhibit 6.2, the new diagnosis of a serious disease (leukemia) warrants intense and invasive treatments that will dramatically affect her life. The treatment for her will include chemotherapy and perhaps a stem cell transplant; these interventions may result in drug side effects, unpleasant symptoms, and changes in appearance, as well as multiple medical appointments and hospital admissions. All this will have a significant impact on her and interfere with her work and social life.

Some medical diagnoses are less disruptive to the patient's life, such as a new diagnosis of hypercholesterolemia in a patient who needs to make changes in his eating habits to decrease cholesterol. Although this patient is not currently facing significant limitations or impacts on his future, he will still need to adjust to the new medical situation. Even a patient without a life-threatening illness could develop new feelings of vulnerability and fears about his future. The adjustment to events that have significant implications for daily activities (e.g., a serious diagnosis, surgery, or amputation) is more difficult than those events that do not have such a significant impact, but all require patients to adjust to the new situation to function adaptively in the context of a new medical problem.

The absolute number of changes a patient needs to make to manage the medical problem can also play a role in the patient's adjustment. One change in a patient's routine is much simpler behaviorally, and also emotionally less stressful, than multiple changes that affect a variety of important aspects of the patient's life. For Ms. T, as she goes through the treatment for acute leukemia, she will be unable to work for at least several months, and she will need to curtail other events that involve physical activity (due to decreased energy and concerns about bleeding) and being in crowds (to decrease risk of infection). She may also have difficulties with sleep and fatigue. All of these matters will require some accommodation on her part. Consider another patient who has been diagnosed with Crohn's disease. Although this disease is generally not life-threatening, the problem of unexpected diarrhea can create great difficulty for a patient with an active work and social life.

Some symptoms and changes in medical status are temporary, such as fatigue and decreased appetite after chemotherapy, while others are permanent, such as new physical limitations after an amputation. It is less stressful for patients to deal with temporary impairments, although many times it isn't clear whether the impairments or changes are temporary or permanent (as in the case of Mr. R), creating a significant amount of worry and anxiety for patients as they wait to discover the permanent impacts of the medical problem. Ambiguity about the permanence of current limitations can be stressful, and the ultimate outcome of the disease may also be unknown. For Ms. T, if the leukemia treatment is successful, she may enjoy a relatively normal life for a long time. If not, she could be dead in 6 months. It is quite a different experience for a patient who has a knee replacement and is told that it is likely that surgery will "fix" the problem, that he will need to undergo physical therapy, but will soon be "good as new."

Regardless of the permanence of the change in medical status or the severity of any associated limitations, the patient needs to come to terms with the changes to accomplish the best adjustment possible. Adjustment can be conceptualized as a continuum, with complete denial of the medical problem or limitation at one extreme, and a complete adoption of an invalid role at the other; the healthiest adjustment is between the two extremes. Consider a patient with sickle cell disease who is at risk for acute pain crises. The patient will need to avoid strenuous exercise and heat and will need to eat and hydrate properly in an attempt to avoid pain crises. If this person is a construction worker in a warm climate, the strenuous exercise and heat are likely to result in repeated episodes of sickle cell pain, missed work, and perhaps hospital admissions. Denial of the illness and its implications can exacerbate the medical symptoms because the patient may not take the necessary steps to promote or maintain his health. At the other extreme, the patient could reorganize his life so that it revolves exclusively around his illness, staying home and in bed in warm weather with an excessive focus on the medical issues. Either extreme is maladaptive, will decrease the patient's quality of life, and could result in frustration, anger, or depression. The best adjustment is typically somewhere between the two extremes: Perhaps the patient can work inside on very hot days, or perhaps he can find work that is less physically strenuous. Either of these work choices would help him to maintain his health, while continuing to manage his employment. He also needs to attend to proper health behaviors, including adequate sleep, nutrition, hydration, and exercise. The patient's challenge is to determine what changes to make in his life to allow him to maintain the best quality of life possible.

Theories of Adjustment

One of the more popular theories of adjustment to new life events and stressors has been proposed by Lazarus and colleagues (Folkman & Lazarus, 1985; Folkman, Lazarus, Dunkel-Schetter, DeLongis, & Gruen, 1986; Lazarus & Folkman, 1984). This model of stress and coping involves a several-step process in which an individual first evaluates what is at stake (primary appraisal) and then considers what can be done to address the problem (secondary appraisal). People then use coping strategies that are intended either to have an impact on the problem (problem-focused coping) or to regulate the emotions associated with the stressor (emotion-focused coping). This process has been studied extensively in relation to a wide variety of stressors, including coping with illnesses such as prostate cancer (Roesch et al., 2005), diabetes, (Duangdao & Roesch, 2008), and HIV/AIDS (Pakenham & Rinaldis, 2001).

Maes, Leventhal, and de Ridder (1996) provided an expansion of the stress and coping model for specific application to coping with chronic illness, see Figure 6.1. In the Maes et al. expanded model, additional variables contribute to the coping behavior that is undertaken by the patient, and the coping behavior results in psychological, social, and also physical outcomes. Specifically, life events that are seemingly extraneous to the medical illness, such as divorce or job loss, as well as events associated with the disease, can influence the individual's appraisal of the illness; for example, a new diagnosis of MS may be appraised significantly more negatively by an individual who is recently divorced than by someone in a stable relationship. Demographic characteristics, disease and treatment characteristics, and the individual's internal (e.g., energy, optimism) and external resources can all affect coping in complicated ways. For example, a person who lives alone and is facing chemotherapy that will likely make him sick and weak may perceive this very differently from someone who has good social support to help him manage the side effects. Each of these factors play

FIGURE 6.1

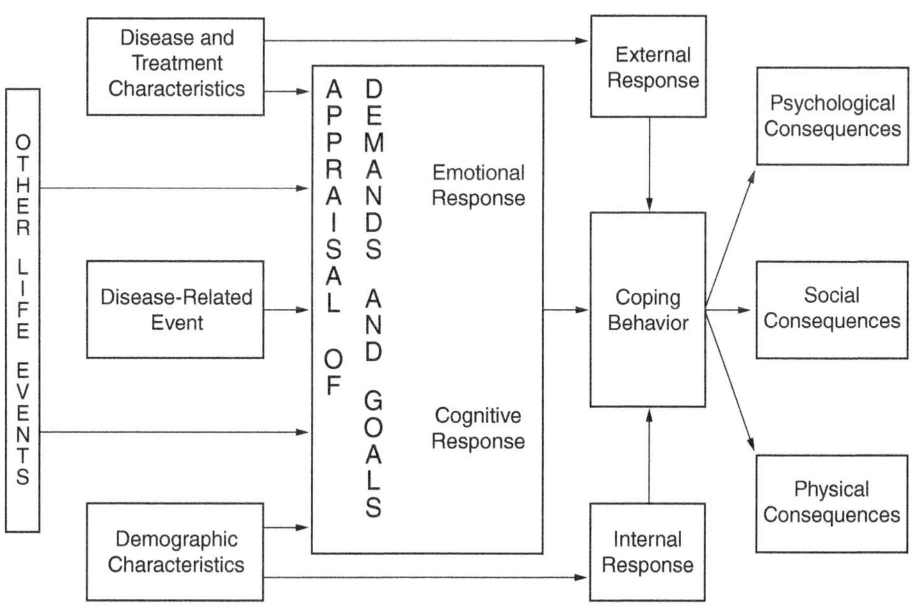

Model for coping with chronic disease. From *Handbook of Coping: Theory, Research, Applications* (p. 229), by M. Zeidner and N. S. Endler (Eds.), 1996, New York, NY: Wiley. Copyright 1996 by John Wiley and Sons. Reprinted with permission.

EXHIBIT 6.3

Conceptualizations of Successful Adjustment to Chronic Medical Illness

Mastery of tasks associated with illness
Lack of psychopathology
Low negative affect or high positive affect
Good functional status
Satisfaction, well-being, positive quality of life

Note. Data from Hoyt and Stanton (2012).

a role in determining the patient's general approach to coping as well as the specific coping behaviors chosen by the individual to address the illness.

Hoyt and Stanton (2012) reviewed the empirical literature on adjustment to chronic medical illness and noted that successful adjustment has been conceptualized by researchers in several ways (summarized in Exhibit 6.3). One conceptualization of successful adjustment involves adequate performance of aspects of the treatment regimen (e.g., taking medications, exercising, attending medical appointments) and requires an understanding of the illness and factors that will influence its course as well as adequate management of symptoms. Others have defined successful adjustment as the absence of significant psychopathology such as anxiety, depression, or adjustment disorders. Patient reports of positive affect or the lack of negative affect have also been used as indicators of successful adjustment to an illness, whereas other researchers have used measures of functional status to reflect adjustment, such as return to work, mobility, and treatment adherence. Finally, patient appraisals of quality of life or satisfaction have been used as markers of adjustment in chronic illness patients.

Although each of these theories and conceptualizations of adjustment to chronic illness have relevance to the adjustment required of patients in the hospital, the inpatient hospital experience is often dramatically different from the experience of a chronic illness in the outpatient setting. In the hospital, the new limitations may be acute, unexpected, and more severe than those associated with chronic illness in the outpatient setting. For example, the adjustment to chronic lung disease in the outpatient setting may involve coping with shortness of breath and limitations on physical activities that increase slowly over time as the disease progresses. In the inpatient setting, a patient may have felt completely healthy yesterday but wakes in the hospital today with significant physical and cognitive impairments poststroke. Although both situations will require the patient to cope adaptively and make lifestyle changes, the patient with the unexpected and catastrophic medical crisis is less prepared emotionally for the situation in which he finds himself.

Adjustment Tasks and Interventions

The psychologist can use markers of successful adjustment (Exhibit 6.3) to assess the adjustment of a specific inpatient to a specific disorder. The psychologist can then intervene to help a patient move toward successful adjustment if the process is only beginning or if the current adjustment is less than optimal. Exhibit 6.4 provides a list of specific tasks that will aid patients in moving toward successful adjustment to their medical illness or limitations. Each of these specific tasks plays a role in promoting successful adjustment to the illness, consistent with the more global adjustment outcomes noted in Exhibit 6.3.

The activities relevant to a patient's successful adjustment include (a) psychoeducation regarding the adjustment process, the illness, specific medications or procedures, as well as strategies to communicate effectively with providers; (b) successful management of emotions; (c) coping with the new limitations and changes associated with the medical diagnosis; and (d) developing feelings of control and efficacy to successfully manage the illness, symptoms, and limitations. Others have reported that the best psychological adjustment to chronic illness is associated with the individual remaining as active as possible, expressing emotions and taking control of the illness, learning to manage the illness, and developing a focus on positive outcomes (de Ridder, Geenen, Kuijer, & van Middendorp, 2008). There is significant overlap among these tasks; Exhibit 6.4 is simply one method of categorizing them to focus the health psychology consultant on areas to be addressed in the treatment of individual patients.

Most interventions to facilitate adjustment to a new diagnosis or transition in medical status would be characterized as psychoeducational or as cognitive or behavioral interventions. A cognitive–behavioral approach fits well in the inpatient medical setting because patients are present-focused and realize they need to learn new skills to help them manage a new problem. Overall, the goals of cognitive–behavioral therapy for use with medical patients include helping individuals to change the way they think about the illness, improving health behaviors, and teaching patients to take control of their illness and improve their health wherever they can. These goals mesh well with the adjustment tasks in Exhibit 6.4. Clinicians choose specific cognitive or behavioral interventions that address these adjustment tasks as needed, given the particular concerns presented by a specific patient. It is not necessary to specifically address each of these tasks with every patient; the most pressing problems for the patient are usually readily apparent after a general discussion about the patient's reactions to and management of their medical problems. Attention to these adjustment tasks can help patients accept their new situation and move toward developing the best life they can. Following is a description of specific interventions used to address these areas of focus when treating individual patients with the goal of facilitating adjustment to new medical issues.

EXHIBIT 6.4

Specific Tasks to Facilitate Adjustment

Psychoeducation
Management of emotional reactions
Coping with limitations and changes
Developing feelings of control over symptoms or limitations and efficacy to manage disease

PSYCHOEDUCATION

Education permeates all of the work done by health psychologists in the medical setting, and it plays an especially important role in facilitating the patient's adjustment to new medical concerns. Education can provide patients with relevant information about the medical and psychological issues associated with the illness, helping them to improve their decisions on how to manage the illness and its implications. Patients who are educated about the medical illness have greater feelings of mastery and control over the medical issues, as well as greater motivation to participate in healthy behaviors to treat the illness. They report greater satisfaction with their medical care and also better quality of life (C. O. Larson, Nelson, Gustafson, & Batalden, 1996).

Educating medical patients generally takes the form of brief didactic discussions that are tailored to the psychological needs and medical problems of the specific patient and are often characterized by cognitive therapy or motivational interviewing components. Although it is to the patient's benefit to be informed about the medical matters, the psychologist will need to determine how much information is appropriate for a particular patient. Patients differ in their need for information, and some research has demonstrated that needs for information change over the course of an illness (e.g., Fletcher, Flight, Chapman, Fennell, & Wilson, 2017). Clinically, some patients have high needs for information, others are easily overwhelmed by too much information, and still others avoid becoming informed, expecting family members to make decisions on their behalf. There may also be cultural and age differences in a patient's ideas of how active in his own care he should be. Yet even for those patients who prefer less information, it is to the patient's benefit to be at least minimally informed about the new medical diagnosis or limitations. Several of the most relevant areas for patient education are described next. The health psychology consultant will need to balance the patient's wishes for more or less information with the benefits of information, and then provide patients with what is most useful.

The Adjustment Process

It is often a struggle to deal with new medical issues, and patients may worry there is something wrong with them as they try to come to terms with bad news about new limitations on their lives and recommended medical treatments. Patients need to understand that adjustment takes time. In many cases, they will also need to understand that additional adjustments may be needed as the disease progresses. Education regarding the adjustment process itself helps to normalize the experience and provides support for patients to give themselves space and time to come to terms with their situation. Talking with patients about the fact that there will be ups and downs in the adjustment process can help them to relax and work at the issues more effectively. It is often helpful for them to understand more about the tasks of adjustment (see Exhibit 6.4) and to realize that their experience is normal, expected, and similar to that of others who are adapting to new medical issues. A discussion of the adjustment process is also a good time to evaluate a patient's social support as well as how they can use it to help them cope.

For Mr. R (the patient with the new stroke whose case is described in Exhibit 6.1), it will be important to have a discussion of how his physical recuperation will take time and include ups and downs, and that his emotional adjustment process will be similar. He could be encouraged to track his physical rehabilitation progress weekly rather than daily because progress is often slow and difficult to see if evaluated too frequently. He could also be made aware that he will likely continue to recover for many months and that his progress may involve plateaus during which it feels like not much progress is being made. He may experience frustration about the recovery process, sadness regarding limitations and losses, and anxiety about what the future holds, and he may feel overwhelmed by the challenges he will face. However, knowing that all these experiences are normal and to be expected will likely help him to persevere.

Communication

Most of a patient's information regarding her disease and its treatment comes verbally from the primary medical team, so clear communication is important. Although seemingly simple, communication is often poor in the medical setting, and many patients can benefit from intervention regarding strategies to improve their communication with their medical providers.

Good communication between patients and their doctors has been consistently associated with patient satisfaction, adherence with treatment recommendations, and also with health outcomes (e.g., Haskard Zolnierek & DiMatteo, 2009; King & Hoppe, 2013; Oliveira et al., 2012) and therefore has significant implications for a patient. Those patients who misunderstand medical information may be unable to adequately adhere to medical recommendations both while in the hospital and after discharge.

There are many reasons for poor communication in the hospital setting. Physicians are often not clear in their explanations to patients, talk too fast, or use terms that patients do not understand. Patients may be too intimidated to ask questions, or too sick or anxious to comprehend and retain information effectively. Some patients are motivated to misunderstand information, especially if the patient's behavior is to blame for the medical problem. Finally, patients and their doctors may have differences of opinion regarding what aspects of treatment are most important as they may have differing goals; for example, a patient may be exclusively focused on short-term pain management, while the physician is more concerned about the longer term prognosis. This discrepancy in focus and goals can create confusion when they discuss the treatment priorities.

The responsibility for effective communication does not fall exclusively on the patient, but there are specific skills that patients can learn to improve their communication with the medical team. Exhibit 6.5 provides some tips for patients in this area and can be used as a handout. It is rare that a psychological intervention with the patient is explicitly focused on "communication" as the goal; rather, communication is usually discussed in the context of the patient seeking more information about the medical illness. At times, especially in the context of a new diagnosis, it is most useful

EXHIBIT 6.5

Patient Tips for Effective Communication With Medical Providers

Be prepared with a prioritized list of questions for the medical team (What is the expected course of the illness? Recommended treatment? Implications for normal activities?).

Have a family member present when meeting with doctors.

Be appropriately assertive in requesting time with doctors for questions.

Understand that doctors don't always have all the answers and that you may not like the answers they can provide.

to schedule a formal meeting with the patient, family, and medical team to review all the new information and to make treatment decisions.

Especially with a new diagnosis, patients may have many questions for the doctor, but it is common for patients to feel anxious and rushed when the doctor comes in to the hospital room, and they forget much of what they wanted to ask. Therefore, it is helpful to have them make a list of their questions so that they are ready for the doctor's visit; this also helps them to collect their own thoughts. Prioritizing the questions makes it more likely that the most important ones will be answered soonest; this is especially important in a complicated medical situation that consists of too many issues to be addressed at once.

Patients often need to be assertive in their requests for information, as the hospital milieu and the fast pace of much of a patient's treatment conspire to make it difficult for patients to get large amounts of time to talk to their medical providers. Most information about a patient's disorder and treatment plan is discussed when the doctors round on their patients (typically daily). These meetings are not scheduled formally, and the patient needs to be ready with questions when the doctors arrive. The patient may also need to ask for more time if the doctors are ready to leave before the patient is finished with his questions. At times, and especially for complicated situations that need repeated discussion as the medical picture changes, a specific resident or nurse can be designated by the medical team to spend additional time providing information to the patient in more detail as the situation unfolds.

Recommending that a trusted family member or friend be present when the patient is meeting with her doctors is also a good idea because it provides the patient with someone who can help to recall the discussion and also provide emotional support. Taking notes can also help patients to remember the information presented.

Patients also need to be prepared for the possibility that their doctors may not know the answers to some of their questions or that the answers may change as the disease or treatment unfolds. It is sometimes difficult for patients to understand that the entire prognosis or treatment plan could change from one day to the next, based on a new laboratory result or the development of an additional symptom. Further, patients may not like the answers they receive in response to their questions, especially if the prognosis is poor. Yet many patients prefer a realistic picture of their situation, even if the news is bad, rather than an unrealistically positive one. Exhibit 6.6

EXHIBIT 6.6

Intervention to Improve Patient Communication and Collaboration With the Medical Team

Ms. S was a 70 y/o woman admitted with a new diagnosis of breast cancer. A health psychology consultation was requested to evaluate her understanding of the medical issues because the medical team felt she was not handling discussions of treatment well. The evaluation revealed no significant psychological history or cognitive deficits, but the patient was overwhelmed with her diagnosis and was not effectively working with her medical team. The psychologist worked with her to manage her emotions and to improve communication with her medical providers. Specifically, the psychologist met with the patient and her daughter to develop a list of their questions about the patient's diagnosis, treatment, and prognosis. They reviewed the list with the patient's nurse, and she answered any questions that she could. They then developed a plan in which the daughter would arrive to visit about the time the medical team rounded daily, and the patient would practice diaphragmatic breathing about this time to help herself relax. They selected the three questions from the list that were most important to ask when the doctors arrived. If the medical team seemed about to leave before the questions were answered, it was the daughter's job to say, "Please wait a minute, we have a few questions." Afterward, the patient and daughter discussed the information they had received and selected their questions for the following day. The psychologist also forewarned the medical team that this plan was being implemented.

demonstrates a case in which the psychologist worked with a patient and her daughter to improve communication with the medical team.

New Diagnostic Information

Many patients have a significant amount to learn if they are diagnosed with a new medical problem, including information about the disease itself, associated symptoms, potential treatments, the expected course of the disease, and the implications of this disease for their lives. Although a great source of information for patients, the health psychologist is not the primary source of information when a patient has received a diagnosis of a new medical condition. The patient's medical team should have delivered the information regarding the disorder, its course, and potential treatments before the psychologist discusses the disease and its implications with the patient. The health psychologist may have a significant amount of objective knowledge of medical disorders but will not have the physician's expertise in this area and will be unable to answer the questions that a patient receiving a new diagnosis is likely to have.

This is not to say that discussing the medical issues with the patient is completely off limits before an official diagnosis from the medical team. Many times patients are impatiently waiting for a differential diagnosis among several disorders and may wish to discuss their concerns about the potential implications of each. In a case like that, the health psychologist will want to be clear with the patient that this is a hypothetical discussion as the answer to the diagnostic question is not yet known.

Yet it is acceptable for the patient to imagine each scenario to begin to anticipate the implications of each for his life. In cases of ambiguity, patients often jump to the worst possible outcomes. It is useful, then, for the health psychologist to use cognitive strategies to help the patient see that there are a variety of possible outcomes and help her avoid settling on one specific (and overly negative) outcome before having data to support that conclusion.

In some cases, the medical team will ask the health psychology consultant to be present when information about a new diagnosis is delivered to a patient; this occurs most frequently if the patient has known psychiatric problems or if the news is especially bad. It is often most useful for the psychologist to listen while the medical team delivers the information and then to stay with the patient after the medical team leaves to help the patient process the new information. At times, the patient is too overwhelmed to know what to think or what questions to ask at this time, and the psychologist can then return later to help the patient process the information or generate a list of specific questions to ask the medical team at their next visit.

Often, a good way to approach a patient's understanding of his illness and diagnosis is to ask generally about his worries and what the doctor has told him about the medical problem. This approach will enable the psychologist to determine whether the patient has asked appropriate questions of the physician and will also expose the patient's understanding of the educational material that has been provided to him thus far. Assuming that the psychologist already knows the patient's diagnosis and understands the relevant issues, he can then help the patient to process the material and to develop additional questions as needed.

When consulted by a medical team to discuss a patient's diagnosis with the patient, be aware that the medical team may have presented the relevant material to the patient, but that does not ensure that the patient has heard and understood it. Beyond the general communication problems that can occur, at times patients are too distressed or confused to process the information adequately, so they have missed the education provided to them. If the health psychology consultant incorrectly assumes the patient is aware of the diagnosis and prognosis, the consultation may not proceed well. One psychologist described an encounter in which she was told by the referring doctor that the patient was aware she had a terminal illness, so the psychologist openly raised the issue with the patient. However, the patient did not understand that she had a terminal illness, so she became distressed and had many questions that the psychologist could not answer. The patient was upset and rapport was damaged because the psychologist had wrongly assumed that the patient understood the information that the physician felt had been presented to her. It is always best to determine what the patient knows about her situation by asking her before proceeding with the consultation.

At times, materials from the Internet can provide a wealth of information to educate patients regarding new medical issues, and physicians will often provide these materials to patients. If handouts on any psychological or medical issues are to be provided to the patient, it will be important to attend to the level at which the material is written. Specifically, the materials should be clear and free of jargon, and they should be written at a reading level that is appropriate to the patient's educational level. The psychologist should also be attentive to issues of illiteracy that will make all written materials irrelevant unless a family member can read them to the patient. Finally, these materials should always come from reputable sites, such as WebMD (https://www.webmd.com), Mayo Clinic (https://www.mayoclinic.org), or Cleveland Clinic (https://my.clevelandclinic.org). It is also a good idea to clear any materials about the medical diagnosis with the medical team before providing them to the patient.

Medical Issues and Treatments

With experience, the health psychologist will develop knowledge of a variety of experiences that patients may have due to different medical treatments. For example, it is quite common for a patient undergoing chemotherapy to experience nausea, vomiting, and decreased appetite. Yet some patients will not be aware of this and may be concerned that something is dramatically wrong if they experience those symptoms. The psychologist can normalize the patient's symptoms and experience as an expected part of the treatment process, while encouraging the patient to discuss the symptoms with his nurse or doctor.

There are many situations in which education regarding medications and side effects can help patients to cope with a specific treatment. For example, a patient who started high-dose steroids within the past few days may complain of anxiety to the health psychologist. After assessment, it may be clear that the symptoms are a side effect of the steroids, rather than anxiety. Similarly, vivid dreams and hallucinations may occur as a side effect of narcotics. Education regarding these experiences as side effects may comfort the patient that he is not "going crazy." The psychologist can work with the patient to develop strategies to help cope with the symptoms, and the medical team should be alerted so that they can help to manage the symptoms or adjust medications.

Many patients are prescribed sleep or pain medications while in the hospital but will avoid taking them for fear of developing an addiction. The psychologist can provide education on the benefits of taking the medication temporarily—that it will make the patient more comfortable and will promote physical healing as well as improved emotional coping, for example. Often this minimal education is all that is needed to enable the patient to comfortably take the medication for the period of time it is needed.

Patients may have ideas and concerns about medical procedures that may or may not be accurate and realistic and that can be addressed by the psychologist to alleviate patient worries. For example, it is appropriate for a patient to have some concern about a cardiac catheterization because the procedure is associated with some serious risks, such as bleeding and stroke. Realistic risks can be discussed with the patient, and anxiety management techniques can be used as needed. In another situation, a patient may be upset and fearful about having an electrocardiogram (ECG). However, this is a pain-free, noninvasive test that poses no significant physical risks. The patient may have serious worries about the results of the procedure and the implications of those for his future, but the procedure itself does not need to be a cause of significant worry. If the health psychology consultant understands the basics of the ECG procedure, the patient's concerns can be addressed and often alleviated.

Patients may request additional information from the health psychology consultant on a new diagnosis at any time during the admission in an effort to educate themselves. The psychologist needs to find a balance in which she works to help patients understand the medical issues without being the main source of information about their illness (which should be left to the medical providers). Although the psychology consultant will discuss many aspects of their illnesses with patients, patients should be referred to their nurses and doctors for answers to specific medical questions. It may also be helpful for the health psychology consultant to contact the medical team to set this up for the patient.

MANAGEMENT OF EMOTIONAL REACTIONS

When initially faced with a new medical diagnosis, or a transition to a different phase of an illness, patients may experience strong emotional reactions, including anger, fear, sadness, or mixed reactions. Patients will also describe feeling "numb" at times, as if the emotions are too strong and they shut down. Patients may be initially overwhelmed with the new limitations and challenges, especially if there are many. They may experience a variety of emotions that switch quickly—from anxiety to sadness to anger, for example. In the new leukemia case in Exhibit 6.2, Ms. T was completely surprised by the diagnosis as she had no inkling that there was anything seriously wrong with her. She was frightened that she would die and leave her young children to be raised by someone else. Her mood was depressed as she felt hopeless, helpless, and powerless to fix the problem.

Anger occurs frequently and may result in the patient blaming himself, his family, or his medical providers for the impairments or diagnosis. Patients may feel the medical problem is due to mistakes on the part of a medical provider or to delays in access to diagnostic testing or initiation of treatment. Frustration can also occur if patients feel powerless to have any impact on changing the situation. Fear or anxiety may be associated with a patient's initial (and sometimes uninformed) ideas of what will be involved as the disease progresses.

One common reaction to the diagnosis of a significant medical problem is the patient asking "why me?" although many patients do not articulate this out loud. (They will, however, typically admit to these thoughts if asked about them.) Because most people tend to believe we live in a just world (Furnham, 2003), they look for reasons why this bad disease would happen to them. Many people are stumped because they feel they have led (or tried to lead) good lives in which they have tried to do the right thing. They may search their history for a time and place in which they did something bad—something that would warrant a punishment such as a terminal diagnosis. Others can find actions in their past for which they feel that punishment might be appropriate. It is important for the psychologist to listen to the patient's description of why punishment is warranted (because otherwise the psychologist's opinion that punishment is not warranted is not credible). The psychologist can then take the position that, regardless of the patient's beliefs, we do not live in a just world, and there is ample evidence of that (e.g., a baby who develops a horrible illness, a murderer who lives a long and happy life). The patient will need to accept the idea that people do not always get what they deserve; one oncologist explained the development of cancer as due to "bad luck" that has no connection to how well the patient has lived his or her life.

The discussion of why the medical issue happened often elicits a discussion of the patient's religious beliefs, and their feelings of how God allowed this to happen. Regardless of the psychologist's own beliefs, helping the patient to work through any challenges this brings to their religious beliefs is useful to them. Referring the patient to her religious leader to discuss these issues further is appropriate when the psychologist does not have the expertise to address a patient's religious beliefs appropriately.

Following a new diagnosis, patients are often frightened about treatments or experiences they may face in the future as a result of the illness or medical treatment. Patients diagnosed with cancer often fear chemotherapy, nausea, pain, and death; patients diagnosed with MS fear losing the ability to walk and cognitive decline. It is important for the health psychology consultant to help patients develop a realistic understanding of the disease without creating an expectation that the worst possible scenario will occur. One of the best ways to combat unnecessary anxieties is to provide patients with information about aspects of the disease and its treatment and prognosis so that they can develop realistic expectations of what the new diagnosis or transition will mean to them. Anxiety management techniques can also be used as needed; these are discussed further in the next chapter.

Patients often need to deal with significant losses due to changes in their medical situation, and they may grieve for these as they would a death, experiencing anger, denial, and other aspects of grief. Patients may experience unexpected and dramatic losses of physical abilities (as might occur with a stroke), or the losses may be more subtle, insidious, and anticipated as those that may occur with a chronic and progressive illness, such as MS or chronic obstructive pulmonary disease (COPD). Patients may lose the ability to engage in many physical activities, such as work, chores, ADLs, sports, and sexual behavior. The lost abilities can have implications for the patient's self-image and identity, especially if they are unable to engage in valued tasks or if their appearance changes. These lost activities can also affect the patient's relationships with coworkers, friends, and family and may result in decreased social support, often because the patient has less social contact and less opportunity to access the social support that is available to him.

Patients may also lose the ability to be spontaneous in their behavior and may need to do more planning of their activities, especially if they are now dependent on others. In the past, a patient may have been able to decide on the spur of the moment to attend an event, but new physical limitations may now require that she make plans for transportation, a wheelchair, and accessible venues if she wants to attend a sporting event. A loss of the ability to be spontaneous can result in frustration, anger, or sadness.

Patients may feel unproductive if they are unable to work or contribute to the household. In the new CVA case (Exhibit 6.1), Mr. R may be unable to return to work, at least for the immediate future. This has implications for his identity as a mechanic as the breadwinner for his family and could also cause serious financial stress. He may also lose important social relationships and the support of his coworkers if he is unable to work. Ms. T may grieve for the loss of her former healthy self, as well as future experiences that she fears she will not be able to have if the leukemia treatment is not successful (e.g., being unable to watch her children grow up and have their own families).

The emotional reactions experienced can be intense, especially if the diagnosis and prognosis are bad. Imagine being given a diagnosis of terminal cancer—and then imagine the strong emotions that may occur when one receives that diagnosis. While experiencing strong emotions, patients are unlikely to be responsive to therapist interventions to provide education or to help the patient develop realistic expectations and plans to face the illness. Patients will need some time to experience and process their emotional reactions and will then be better able to engage in planning and cognitive work. Therefore, the health psychology consultant will need to be aware of the patient's emotional state to determine the proper timing for any interventions.

The management of the intense emotional reactions that occur immediately after diagnosis is similar to the management of any strong emotional reaction that a psychologist would help a patient to address. The most relevant aspects of this process will typically involve a phase in which the patient is encouraged to experience her emotions, followed by a phase in which she decides what, if any, actions should be taken (Greenberg, 2004). Patients may feel there is no way that they will ever "be OK" with the medical issue they are facing. While the psychologist cannot promise the medical issue will be OK, she can reassure the patient that she can learn to deal with it. After the patient has had time to express and process the emotions, cognitive and behavioral strategies can be used to help her make plans to cope.

Interventions to aid the emotional management process involve education regarding the adjustment process, and encouragement for patients to take as much control as they can. One area over which a patient can typically exert a significant amount of control is the management of his own emotions. It is often useful for patients to view their adjustment as a process in which they grieve or express their anger, but then they move on to active planning and coping to help themselves adapt to the situation in the best way they can.

Clinically, it is useful to encourage patients to stay focused in the present as much as possible and to avoid thinking too far into the future. It is not uncommon for people to fear the worst when initially given a bad diagnosis and prognosis, although after they have had a chance to come to terms with the illness, many people then become more optimistic (e.g., "I will be the one in 10 patients who is cured"). A hopeful, but realistic, attitude does much to help a patient manage the stress associated with a new medical diagnosis.

Patients may engage in denial when given a new medical diagnosis, or at any time later, throughout treatment and various stages of the illness. While usually thought of as maladaptive, the literature provides examples of "healthy denial" (Druss & Douglas, 1988); this might be most useful when it allows a patient to delay acceptance of an illness or its implications until she is better able to manage it emotionally. In its extreme, however, denial delays the patient's emotional adjustment and interferes with treatment and adherence, as the individual does not accept that action needs to be taken. In extreme cases the patient may avoid treatment completely.

Denial can take many forms. Consider a woman with metastatic cancer who did not deny that she had cancer but did deny the seriousness of the disease, as well as the fact that the illness was terminal. The patient continued to seek novel treatments, even after she had been told that all were futile. She was a single mother, and because she was certain she would live, she failed to make plans for someone to care for her children after her death. When a patient like this is firm in the denial of the illness or its implications, it is generally not useful to repeatedly point it out to them. Rather, questioning the patient about the symptom or disease (e.g., what is it, what does it indicate, what does this mean for her life and future) may help her to accept the objective data and then to move toward dealing with it.

COPING WITH LIMITATIONS AND CHANGES

Lazarus and Folkman (1984) defined *coping* as "the constantly changing cognitive and behavioral efforts to manage specific external and/or internal demands that are appraised as taxing or exceeding the resources of the person" (p. 141). One aspect of the adjustment process involves patients learning to use appropriate coping strategies to help them to engage in new behaviors, use cognitions that facilitate adaptive behavior, and deal with the emotional aspects of the new illness or medical problem. Coping strategies can be learned, and thus one goal of the psychologist's intervention when helping a patient to adjust to the medical situation is to teach improved coping.

Much research has been dedicated to the delineation of specific coping strategies and the stressful situations in which they are most useful (e.g., Billings & Moos, 1981; Folkman et al., 1986). Coping strategies have been divided into several categories by Lazarus and colleagues, who have done a significant amount of research in this area (e.g., Folkman et al., 1986; Lazarus & Folkman, 1984). These researchers have defined problem-focused coping strategies as those that are designed to have an impact on the current stressor. In the context of adjustment to a new medical illness, this could include making plans to manage the illness, engaging in healthier behaviors, and seeking support from others. Another type, emotion-focused coping, involves activities that are intended to regulate or avoid emotion, such as drug use or exercise. Others have categorized coping strategies somewhat differently; for example, Litman (2006) reported on two coping styles that are approach-oriented (i.e., self-sufficient and socially supported) and one that involves a negative, avoidant style.

Research on coping with medical illnesses such as diabetes, prostate cancer, and HIV has revealed that coping strategies characterized as active, problem-focused, or approach-oriented are associated with better adjustment (Duangdao & Roesch, 2008; Moskowitz, Hult, Bussolari, & Acree, 2009; Roesch et al., 2005; Roesch & Weiner, 2001).

Avoidant strategies have been associated with poorer adjustment (Moskowitz et al., 2009; Roesch et al., 2005; Roesch & Weiner, 2001) and also with psychological distress (Dempster, Howell, & McCorry, 2015). One study of patients with end-stage renal disease reported that avoidant coping was associated with increased mortality (Wolf & Mori, 2009).

Regardless of one's theoretical approach to coping, when intervening with medical inpatients clinically, there are many coping strategies available to help patients manage new medical issues and limitations. Table 6.1 contains a list of some common coping strategies that can be used by patients to cope with new medical issues (selected from Billings & Moos, 1981; Carver et al., 1989; Folkman et al., 1986; Litman & Lunsford, 2009), as well as examples of how they can be used by patients to cope with their medical problems. Some of these coping strategies involve engaging in behaviors to help solve the problem (e.g., active coping) or to enlist social support. Others involve cognitive strategies to either promote healthy behavior (e.g., positive reappraisal) or activities to help manage emotion (e.g., distraction).

One aspect of adaptive coping involves patients assessing their priorities in life, including specific activities that are most important for good quality of life and positive mood. A patient's priorities might include work, sports, relationships, or any activities that help them feel loved, productive, and happy. Some of these priority activities may not be affected by the medical problems, and the patient can then make plans to ensure that they continue. Others may be disrupted by the medical illness, and then patients will need to develop plans to continue these activities in new ways

TABLE 6.1

Coping Strategies and Examples of Their Use With Medical Problems

Planning/problem-solving	Figuring out what changes to make to accommodate new illness; how to manage new medication
Active coping	Take prescribed medication; get a second opinion
Seeking instrumental or emotional social support	Asking informed family/friends for opinions on treatment decisions; talking to cancer survivors; enlist help to decrease physical obligations
Religious coping: positive	"I can manage with God's help"; seek religious support
Acceptance	"This has happened to me and I just need to deal with it now"
Positive reappraisal	"This will force me to make some changes in my life, which I wanted to do anyway"
Denial	Refusing to believe the diagnosis; refusing medical treatment
Disengagement/distraction	Removing oneself emotionally or physically from the situation
Wishful thinking	Unrealistic fantasizing about things being different
Humor	Finding something funny about the situation; making light of it
Substance use; overeating	Overusing drugs, alcohol, or food to avoid addressing the problem
Taking responsibility	Seeing one's role in the problem

or find substitutes. For example, immediately after his stroke, Mr. R lost the camaraderie and social support that he had received from his coworkers. The goal then was to help him find other ways to obtain this support (perhaps by meeting coworkers for lunch once weekly) or by finding other sources of support (make new friends in his rehabilitation program). There may also be activities that Mr. R is no longer able to do at all, and he may need to reassess his situation and learn to be content with what he is able to do, at least for now, as he works to regain his functioning. For now, he may be unable to share yard chores with his son, although he can still help his son to plan the work and can help him collect the proper tools.

The term *coping* has been used to refer to just about anything that a patient does to try to deal with a stressor—there is no assumption that the strategies are either useful or adaptive. Those strategies in Table 6.1 that are associated with active problem-solving (e.g., planning, active coping, seeking support) are most associated with positive adjustment in medical inpatients, based on the literature reviewed in the preceding paragraphs. Some of the other strategies may be useful temporarily or at certain times during the adjustment process, although would not be recommended generally. For example, although distraction is not adaptive if used exclusively, it can be effective at helping patients to titrate information and manage their emotional reactions, especially when they are initially told about a terminal illness. Other strategies in Table 6.1, although commonly used by patients ostensibly to help them cope, are not adaptive and may even be harmful (e.g., substance use, overeating).

When discussing coping with medical patients, it is useful to simply ask them what they do to help themselves cope in general, and to help them manage the medical issue specifically. The patient's strategies can then be discussed in terms of how useful they are. Additional coping strategies can then also be described, and patients can generate ways they might use these to help them progress through the adjustment process. Discussing maladaptive strategies with patients is also important so that they can consider replacing them with more adaptive strategies. (See Jacobsen et al., 2014, for specific examples of interventions to help patients improve their coping.) Following is a summary of the discussion of coping that the psychologist had with Mr. R, the new stroke patient.

Several days after his stroke, Mr. R described working to figure out what he needed to do to manage his physical limitations as well as his financial obligations (active planning, problem-solving). He also reported trying to accept his new situation rather than denying it. He reported a tendency to overuse alcohol when stressed at previous times in his life, but he acknowledged that would not be useful in this situation because it would likely exacerbate his physical and cognitive impairments and delay his recovery (as well as create additional risk of further injury). He was open to the idea of using his social support system to help him manage instrumental tasks, although he was less comfortable seeking emotional support from his social network or his church.

Religious coping is an important strategy for some patients, especially when individuals have significant and life-threatening illnesses (Koenig, Larson, & Larson, 2001), evidenced by frequent use of religious coping in patients with advanced cancer (Balboni et al., 2007; Phelps et al., 2009). Religious coping presents a special case, however, in that patients who do not consider themselves to be actively religious are typically not interested in using religious coping strategies. Therefore, teaching religious coping strategies is not appropriate for all inpatients. Because religious coping strategies can have either positive or negative effects, depending on the specific cognitions or beliefs that patients use, the goal of the psychologist is to help a patient who already uses religious coping strategies to adjust the specific cognitions or beliefs to those who are most healthy and adaptive.

Specifically, positive religious coping involves the belief that God is a benevolent collaborator and may result in the patient seeking religious direction and support from clergy or church members; negative religious coping views God as punishing or unable to answer prayers and may be associated with feelings of abandonment by the church (Pargament, Smith, Koenig, & Perez, 1998). Negative religious coping may also include the idea that the medical illness is God's will, so there is nothing the patient can (or should) do about it, which can have significant implications for adherence to the medical regimen.

Positive religious coping is used more frequently than negative (Pargament et al., 1998) and is associated with better adjustment, less depression, better quality of life, and improved adherence to dietary recommendations (see Gall & Guirguis-Younger, 2013, for a review). It has also been associated with a greater preference for intensive life-prolonging care and also patient receipt of more care of this type when patients are near death (Phelps et al., 2009). Negative religious coping is associated with poorer adjustment (Pargament et al., 2000) and with suicidal ideation in patients with advanced cancer (Trevino, Balboni, Zollfrank, Balboni, & Prigerson, 2014).

DEVELOPING FEELINGS OF CONTROL OVER SYMPTOMS AND EFFICACY TO MANAGE DISEASE

Adjustment is facilitated if patients feel they have some control over the disease and the ability to manage it successfully. Feelings of control are directly related to a patient's understanding of the disease itself, the typical course, expected symptoms, potential treatments and side effects, and other aspects of the medical situation. Even before taking any action to manage the disease, patients report feeling more in control simply because they have received education about the disease—for example, "Now I at least understand what I am dealing with." Therefore, education is paramount in the development of feelings of control.

Once a patient understands the objective facts about the illness, he is better able to determine the personal implications for his life and take stock of what he is dealing with. There may be physical or cognitive limitations to manage, or perhaps new medical activities that need to be undertaken to promote health over the long term. Helping patients to evaluate the personal implications of the disease, including any limitations, is one important role for the health psychology consultant. Although there are some generalities, the personal implications of the disease will be patient-specific. For example, dealing with cognitive impairments that involve slow processing and difficulty manipulating numbers will be difficult for anyone, but this limitation may have more significant implications for an accountant than for a house painter.

Patients need to learn their limits and then develop some sense of efficacy at working within them. Although the benefits of activity—broadly defined to include physical, social, and intellectual activity—are undisputed for medical patients, many cannot spontaneously engage in activities that they could easily do in the past. However, it is important for patients to give up as few activities as possible. Instead, they may need to plan (often extensively) to successfully manage previously simple activities and also realize that the plans may need to change when the day arrives or as the activity unfolds. For example, Mr. R used to enjoy going to the beach with his kids and would spend hours on his beach towel in the sun while they swam and visited with friends. Depending on his status after his recuperation from the stroke, he may still be able to go to the beach, although engaging in this activity may be more complicated. If he has mobility problems, he may need to make plans for a wheelchair, appropriate transportation, and an accessible entrance to the beach. He may need to find a place that is not sandy and that has shade. He may also need to be sure he has a family member along to help him physically. The goal is to continue to enjoy the activity if it is at all possible and to be sure he is safe in the process. Many patients will complain that all the planning is frustrating and detracts from the experience, but doing the activity with the new limitations is preferable because activity restriction has been associated with depression in medical patients (e.g., Mausbach et al., 2011; Williamson, 1998, 2000). If there are activities that a patient is no longer able to engage in at all, the patient should seek other activities to replace them.

The patient's doctor can usually provide basic information about physical limitations that are associated with a patient's disease. Depending on the severity of the disease, a patient with lung disease may be able to engage in household chores such as cooking, washing dishes, and folding laundry, but she may not be able to carry a laundry basket downstairs or change bedding because these activities involve more exertion. In addition, the activities that a patient can comfortably manage may change over time if a disease progresses, for example, a patient's COPD may progress, and she may experience increased shortness of breath with less exertion; then she has to adjust her physical activity further. Even when stable medically, a patient's abilities may fluctuate from day to day, often for no clear reason. Patients with MS often have good days when they have energy and bad days when they are completely fatigued; there may be no pattern to what each day will turn out to be. When patients have energy ("a good day"), there is a tendency to overdo activities and then pay for it with decreased energy and increased fatigue the next few days. Because of the idiosyncratic nature of much of this, patients may need to monitor their own responses to various activities to determine their own personal limitations. It is in a patient's best interest to engage in physical activity because its lack is associated with depression (Jensen, Molton, Gertz, Bombardier, & Rosenberg, 2012). Physical rehabilitation programs can help patients to determine their physical limitations as well as teach them behavioral strategies to compensate for them.

Patients may also need to adapt to the idea of using aids (e.g., canes, walkers, wheelchairs, oxygen) to help them be as functional as possible. For many people, beginning to use an aid is difficult emotionally because they may feel stigmatized or inadequate as a result. Many will refuse completely or will avoid using aids until they have a scare that helps them realize they need the aid for safety reasons. It is useful for the psychologist to have a discussion with the patient about the goal of making her quality of life as good as it can be. Specifically, if the use of an aid enables the patient to engage safely in enjoyable activities, it is preferable to use the aid rather than miss the activity or risk harm by doing it without the aid. Some patients make healthy efforts to decrease the negative connotation of the aid; one patient bought several canes and covered them with colorful paper to make them fashionable accessories to complement her outfits. Others commented on them often, and this allowed her to address her mobility limitation openly and begin to accept it as part of her life, in the context of social support.

Pacing is an important skill for patients to learn and involves breaking an activity into smaller parts with breaks in between them. Patients often use pacing to help them accomplish chores at home. For example, a patient does chores for 30 minutes, then rests for 15 minutes, and then repeats the process. She works for a total of 3 hours per day at these chores so that she doesn't become overly fatigued. Several times during the process, she stops to reevaluate how she is feeling and adjusts her plans accordingly.

Pacing is often foreign to patients, and they may resist the idea, complaining that the activity isn't the same if they can't do it the way they always have done it. It may not be "the same," but new arrangements are necessary, or the patient may not be able to do the activity at all; a discussion of this can often help move the patient toward acceptance of a new routine. Patients may try it the old way, and after either being unsuccessful at accomplishing the goal or being exhausted for several days afterward, they may understand the benefits of pacing and begin to make changes. Pacing is a particularly useful concept for patients with medical problems that can be exacerbated by activity, such as COPD, sickle cell disease, or MS. It is important emotionally for patients to maintain as much activity as possible to decrease the risk of developing depression or anxiety (e.g., De Mello et al., 2013; Mammen & Faulkner, 2013); pacing and planning are skills they can use to remain active and exert some control over the physical limitations caused by the disease. Exhibit 6.7 is a patient's description of using

EXHIBIT 6.7

A Patient's Description of Adaptive Coping

"I would say I am well adjusted to my emphysema now. I know how to pace my daily activities so that I don't get short of breath. I can do much of what I want to do, although not the same way I did it before. I am still sad about those activities I can no longer do, like mowing the lawn, golfing with my buddies, and playing football with my grandkids. Mostly I am able to do other (less strenuous) activities with my grandkids and my friends, and I just rest more along the way, and that is better than nothing. I wouldn't say I'm happy about my situation, but I am mostly content and my quality of life is OK. My expectations have just had to change."

pacing and its effect on his quality of life; Exhibit 6.8 is from a patient who is unwilling to make changes in his activity.

A major focus for the psychologist is to encourage behavioral activation, so that patients can do all they can safely do and avoid closing down their lives. As patients reevaluate their lives and make changes to their behavioral patterns and also their thinking and expectations, they need to work to re-create their roles and activities, rather than simply discontinuing activities they are no longer able to do. A patient who stops engaging in previously pleasurable activities, without replacing those activities with others that are satisfying, is at risk for depression. It has long been known that engaging in pleasurable events is associated with improved mood and less depression (Lewinsohn & Graf, 1973). While patients may need to give up certain activities or roles at home, they need to develop others so they can continue to feel they are productive and contributing to the family. After discharge, Mr. R will likely be unable to mow the lawn and to fix the family cars, but perhaps he will be able to fold the family's laundry and help his granddaughter with her homework. Activity, defined broadly to include social, intellectual, and physical activity, can result in improved mood and successful adjustment. Activity can decrease rumination and worry and can focus patients on issues beyond themselves and their illness.

Another way that patients gain some feeling of control over their disease or symptoms is by engaging in behaviors that have an impact on it. These activities may involve attendance at medical appointments, treatments, or hospital admissions; medication adherence; or changes in diet and exercise. Some aspects of the medical regimen may be linked closely to a corresponding change in symptoms; for example, a patient with COPD who experiences shortness of breath and then uses an inhaler should see a quick reduction in symptoms. The immediate reinforcement will help to maintain the behavior. Other health behaviors, however, are less clearly related to the patient's immediate symptoms—eating a heart-healthy diet does not immediately (and may never) result in a cardiac patient feeling better. In cases like this, patients need to consider the objective benefits of the diet and then motivate themselves to follow it, even if there is no clear short-term reinforcement for the behavior. Adherence to recommendations can be a significant problem with medical patients and is discussed more fully in Chapter 12.

It may seem that there is little the individual can control in the face of devastating medical problems, but typically there is *something* they can do. Patients may be unable to control the actual disease process, but they can usually exert control over some

EXHIBIT 6.8

A Patient Who Does Not Yet Accept His Medical Condition

"Adjustment? No, there is no adjusting to this. I just continue to do what I always did because I won't give in to this disease. My wife says I do too much, and then I pay for it with discomfort, shortness of breath, and fatigue—but I'm not willing to change my lifestyle because of this disease."

symptoms or over their own emotional reactions. They can work on their health generally by exercising, eating properly, and getting sufficient sleep. They can also work to keep their spirits up to avoid additional problems associated with emotional distress or negative mood. Monitoring one's mood and taking action to improve it if needed, are other important ways for a patient to exert control over the situation. About a week after his stroke, Mr. R was feeling powerless to help himself recover. The psychologist raised the issue of control, that is, that some aspects of his illness were out of his control, but there were others over which he could have some impact. Specifically, he was able to see how he could exert some influence over his recovery by (a) attending to his nutritional status by following food intake recommendations; (b) engaging consistently in occupational therapy, physical therapy, swallowing sessions, and associated homework assignments; and (c) improving his spirits by asking his family to bring him some activities from home and also to spend more time with him at the hospital. This discussion gave Mr. R some specific activities to perform to improve his medical and emotional situation, as well as a greater feeling of control.

A patient can also exert control by managing her own expectations and developing a realistic and adaptive approach to the illness, learning to integrate the illness as one part of an otherwise full and varied life. An adaptive attitude toward a medical illness is characterized by a willingness to learn and to take appropriate action to manage the illness and limitations to the best of one's ability (e.g., "I need to do what I can to deal with this"). Those patients who actively take on the illness and do all they can to fight or manage it are usually quite open to suggestions from the health psychology consultant regarding ways they can adhere to treatment, manage their mood, and generally do what they can to promote their own health. Part of an individual's initial reaction, especially to a particularly devastating illness, may involve feelings of giving up and of feeling powerless to have any impact on the illness. Patients may feel beaten by the illness or a new medical development and may give up on doing anything to help change its course. Although not unexpected as an initial reaction to a devastating diagnosis, this approach will be maladaptive in the longer term. One goal of psychological intervention is to increase a patient's willingness and ability to manage the illness and to maintain a good quality of life. A patient's approach to the illness may also fluctuate in response to new developments or perceived successes and failures as they go through the process.

Patients have expectations about health and illness and need to integrate the new illness into their lives and identity. Those who have been ill previously or throughout their lives may have already successfully integrated the medical problem into their lives, but for those patients without a significant medical history, a new diagnosis may present a major challenge. Patients may complain that they are "no longer the same person" now that they have the disease, and they will need to be encouraged to accept the disease as a part of their multifaceted identity (not as something that defines them completely). Often a discussion of others in the patient's social network who have chronic medical issues can help the new patient to see how one can learn to live with and manage a disease without allowing it to take over her life completely.

Factors That Influence Adjustment

Several factors can influence the patient's adjustment to the medical problems, including premorbid stressors, the individual's personal capabilities, and external resources. These are reviewed in this section.

PREMORBID STRESSORS

Many patients have ongoing social or psychological issues that escalate when the patient and the family are faced with serious medical problems. A common scenario involves that of a patient who is usually overly attentive to her family's needs but is now in the hospital with a serious medical problem; yet her family continues to expect her to take care of their needs. For example, the patient may have developed lung disease and requires a lung transplant. She is in the hospital dealing with shortness of breath and new treatments, including a nebulizer and steroids, and an extensive medical workup for possible lung transplant listing. Her husband drops off the bills and checkbook so that she can continue to manage the family's finances, and her teenagers call repeatedly throughout the day, expecting her to resolve disagreements among them. Although in some cases, activities from home can distract the patient from worry and normalize the hospital admission, most times the family conflicts increase the patient's stress level, making it more difficult for her to come to terms with her medical situation. In many cases, the stress associated with the new medical crisis exacerbates the ongoing social stressors.

In the inpatient setting, the health psychology consultant will want to address the ongoing social issues to the extent that they impact the management of the current medical situation. For this patient with lung disease, the intervention might involve encouraging the patient to set limits with her children, enlisting someone else to pay the bills for now, acknowledging the difficulty of letting go of some of these family responsibilities, and encouraging her to make her health her top priority for now, because this is ultimately in her family's best interests also. Patients can then deal with the ongoing social issues more extensively on an outpatient basis if they wish.

Ms. T, the patient with newly diagnosed leukemia (Exhibit 6.2), had a conflictual marriage, and her husband had been involved in an extramarital affair for the past 2 years. After the patient's leukemia diagnosis, he announced that he would no longer be sexually intimate with his wife because he didn't want to "catch it." In a healthier relationship, providing the couple with information about how leukemia develops (and that it is not spread through sexual activity) would likely resolve this problem, but there were other factors at play in this marriage, and Mr. T continued to assert that he was protecting his own health by avoiding sexual activity with his wife. As education failed to resolve this issue, the psychologist worked with Ms. T to help her develop a plan to manage the relationship issues while she was in the hospital. Because many aspects of the marital relationship warranted intervention, referrals were made at discharge for outpatient treatment.

PERSONAL RESOURCES

A patient's own personal resources also affect her ability to successfully adjust to new medical issues. Patients who are intact cognitively have an advantage because they are more likely to understand the issues associated with the illness and its treatment, make realistic plans to manage the medical problem, and be able to follow through with those plans. Education and health literacy are factors that also improve a patient's ability to manage and adjust because they are associated with better understanding of the medical matters. Similarly, patients without physical limitations are able to do more instrumentally to help themselves and adhere to appointments and treatments.

Dispositional optimism is a trait that "reflects the extent to which people hold generalized favorable expectancies for their future" (Carver, Scheier, & Segerstrom, 2010, p. 879). Optimism has been studied in the context of a variety of medical problems, such as coronary artery disease and bypass surgery, cancer treatment, in vitro fertilization, ischemic heart disease, and adjustment to AIDS, and has been associated with decreased distress, improved mood, less depression, increased life satisfaction, and good adjustment to medical problems (Carver et al., 2010; Helgeson, Snyder, & Seltman, 2004; Rasmussen, Wrosch, Scheier, & Carver, 2006). Optimism seems to affect these positive adjustment outcomes through its association with coping. That is, optimism is positively correlated with approach and problem-focused coping strategies and negatively associated with avoidance and emotion-focused coping strategies (Nes & Segerstrom, 2006). Optimism has also been associated with flexible coping strategy use in different contexts (Nes & Segerstrom, 2006) and is especially beneficial when the medical disease is controllable (Fournier, de Ridder, & Bensing, 2002).

Patients with a history of successful coping with other life stressors have already developed some skills to help them navigate and cope with the new medical stressors. They often report a sense of control and efficacy at dealing with the current problem, reporting confidence and motivation to successfully master the new medical issue. Mr. W was a 62-year-old Caucasian man who had a history of drug and alcohol abuse from ages 18 to 36. He successfully quit using substances and had remained abstinent for more than 25 years. When he was diagnosed with a serious and difficult-to-treat cancer, he remained confident and immediately developed a plan to manage any and all aspects of the treatment that he could handle himself (e.g., diet, exercise, scheduling chemotherapy appointments, social activities to lift his spirits). He reported that beating the substances had thoroughly prepared him for beating the cancer, and he had no doubts that he would do so.

Posttraumatic growth refers to "positive change that the individual experiences as a result of the struggle with a major loss or trauma" (Calhoun & Tedeschi, 2001, p. 158). A similar construct, *benefit-finding,* refers to the "discovery of benefits from living with adversity" (Affleck & Tennen, 1996, p. 899). Many difficult medical diagnoses, such as cancer, HIV, and rheumatoid arthritis can result in posttraumatic growth (see Tedeschi & Calhoun, 2004, for a summary); benefit-finding has been reported in breast cancer, spinal cord injuries, diabetes, and stroke (see Affleck & Tennen, 1996, for a summary). The benefits or growth that patients report can involve major aspects of their lives, such as improved family relationships; positive changes in personality, such as personal strength or patience; changes in life priorities and goals; and also increased spirituality (Affleck & Tennen, 1996; Tedeschi & Calhoun, 2004). One patient described himself as a workaholic who had spent little time with his kids, but after being diagnosed with lung cancer, he was unable to work and spent more time with his family. When back to work later, he still made time with them a priority and credited this to his diagnosis of lung cancer. Individuals who feel they have experienced positive changes as a result of their medical diagnosis use this to enable further coping. Personal experiences involving benefit from the medical situation are most likely to affect ongoing coping as a disease progresses, rather than at the time of the initial diagnosis (because individuals have yet to experience any benefit or growth).

EXTERNAL RESOURCES

External resources also play a role in a patient's adaptation to a new medical situation. The patient's social network can provide support to help with the emotional issues, as well as instrumental support in dealing with practical matters (especially in the case of a patient with cognitive or physical limitations). Patients with good support have people in their lives who are willing to help them manage the inpatient hospital stay and also any relevant adjustment tasks. However, family and friends frequently do not know specifically what to do to help the patient. Many patients need to be encouraged to explicitly tell family members what would be helpful to them, such as more frequent visits, playing cards, caring for the patient's cat, or ending a visit if the patient is tired. Many friends and family members will do all that they can to help and support the patient if they are made aware of the patient's needs. In cases in which social support is poor, the patient can give family members the opportunity to be useful by making a request of them and can then seek other ways to get what she needs if they are not responsive.

Socioeconomic status also plays a role in a patient's adjustment to a medical illness. Specifically, patients with greater resources (such as finances and access to health care services) can use those to provide additional instrumental help as they work to adjust to the medical stressor. Patients with financial and other economic problems face additional challenges that can complicate and delay the patient's adjustment to the illness. Social workers are often a valuable resource to help patients address these problems.

Summary and Case Example

Overall, the health psychology consultant should approach the patient's adjustment with an encouraging attitude that normalizes the patient's emotional reactions and concerns. Education should focus on objective facts and a realistic perspective regarding what the patient is dealing with. Practical interventions can be used to help the patient to make behavioral changes to address any lifestyle factors that can affect the medical illness. Patients can be helped to develop a positive and realistic attitude toward the illness and its implications, as well as reasonable expectations for themselves. It is useful to keep patients focused on the current situation, while avoiding too much of a focus on additional problems that could happen later. Exhibit 6.9 describes a case that demonstrates some of these factors.

EXHIBIT 6.9

Adjustment to Crohn's Disease

Ms. C is a 23 y/o woman who is working on her master's degree in sociology. She was diagnosed with Crohn's disease a year ago and spent a week in the hospital at that time, with diarrhea, abdominal pain, and dehydration. As she had no significant past medical history, she had difficulty accepting the diagnosis of a chronic illness and was overwhelmed by the new medical symptoms. After discharge, the patient did not follow dietary recommendations and had several significant episodes of diarrhea and abdominal pain. These had also occurred at social events, and she was embarrassed by episodes of bowel incontinence and diarrhea. After that initial period of denial and nonadherence, she began to work with a dietician to develop a diet that would help her to avoid diarrhea and discomfort. With the new dietary plan, she experienced a few episodes of diarrhea, but all were brief and mild.

The patient was again admitted to the hospital 4 days ago with significant diarrhea, fatigue, and abdominal pain. Her doctors prescribed a new drug to suppress her immune system that was expected to decrease her symptoms over the long term. At present the patient is weak and experiences frequent diarrhea. She is frustrated because she felt she had gained some control over her symptoms as a result of dietary changes, but this does not seem to be having a positive impact on her symptoms currently. Patient is now talking about dropping out of graduate school, stopping her volunteer work, and decreasing her social activities because she wants to avoid either cancelling them due to diarrhea or embarrassing herself with episodes of incontinence if she does attend classes and activities. Ms. C has been talking to another Crohn's patient who has recommended that she not eat or drink for 24 hours before going out. Even though the patient's doctors are against this strategy, Ms. C would like to try it. She isn't sure how to implement it, though, because she is used to being out of the house daily for various activities (so it would mean not eating or drinking at all). Her mood is low, and she feels she will not be able to date, marry, or have a family as the Crohn's symptoms will interfere with any potential relationships.

Intervention with Ms. C began with a discussion of her knowledge of Crohn's disease. She could report that it was a chronic illness characterized by abdominal pain and diarrhea. She understood there could be periods in which she would be symptom free, followed by periods of significant symptoms with no apparent cause. She understood that stress and spicy foods could exacerbate Crohn's symptoms. She feared needing a surgery to treat the Crohn's someday, although her doctors had never described this as a treatment option for her.

Ms. C understood that her current symptoms could continue for a while but that her doctors were optimistic about the new medication decreasing them (although they stressed there were no guarantees). The patient was aware there could be some side effects of the medication, such as kidney or liver damage, as well as serious infections; she was minimally concerned about but accepting of those risks if it meant her gut symptoms would decrease.

EXHIBIT 6.9 (*Continued*)

Adjustment to Crohn's Disease

In terms of managing the symptoms, Ms. C had demonstrated healthy and active coping before this hospital admission, but now she was discouraged that her dietary efforts hadn't enabled her to avoid her current symptoms. Despite that, she did have some optimism that the new medication combined with her efforts to eat right and avoid stress would help her to decrease or avoid symptoms in the future.

The patient felt she would not be able to return to graduate school, her volunteer job at a zoo, or to date and engage in social activities with her friends. She did understand, however, that limiting her activities so dramatically could negatively affect her mood and quality of life. She was "stuck" in terms of how to continue her normal activities in the context of Crohn's disease. The psychologist discussed with her the idea of planning and organizing her activities to avoid embarrassing or difficult situations. Therefore, although she would lose some spontaneity, she might still be able to engage in many of her typical activities if she planned properly. Ms. C warmed to this idea and within a few days had developed plans to continue with her school and social activities. She planned to eat small portions and foods that her body tolerated well, and she became aware of bathroom locations in the buildings in which she had classes. She realized she had fewer symptoms early in the day, so planned to schedule morning classes as much as possible. She also planned to take a few online classes from home, while realizing that she would miss some important social interaction if she did online courses exclusively. Ms. C also enlisted the support of her two best friends to plan social activities that did not involve eating out and that occurred at locations that had accessible bathrooms in case she needed one.

As the medication began to take effect, her symptoms began to subside, and Ms. C again began to believe that she might be able to manage them and to have the life she had hoped for. She was aware there would be ups and downs in the adjustment process but demonstrated a healthy attitude toward coping. She was discharged from the hospital and made plans for outpatient treatment to continue to work on the management of her symptoms and her emotional reactions to the disease.

Anxiety 7

Anxiety occurs frequently in the inpatient medical setting. It may be demonstrated in a variety of ways and occur due to a variety of causes. Some patients may experience a lone symptom, such as an inability to relax; others may experience a constellation of anxiety symptoms, such as shortness of breath (SOB), heart palpitations, chest pain, decreased concentration, worry, and muscle tension. The symptoms may be intermittent or continuous, and they may range from very mild to extremely intense episodes. Some may result in *Diagnostic and Statistical Manual of Mental Disorders* (fifth ed.; American Psychiatric Association, 2013) diagnoses; other presentations may not meet criteria for a formal psychiatric diagnosis, but they are no less important and also warrant appropriate intervention.

Sources of Anxiety

In the medical inpatient setting, anxiety symptoms can occur due to a preexisting anxiety disorder that occurs independently or is comorbid with a chronic medical condition. Some medical problems present with anxiety symptoms that can be confounded with psychological causes of anxiety, creating difficulty distinguishing a medical from a psychiatric diagnosis. Anxiety

http://dx.doi.org/10.1037/0000108-008
Health Psychology Consultation in the Inpatient Medical Setting, by S Labott

can also be a side effect of medications or other medical treatments intended to treat the medical problem. Finally, new-onset anxiety for purely psychological reasons can occur if a patient is diagnosed with a new medical disease or is facing frightening medical procedures or treatment.

Although each of these scenarios involves anxiety symptoms, the etiologies differ, and the anxiety-management interventions need to be tailored to the specific etiology to achieve the best outcome. For example, SOB associated with a medication will be less effectively treated with cognitive therapy than will anxiety that is associated with fears and worries about a new medical diagnosis. Each of these etiologies of anxiety and relevant treatments are described in more detail in the following sections.

PREMORBID ANXIETY

Patients with preexisting anxiety disorders may develop medical issues that are completely independent of the anxiety, or they may present with chronic medical conditions that are frequently associated with anxiety disorders. In either case, the anxiety and the medical issue can exacerbate each other, warranting appropriate treatment for both. Consider three patients: One has a preexisting generalized anxiety disorder (GAD) and is admitted to the hospital for workup of unexplained gastrointestinal symptoms; the second patient has no history of GAD but the same gastrointestinal complaints; and the third patient has a history of GAD and previously diagnosed irritable bowel syndrome (IBS) and is admitted with symptom exacerbation. Each of these patients represents a different mix of psychological and physiological symptoms that will need to be considered when treating the patient's anxiety in the hospital.

Patients with a preexisting anxiety disorder may have more difficulty coping with the medical issues and the hospital admission. When caring for patients with premorbid anxiety or any preexisting psychiatric issues, it is important to obtain a thorough psychiatric history because this will dictate the appropriate treatment during the inpatient admission. This history will also inform referrals for ongoing treatment after discharge.

Information about the patient's outpatient treatment for anxiety (both medications and therapy) is extremely relevant. Anxiolytics prescribed for outpatient use will need to be continued while the patient is in the hospital unless they are contraindicated due to the current medical problem. Patients may have information on their psychotropic medications and dosages, and the primary medical team will often order these. If patients cannot provide sufficient detail or documentation regarding their psychotropic medications, then the outpatient prescriber will generally need to be contacted for that information, especially if the prescriber is a psychiatrist. (This task is often performed by a psychiatrist who is consulted to address the patient's psychiatric medications while in the hospital.) If the psychiatric mediations are prescribed by a nonpsychiatrist (e.g., a primary care provider or oncologist), an inpatient psychiatrist may complete a new evaluation to assess the patient's current need for psychotropic medications. A new inpatient medication evaluation may also be performed if the patient has a history of a serious mental illness but has not been in any treatment or on any psychotropic medications recently, especially if psychiatric symptoms are currently present.

It is also important to know if a patient is currently engaged in outpatient psychotherapy. For a patient who is engaged in therapy, the health psychology consultant will intervene to deal with the specific issues relevant for this medical admission but will need to avoid interfering with the ongoing outpatient treatment. If patients have a history of anxiety and have been in therapy to address it, they may have a variety of skills (e.g., relaxation techniques, cognitive strategies) that can help them to manage the anxiety associated with this hospital admission. Existing skills can also form the basis for additional strategies to target the specific anxieties the patient is experiencing this hospital admission.

Some patients may need ongoing outpatient psychological or psychiatric treatment but may not have a current provider. If they have a past therapist or psychiatrist to whom they can return, this may be the best option. If not, the health psychology consultant can facilitate a new referral to an appropriate therapist or psychiatrist when the patient is discharged. Depending on the setting, availability of providers, and insurance requirements, finding an outpatient provider may be difficult, so the psychologist will need to discuss the outpatient referral with the patient early in the admission and then begin working so that proper referrals are ready for the patient at the time of discharge. Sample 7.1 shows an example of an initial consultation with a patient with a history of anxiety, as well as a summary of the follow-up treatment while the patient was in the hospital.

NEW-ONSET ANXIETY WITH PSYCHOLOGICAL ETIOLOGY

Anxiety is common in the hospital setting, even in patients with no premorbid history of anxiety. Much research has documented increases in anxiety when patients are newly diagnosed with a serious disorder (e.g., Giordano et al., 2011; Tavoli et al., 2007). The stage of the disease can also be associated with increased anxiety: The more severe the disease, the more intense the anxiety (Vodermaier, Linden, MacKenzie, Greig, & Marshall, 2011). However, the presence and degree of anxiety is quite variable across patients, underscoring the need for screening or evaluation of individuals to determine their particular reaction to a new diagnosis and resultant psychological needs. For many, the intensity of anxiety decreases over time after the initial medical diagnosis, with upsurges in anxiety symptoms that are triggered by new medical symptoms, medical appointments, or hospital admissions. It is common for patients, even those doing well physically and emotionally, to experience increased anxiety before an outpatient appointment with the doctor. If all then goes well, the anxiety may subside quickly but may occur again before the next outpatient visit.

Similarly, patients may have received bad news about a chronic medical problem, such as chronic kidney disease that now requires dialysis and possible kidney transplant. Although these patients may have previously adjusted to the fact that they have a chronic disease, the new problems associated with that disease can result in an increase in anxiety. This change in their medical status may require additional adjustment as they learn to accept and cope with their situation.

Patients with medical symptoms that are as yet undiagnosed may also experience significant anxiety. Most people have little understanding of medical issues, but they often know enough to realize that the symptoms they are experiencing could be associated with a life-threatening disease. Of course, the symptoms could also be associated with a benign disorder, but that is typically not foremost in the patient's mind. Being admitted to the hospital to confirm a diagnosis is more anxiety-provoking than outpatient testing (although that can also result in significant anxiety).

During the diagnostic process, patients may have experienced various tests and procedures, and the results of the testing may then require additional testing to confirm a diagnosis. All this can result in a significant amount of time for individuals to wait for results. The wait can be associated with intense anxiety and worry because patients may feel the results of the tests will significantly change their lives, and yet there is nothing to be done at present besides wait.

Patients in the hospital may also experience anxiety about undergoing specific tests or procedures. Many patients have needle phobias, making blood draws, biopsies, and infusions of any kind stressful. They may be claustrophobic about magnetic resonance imaging (MRI) and other scans. They may experience anxiety about the physical risks associated with specific medical tests and procedures because many common procedures (e.g., placement of intravenous lines and catheters) can result in infections. Patients may also be facing more serious procedures, such as cardiac catheterization or surgeries that carry additional risks of blood clots, stroke, or death. Although some degree of anxiety is to be expected in these situations, anxiety management is still appropriate to help patients be as comfortable as possible.

Even after patients have been through the medical testing, have a confirmed diagnosis, and then have a treatment plan, the anxiety may not subside. The treatment for many medical problems includes some level of uncertainty regarding how well the treatment will work, as well as concerns regarding what happens next if the current treatment is not successful. Patients may experience fears of pain and a decrease in quality of life. They may experience anxiety about physical limitations or unknown life changes they will need to make in the future (e.g., quitting work, using a walker). They may be fearful of unknown treatments in the future, and they may also fear death.

The hospital milieu itself may be a source of anxiety; patients may not know what to expect during the hospital admission and may feel out of control of the situation. Patients are typically unable to maintain their normal routine when in the hospital, there is little privacy, and it may be difficult to maintain one's dignity. Personal relationships may be stressed and changed as a result of the hospital admission. Family members may be forced to take on new roles, especially if the patient becomes dependent on others for personal needs, such as feeding and toileting.

It is not uncommon for people to try to avoid either a hospital admission or outpatient treatment due to anxiety, even if they know they have a serious medical problem and need treatment; this can result in the medical issue being significantly worse, and more difficult to treat, when the patient does finally seek treatment for it. Mrs. S was a patient who had a noticeable mass on her neck, and her physicians recommended surgery to remove it and test it for malignancy. She was anxious about the possibility of a cancer diagnosis and avoided scheduling surgery for 2 years. When she finally was willing to engage in treatment, the mass was so large that she was unable to move her head, and the tumor had metastasized to her brain, liver, and lungs. Despite both surgery and chemotherapy, she died 6 months later. Had she undergone treatment when the mass was smaller, perhaps the outcome would have been different.

The case described in Sample 7.2 provides an example of an initial consultation with a patient with a new diagnosis of acute leukemia, as well as a summary of the psychological inpatient treatment during this admission. This patient would never have been seen by psychology if she had not developed a catastrophic medical problem (acute leukemia) and been admitted emergently to the hospital. Because she had not experienced problems with anxiety before, she had few skills to help her manage her symptoms, but she was bright and motivated to do what she could to cope with her symptoms and feel better. As might be done in any outpatient anxiety treatment, the patient was taught behavioral and cognitive skills to help her manage the anxiety symptoms. The difference is that, for this inpatient treatment, the training in the use of these techniques was much abbreviated. The plan was to spend a minimal amount of time providing the patient with basic training in the use of several anxiety management techniques that she could begin to practice and use immediately. During follow-up visits, the psychologist monitored what worked for her and helped her to improve her skills at using any of the strategies that were working. Additional interventions were added as needed.

MEDICAL DISORDERS PRESENTING WITH ANXIETY SYMPTOMS

Some medical disorders present with symptoms that are largely indistinguishable from anxiety symptoms, even though anxiety per se may not be present. Exhibit 7.1 lists some medical causes of anxiety. For example, patients with hyperthyroid (overactive thyroid) problems, especially before formal diagnosis and treatment, may present with anxiety symptoms such as nervousness, moodiness, jitters, increased heart rate, shortness of breath, increased sweating, and weight loss. If the patient initially presented to a psychologist for diagnosis and treatment of these symptoms, treatment for anxiety or depression might be started, but that treatment would not be very effective because the physiological cause of the symptoms was not addressed. If the patient initially presented to a physician with these symptoms, a simple blood test could confirm the hyperthyroid diagnosis, and medication could treat the problem successfully, often without the need for additional psychological intervention.

In the context of chronic obstructive pulmonary disease (COPD; i.e., emphysema or chronic bronchitis), patients commonly experience dyspnea (SOB). It may occur with exertion but is often not life-threatening if managed properly; nonetheless, this can be frightening for patients. If a patient with COPD (unknown to the psychological provider) was seen in an outpatient psychology clinic and reported SOB, this could be interpreted as a symptom of anxiety. The psychologist might begin traditional anxiety treatment, but it would likely have only minimal impact because the SOB is due to poor lung function and not anxiety per se.

EXHIBIT 7.1

Possible Medical Etiologies of Anxiety

Neurological
Delirium
Dementia
Huntington's disease
Migraines
Multiple sclerosis
Other degenerative neurological disease (e.g., Creutzfeldt–Jakob disease)
Seizure disorders
Sleep disorders
Transient ischemic attacks

Endocrine
Addison's disease (hypocortisolism)
Cushing's syndrome (hypercortisolism)
Hyperparathyroidism
Hyperthyroidism
Hypoglycemia
Hypothyroidism
Pheochromocytoma

Cardiopulmonary
Angina
Asthma
Cardiac arrhythmias
Chronic obstructive pulmonary disease
Mitral valve prolapse
Pulmonary embolus

Toxins/poisons
Lead
Manganese
Mercury
Organophosphates

Infections
Meningitis
Neurosyphilis

Medications and drugs
Alcohol intoxication/withdrawal
Antidepressants
Antihypertensives
Benzodiazepine withdrawal
Corticosteroids
Cough and cold medication (may contain ephedrine or caffeine)
Insulin
Marijuana
Monosodium glutamate
Oral contraceptive pill
Stimulants (intoxication/withdrawal)
Sympathomimetics
Thyroid supplements
Weight loss products

Note. From *Comprehensive Textbook of Psychiatry* (9th ed., p. 1907), by B. Sadock, V. Sadock, and P. Ruiz (Eds.), 2009, Philadelphia, PA: Wolters Kluwer/Lippincott Williams & Wilkins.

Some patients with breathing problems due to medical disorders may also develop anxiety as a result of the physiological breathing problem, and this anxiety can exacerbate the underlying breathing problem. The patient may then develop an anxiety disorder that interacts with and complicates the initial breathing problem. For example, it is not uncommon for a patient to feel SOB due to poor lung functioning, then to get scared and have thoughts such as "oh, no, I can't breathe, I could die from this." These types of cognitions create anxiety, which exacerbates the SOB. Anxiety was not the original problem, but the fearful cognitions then elicited anxiety that exacerbated the original medical problem. Intervention in this case could involve both psychological and medical treatment. That is, cognitive strategies could be used to help the patient manage the anxiety-provoking cognitions and behavioral strategies developed to decrease physical exertion and SOB in the first place. At the same time, the patient's physician could treat the lung disease with medical interventions, such as oral medication, inhalers, nebulizer treatment, or a combination of these.

Cardiac problems can also present with anxiety-like symptoms, such as increased heart rate, palpitations, or chest pain. Similar to the COPD patient just discussed, if a patient with cardiac problems presents to an outpatient psychologist with complaints of increased heart rate and chest pain, and if the psychologist is unaware of the cardiac issue, the misdiagnosis of an anxiety disorder could occur, but psychological treatment will have little impact on the underlying cardiac problem. Further, psychological symptoms can at times exacerbate cardiac problems (e.g., when a panic attack triggers angina).

A cardiac patient may also develop anxiety about symptoms associated with the cardiac problem, such as increased heart and respiration rate, and the anxiety may then exacerbate the cardiac symptoms or impact the patient's treatment adherence. Consider a cardiac patient who is recuperating from a recent myocardial infarction (MI). Part of his regimen involves making healthy changes to his lifestyle, such as improving his diet and beginning an exercise regimen. The patient is agreeable with the treatment plan, but when he begins to exercise, his heart rate increases, and this feels similar to his experience of the heart attack he had recently, so he becomes anxious. He then begins to avoid exertion so that he does not experience these physiological symptoms, and he becomes nonadherent with this aspect of his treatment plan. The psychological treatment for this patient would include education on the physiological symptoms associated with exercise and also those associated with cardiac problems, as well as their similarities and differences. The patient should also be educated on his current cardiac status—that his doctor has run the appropriate tests and determined that it is safe for him to undertake this exercise regimen. The patient could then begin to exercise slowly and can be desensitized to the symptoms of exertion as he monitors his heart rate to be sure he is safe. Over time, he can learn to tolerate an increased heart rate without fearing that he is having another heart attack.

Anxiety symptoms also frequently play a role with patients who have an automatic implantable cardioverter defibrillator (AICD) implanted to prevent sudden cardiac death due to malignant arrhythmias. The AICD senses an arrhythmia and shocks the heart to cause it to return to a regular rhythm. These shocks may be painful, and some patients develop symptoms of anxiety and avoidance that are similar to those seen in panic patients (Pauli, Wiedemann, Dengler, Blaumann-Benninghoff, & Kühlkamp, 1999). Education, relaxation strategies, and cognitive restructuring can all be used to help manage the anxiety.

Hypoglycemia (low blood glucose) can occur for a variety of reasons and can also result in symptoms that can be confused with anxiety, such as sweating and jitters. As with other physiological problems of this type, treatment with psychological methods will not improve the medical symptoms, but medical treatment to increase blood glucose will successfully manage the problem.

CO-OCCURRING ANXIETY AND MEDICAL DISORDERS

Although anxiety and medical disorders can interact with and exacerbate each other, there are some medical problems that have a stronger association with anxiety than others; these tend to co-occur frequently. It is often impossible to determine whether the anxiety could have caused the medical disorder or the medical disorder caused the anxiety. Comorbid anxiety is most frequently found in gastrointestinal (IBS, peptic ulcer), respiratory (asthma, COPD), and endocrine (thyroid, diabetes), cardiovascular, and pain (arthritis, back pain) disorders. (For reviews of anxiety and these comorbid medical conditions, see Culpepper, 2009, and Muller, Koen, & Stein, 2005.) Although anxiety will frequently occur when individuals are newly diagnosed with a medical problem, ongoing anxiety has been associated with greater disability, increased health care utilization, and decreased quality of life in patients with a variety of chronic medical illnesses (Roy-Byrne et al., 2008).

Härter, Conway, and Merikangas (2003) studied individuals from the community and clinics to determine the association between anxiety disorders and medical illnesses. Anxiety disorders were significant predictors of cardiac, gastrointestinal, and genitourinary disorders, as well as migraines, when controlling for gender, substance use, and depression. Individuals with anxiety disorders were also 3 times more likely to report they were in poor health compared with those without anxiety disorders.

In a meta-analysis of studies of IBS patients, Fond et al. (2014) reported significantly higher anxiety and depression (measured by standardized rating scales) in IBS patients compared with control participants, although the results were less clear for IBS subtypes. Popa and Dumitrascu (2015) also reviewed the literature and reported that more than 50% of IBS patients reported anxiety or depression.

While physiological causes have been clearly documented in the development of ulcers, there remains evidence that anxiety also plays a role. Specifically, Goodwin and Stein (2002) have reported that the likelihood of the development of peptic ulcer disease was 5 times higher in individuals with GAD. Taha et al. (2014) have reported that panic attacks and generalized anxiety disorder were associated with an increased prevalence of recent ulcer and also increased risk of ulcer over the next 10 years. Others have also reported that anxiety disorders were associated with the diagnosis of peptic ulcer over a 10-year period (Goodwin et al., 2013).

Pain has also been associated with the presence of anxiety and depression. In a sample of more than 3,000 adults, McWilliams, Goodwin, and Cox (2004) studied arthritis, migraine, and back pain. In regression analyses that adjusted for demographic variables and other pain conditions, significant correlations were found between GAD and panic and all three of the pain conditions. Further, the association between the anxiety disorders and the three pain conditions were stronger than between the pain conditions and depression (although those were also positive and significant).

Researchers have also reported that 30% to 70% of adult asthma patients have problems with anxiety (Cordina, Fenech, Vassallo, & Cacciottolo, 2009; Fernandes et al., 2010; Urrutia et al., 2012), and patients with uncontrolled asthma report significantly higher levels of anxiety and depression than do patients with controlled asthma (Di Marco et al., 2010; Vieira, Santoro, Dracoulakis, Caetano, & Fernandes, 2011). Anxiety is associated with decreased quality of life in asthma patients (Urrutia et al., 2012), as well as with increased use of medications and health care utilization (Cordina et al., 2009; Di Marco et al., 2010; Fernandes et al., 2010). GAD and panic are also associated with COPD (Muller et al., 2005). Results such as these provide good motivation for the addition of a psychological anxiety management component to asthma management programs.

Thyroid dysfunction has been associated with anxiety, with the most severe symptoms in those with overt hyperthyroidism; successful treatment results in significant improvements in anxiety symptoms (Gulseren et al., 2006). Thyroid dysfunction has also been associated with an increased lifetime prevalence of GAD and panic disorder (Simon et al., 2002).

Culpepper (2009) provided an example of one way that anxiety can interact with medical illness, using cardiovascular disease as an example. Specifically, individuals with anxiety may be more sensitive to heart rate and may interpret minor changes as significant medical issues, increasing their anxiety and then further increasing their heart rate. The perception that a symptom is of concern creates more anxiety, which exacerbates the symptom. Ultimately, then, the perception that the increased heart rate is a problem can further increase heart rate and could lead to a more intense symptom that *is* medically significant. A similar type of interaction has been described between anxiety and IBS symptoms (Popa & Dumitrascu, 2015): IBS symptoms can increase anxiety and distress, which can then increase physical symptoms in a cyclic fashion.

Sample 7.3 describes a patient with COPD and associated breathing problems who developed anxiety after a traumatic experience. A summary of the psychological intervention follows the consult.

ANXIETY SYMPTOMS SECONDARY TO MEDICATIONS

Many medications used to treat medical or psychiatric problems can result in anxiety symptoms as side effects. Exhibit 7.2 provides a list of medications that can elicit anxiety (from Colón & Popkin, 2002); some are also noted in the bottom section of Exhibit 7.1. These are not comprehensive lists, but they demonstrate that medications are an important consideration when treating psychological issues in medical inpatients. Psychologists in the inpatient setting may most often see anxiety that is associated with bronchodilators or steroids (described in more detail subsequently).

EXHIBIT 7.2
Medications Associated With Anxiety

Anesthetics/analgesics
Antidepressants (tricyclics, selective serotonin reuptake inhibitors, bupropion)
Antihistamines
Antihypertensives
Antimicrobials
Bronchodilators
Caffeine preparations
Calcium-blocking agents
Cholinergic-blocking agents
Digitalis
Estrogen
Ethosuximide
Heavy metals and toxins
Hydralazine
Insulin
Levodopa
Muscle relaxants
Neuroleptics
Nonsteroidal anti-inflammatories
Procaine
Procarbazine
Sedatives
Steroids
Sympathomimetics
Theophylline
Thyroid preparations

Note. From *The American Psychiatric Publishing Textbook of Consultation-Liaison Psychiatry: Psychiatry in the Medically Ill* (2nd ed., p. 400), by M. Wise and J. Rundell (Eds.), 2002, Washington, DC: American Psychiatric Association. Copyright 2002 by the American Psychiatric Association. Reprinted with permission.

Bronchodilators are drugs used to treat COPD, asthma, bronchitis, and other pulmonary disorders. They relax the airway to facilitate breathing. These medications are frequently delivered through inhalers but can also be taken in other ways. They can be used for either short- or longer term treatment and include anticholinergics, beta-agonists, and theophylline. Although quite effective for improving the ease of breathing, they can be associated with side effects that include anxiety symptoms, such as rapid (or irregular) heart rate, restlessness, jitteriness, and tremors, as well as poor sleep and irritability.

Corticosteroids, such as prednisone, prednisolone, cortisone, methylprednisolone, and dexamethasone, are used to decrease inflammation and activity of the immune system. These medications are important in the treatment of many medical issues, such as breathing problems, allergies, arthritis, skin disorders, cancer, lupus, and colitis. However, many patients will experience side effects from corticosteroid use. Physical side effects include osteoporosis, diabetes, cataracts, weakness, bruising, blurred vision, acne, water retention, and facial puffiness (Cushingoid appearance). Psychological and neurological side effects include increased appetite and weight gain, insomnia, restlessness and anxiety, mood swings, jitteriness, psychotic symptoms, mania, depression, and delirium. These symptoms are associated with high doses of steroids (generally greater than 40 mg prednisone per day; West & Kenedi, 2014), and the symptoms often begin within a few days of starting the high-dose steroids. The physical and psychological side effects may present with mild to severe symptoms (e.g., osteoporosis noted only on x-ray vs. ribs that crack when the patient sneezes). Milder versions of side effects may be manageable for patients, but more intense side effects can be debilitating.

Nervousness and jitters are common, and although these symptoms reflect no serious medical issues, they can disrupt the patient's quality of life. One lung transplant patient was on high-dose steroids to treat an episode of acute organ rejection. Her hands shook so badly that she was unable to drink from a coffee cup without spilling. She also experienced the same jittery feeling in her stomach, which was very unpleasant for her.

Most striking of the psychological side effects of steroids is a steroid psychosis. Steroid psychosis is rare; the usual presentation includes restlessness, agitation, emotional lability, insomnia, hallucinations, and delusions (see Chapter 9, this volume, for more detail on this).

Anxiety, psychosis, and other psychological symptoms that result from steroid and other medication use are only minimally responsive to typical psychological interventions. These are reactions that are physiologically driven, and so relaxation and other traditional strategies are less useful than for anxiety symptoms of a psychological etiology (e.g., fears about undergoing a medical test). The main treatment for psychological side effects due to steroids involves tapering and then discontinuing the steroids. The symptoms should clear after the drug is discontinued. However, if the steroids are necessary to treat the medical problem and discontinuing them is not feasible, antipsychotics and mood stabilizers may help to manage the psychotic symptoms (Kenna, Poon, de los Angeles, & Koran, 2011). The less serious symptoms (e.g., moodiness, jitters) are best managed with education (as described in the next section).

Anxiety Management in the Inpatient Setting

The etiology of a patient's anxiety symptoms is critically important in determining the appropriate treatment. The most common interventions to address anxiety symptoms in the inpatient setting involve education, anxiolytic medications, relaxation and breathing strategies, and cognitive interventions, all of which are described in this section.

Generally, for anxiety symptoms due to physiological causes or medications, treatment is likely to involve additional medical interventions. These interventions may involve changes to the current medication regimen with the hope of decreasing anxiety symptoms, or the addition of medications designed to treat the anxiety symptoms specifically. For anxiety due to psychological etiologies (e.g., fears of illness, hospitalization, medical procedures, or death), psychological treatments are the primary intervention. As many anxiety symptoms are multidetermined and involve both physiological and psychological etiologies, combination treatments are useful. Exhibit 7.3 lists issues to consider when differentiating between premorbid anxiety disorder, anxiety that is comorbid with a medical disorder, anxiety due to medications, a medical disorder presenting as anxiety, or new-onset anxiety due to medical stressors.

EDUCATION

For patients with anxiety symptoms of any etiology, education is one of the most powerful interventions. Most medical patients have experienced anxiety previously in their lives (e.g., when at a job interview or giving a speech), but most have not experienced prolonged anxiety symptoms, and, as a result, they have little understanding of the symptoms, their triggers, or strategies that can be used to manage them. Even patients with preexisting anxiety disorders often have little understanding of them. Therefore, it is useful to provide patients with (a) a description of anxiety symptoms, to include overlap with the symptoms of some medical disorders; (b) examples of ways in which anxiety can exacerbate a medical problem; and (c) education about anxiety as a frequent occurrence in the hospital, as a result of either psychological or medical issues. Especially for those patients without a psychiatric history, normalizing the occurrence of these symptoms in the hospital can help to alleviate a patient's concern that she is "going crazy." Providing information about various treatments for anxiety is useful, as is a discussion that is tailored to the role of anxiety in the patient's specific medical situation. A patient with anxiety about medical procedures and a new diagnosis can achieve a fair amount of control over the symptoms using psychological techniques and can learn to successfully manage them when they occur. However, a patient with anxiety as a side effect of a specific medication that can't be discontinued

EXHIBIT 7.3

Differentiating Anxiety Symptoms Due to Drug Effects, a Primary Medical Disorder, a Primary Anxiety Disorder, or Comorbid Anxiety and Medical Diagnoses

Is there a history of anxiety, a medical disorder, or both? Which occurred first? Does one seem to exacerbate the other?

What triggers the anxiety symptoms (worry, exertion)?

Has a new medication been started recently that could account for new anxiety symptoms?

Are there new stressors in the patient's life that seem to account for the new symptoms?

What treatments have helped to decrease the symptoms (medications intended to improve breathing or cardiac functioning, relaxation or cognitive strategies)?

What interventions have not helped to relieve the symptoms (relaxation)?

What are the specific symptoms the patient experiences (e.g., worry is more likely psychological, but jitters could be either psychological or physiological)?

will have less success at controlling and managing the anxiety symptoms through her own efforts, although education may decrease her concern about the symptoms and enable her to tolerate them more successfully. In this manner, each patient gains some basic education about the symptoms of anxiety, as well as specific information about the cause of and treatment for anxiety given her specific medical situation.

PSYCHOTROPIC MEDICATION

As with any outpatient anxiety disorder, medications may be helpful to manage the anxiety symptoms experienced by medical patients. Many nonpsychiatrist physicians are comfortable prescribing low doses of anxiolytics to their inpatients who are experiencing anxiety symptoms, and they may have expertise in the use of certain anxiolytic medications in the context of a specific medical issue. For example, it is common for patients who are on ventilators and not sedated to experience some symptoms of anxiety because it is a frightening experience to be dependent on a machine for breathing, and the patient may have difficulty working with the machine to achieve regular and comfortable breathing. Further, when a patient is to be weaned from the vent, there is often anxiety about one's ability to breathe and fears of suffocation if unable to breathe independently of the ventilator. In these cases, it might seem obvious that an anxiolytic could help a patient to manage the anxiety associated with these situations. However, anxiolytics can suppress the respiratory drive in a patient with breathing problems, and that could decrease his ability to breathe independently, making it more difficult to wean the patient from the ventilator. Pulmonologists are aware of these issues in patients with breathing problems and can determine whether and when an anxiolytic is appropriate. Similarly, most cancer patients respond to psychotropic medications at lower doses than do their healthy counterparts, a fact known to oncologists.

For those patients for whom a psychotropic medication might prove useful, a consult with psychiatry will often be the best option. (At times, there may be some pressure for the health psychology consultant to take an active role with medication management; Chapter 15 discusses ways to stay within the psychologist's area of expertise.) Most consultation psychiatrists will complete an evaluation and provide medication recommendations. They frequently provide minimal follow-up, so the primary physician and the psychologist may need to monitor the patient for any new symptoms or side effects that would warrant another visit from psychiatry as the hospital admission proceeds.

Colón and Popkin (2002) provided a good description of the management of anxiety in the hospital setting. Before starting medication, any medical causes of the anxiety should be addressed. Benzodiazepines are one of the most common medications used to treat anxiety in the medical setting, and antidepressants and nonbenzodiazepine anxiolytics are other good options. These authors also note the importance of considering the onset of action, duration of action, side effect potential, interactions with other drugs, and abuse potential when selecting a medication to treat anxiety in medical inpatients.

COGNITIVE AND BEHAVIORAL TECHNIQUES

Many cognitive and behavioral strategies used in the outpatient setting can be adapted for use in the inpatient medical setting. Some, such as diaphragmatic breathing, imagery, desensitization, and distraction, are beneficial in helping medical patients to manage anxiety. Others, such as progressive muscle relaxation and anxiety symptom induction, are less useful because they may tax the patient physiologically. These and other techniques are discussed next.

Relaxation, Breathing, and Imagery

In the inpatient hospital setting, relaxation strategies are one of the most useful tools that patients can use to cope with anxiety. The hospital milieu is not conducive to relaxation, but it is generally easy to find something that a patient can use to relax. This may include anything from simple activities to more formal relaxation strategies. At times, anxiety-management training can be done with a patient and significant other together. If both are experiencing anxiety, they can support each other as they learn to cope with the anxiety.

Patients can learn a variety of strategies to promote relaxation, including progressive muscle relaxation (PMR), diaphragmatic breathing (DB; also called abdominal breathing), and imagery of various types. Exhibit 7.4 provides an overview of steps to follow when teaching relaxation strategies to medical inpatients. PMR is popular in the outpatient setting and involves the tensing and relaxing of muscles and muscle groups to achieve relaxation. Bourne (2015) provided step-by-step instructions for the tensing and relaxing of muscles that can be used by either the therapist or client to achieve relaxation through this method. As in any setting, the psychologist would teach the patient the procedures and encourage practice to improve relaxation skills over time. It is often useful to provide an audio recording to facilitate practice. Some patients are comfortable with mobile devices and prefer apps to help them with relaxation and other coping strategies. As with any materials provided to patients, the

EXHIBIT 7.4

Teaching Relaxation Strategies

- Explain the rationale for the strategy, especially how it will help the patient to relax, as well as the benefits of relaxation in terms of decreased anxiety and physical healing.
- Demonstrate or explain the task.
- Instruct the patient as she attempts the task herself, coaching on how to improve.
- Assess the level of successful relaxation and how the patient felt about the task.
- Adjust the intervention as needed to fit the specific patient and situation.
- Collaborate with the patient to determine when and how much to practice, expectations, and plans to adjust the plan as needed.
- Next visit: Review all and reinforce practice and progress, troubleshoot problems, review techniques and make adjustments as needed, and introduce additional relaxation techniques if warranted.

psychologist will need to research specific apps thoroughly before recommending them. If Internet connectivity in the hospital is poor, apps should be avoided.

The inpatient psychologist is unlikely to use PMR as the first line of treatment because the tensing of muscles may exacerbate many medical conditions. For example, a patient with pain of any type would be ill-advised to tense muscles associated with the painful area. Similarly, postsurgery patients will need to avoid stressing the area around an incision, and patients who are deconditioned and weak may experience muscle cramping and difficulty following the PMR procedures. A thorough review of the patient's medical record should explicate any issues of concern. In some cases, the PMR procedure can be adapted to avoid working with a specific area of the body, but often it is best to avoid PMR altogether and intervene with a less risky strategy.

DB is a useful relaxation strategy because it does not involve tensing muscles as PMR does. It can be used by most medical patients but should be avoided in patients with breathing problems (e.g., those with pulmonary disease, on a ventilator, or with SOB). DB is easy for most patients to learn and use, and although practice is still important to improve the onset and duration of relaxation, most patients can achieve some benefit quickly. This is also a technique that can be easily used in the course of normal daily activities once patients have developed the relevant skills. When teaching patients DB, it is useful to provide some information about the diaphragm and how it works and to demonstrate abdominal breathing by placing one hand on the chest above the diaphragm and one hand below it so that patients can see the effect of differential breathing from the bottom versus the top of the lungs. Patients can be taught to inhale and exhale slowly, holding both the inhale and exhale positions briefly (see Bourne, 2015, p. 91, for step-by-step procedures). Be aware that some patients will hold their breath or breathe deeply and quickly; those behaviors should be avoided because they will not facilitate relaxation.

Imagery (generally guided) is also a useful relaxation technique on its own, or it can be combined with other relaxation techniques, such as DB. The psychologist should first explain the rationale for using imagery (i.e., to promote relaxation, decrease anxiety, and improve overall comfort). The patient should then be asked to select a relaxing time and place. Some patients may have difficulty choosing a setting, and the psychologist can provide some examples of settings that are commonly associated with relaxation (e.g., a beach). Some patients may select a setting that does not appear relaxing, and the psychologist should then question her to be sure it meets the criteria for a relaxing situation. (One patient selected a civil rights march with Dr. Martin Luther King. Although this did not appear to be a physically relaxing event, for this woman, it was emotionally the most at peace she had ever been, and she was able to achieve good relaxation while using it as her image.) Once the setting is selected, the patient will need to describe specifics of the situation, including what it looks like, who was there, and what they felt emotionally and physically, so that the psychologist can (at least initially) guide them through the imagery process. Before beginning the imagery exercise, the patient should be comfortable in bed. The psychologist can then present the image, using a quiet and soothing voice, and directing the patient's attention to any sights, sounds, or feelings that will help them to get back into the situation as if it was happening now. Afterward, the success of the procedure should be assessed, and improvements to the induction discussed, with the hope that the patient can use these when he engages in the imagery task on his own.

The procedure just described is a basic imagery technique that can be used with almost any patient with any medical condition. There are some guided imagery procedures that have been developed for specific situations (e.g., for cancer patients). These techniques generally involve either (a) something attacking the cancer, such as blood cells that swim through the body and attack and destroy cancer cells, or (b) something that circulates through the body spreading strength and healing (H. Hall, 2003). These specific strategies are useful with some patients, but it should be made clear to the patient that this is a relaxation strategy and not a cancer treatment. Although these techniques may be useful in helping the patient to cope with treatment and to feel healthier and stronger, they should not be misunderstood as a treatment for cancer per se.

Systematic Desensitization

This is a useful strategy when the patient is anxious about a specific object or situation, such as a needle phobia or claustrophobia. Systematic desensitization (SD) involves developing a hierarchy of situations that gradually approximate the feared stimulus and then allowing the patient to pair images of those items with relaxation. Starting with the least anxiety-provoking item in the hierarchy, the patient then learns to manage the anxiety in graduated steps until she is able to relax with the most anxiety-provoking item.

In the inpatient medical setting, SD can be performed as it would be done in the outpatient setting but with one major exception: All procedures must be abbreviated because the feared test or procedure will likely need to occur quickly. For a blood draw, the patient may have only a few hours to prepare, and other procedures (e.g., MRI) may occur within a day or so. The psychologist may have only one visit to work with the patient. This time frame will typically influence the goals; rather than helping the patient to achieve complete relaxation and comfort with the situation, the goal is to help the patient to manage it with as much comfort as possible. (If there will be repeated procedures, more work can be done along the way.)

Table 7.1 contains an example of a hierarchy that could be used for a patient with a needle phobia. Although patients typically generate the items and distress ratings themselves with the help of the therapist, having a basic structure to begin with will facilitate the process in the inpatient setting. Auerbach and Gramling (1998) presented another example of a hierarchy used by a patient with anxiety about a MRI procedure.

Exposure Treatment

At times, it is possible to expose the patient to the feared stimulus before the actual test or procedure. As with a classic spider phobia treatment, perhaps a patient can be

TABLE 7.1
Sample Needle Phobia Hierarchy for Systematic Desensitization

Subjective units of distress	Stimulus
100	View own blood entering the test tube
95	Venipuncture technician sticks the needle into the vein
80	Technician feels arm, selecting best vein to draw from
70	Technician puts tourniquet on arm in preparation for blood draw
50	Technician unpacks supplies for blood draw
40	Technician enters the room
25	Waiting for venipuncture technician to arrive
20	Informed by doctor that blood draw is necessary

taken to a procedure room, to learn to relax while gradually approaching the feared stimulus. Often it is not feasible, however, to move a patient or to have an empty procedure room available to practice these skills.

Alternately, at times the psychologist can go to the procedure with the patient and can help him to use the previously learned relaxation strategies while the actual procedure is being performed. If a patient needs to spend time in a hyperbaric chamber or an MRI machine, it is sometimes possible for the psychologist to be outside, providing relaxation instructions through a speaker to the patient in the chamber. Although these interventions often are successful, there can be challenges associated with infection control or the psychologist simply being in the way.

A special use for in vivo exposure and relaxation occurs in the intensive care unit when a patient is anxious about being weaned from a ventilator. The weaning process involves the medical team adjusting the ventilator settings to provide less support for the patient's breathing. Patients have a weaning trial during which they are monitored to see how they are doing with decreased ventilator support. If they are doing well, the trial will continue with another change in settings to decrease respirator support, either right away or after the patient has had time to rest with the ventilator back to full support. Anxiety will interfere with the patient's ability to wean from the ventilator successfully, but the psychologist can visit the patient during the weaning trial (as it happens in the patient's hospital room) and can coach the patient in behavioral, cognitive, or distraction strategies as the weaning trial progresses. Previous work with the patient on relaxation is useful, but if that is not possible, many of the relaxation strategies can be simplified and used successfully while the weaning trial is underway.

Challenging Maladaptive Cognitions

One of the mainstays of cognitive treatment is the challenging of a patient's unrealistic or maladaptive cognitions. When facing a medical procedure, patients will often catastrophize or demonstrate other cognitive distortions. After providing a patient with education about the specific procedure, her cognitions can be evaluated and then adjusted to more adaptive versions. In the inpatient medical setting, the stimulus for the patient's anxiety is likely to be unpleasant or uncomfortable (maybe even painful), but (a) it can be managed, and (b) there is likely to be some benefit of undergoing the procedure. Patients can be provided with cognitions that will help them to master the situation, such as "I can get through this," "It is time-limited," "I have been through worse," "It will help my doctors to get the information they need to develop the proper treatment for me," or "This treatment will help to improve my condition." Coaching patients in challenging their own maladaptive cognitions and then replacing them with more adaptive ones is the goal of this intervention.

When utilizing strategies such as this, psychologists should be aware of catch phrases that were perhaps learned in the context of treating irrational anxiety in graduate school, but that may not be useful in the inpatient medical setting. One example of this involves asking an anxious patient, "What is the worst that could happen?" In the outpatient setting with a patient who is socially anxious, for example, the worst outcome could be shame or embarrassment; the psychologist can then work with the patient to realize these outcomes are not horrible or impossible to manage. In the hospital setting, the worst outcome for a patient is death and associated losses, like not being able to see his children grow up and have their own kids. Convincing anxious patients that this is an acceptable and manageable outcome is close to impossible, so asking for the worst possible outcome is not useful.

Thought-Stopping

This technique involves allowing the patient to envision the anxiety-provoking stimulus. Initially, the clinician interrupts the thoughts, but then the focus is shifted to the patient doing so. The patient learns to envision a stop sign and says "Stop" when the targeted thoughts occur. He then directs his attention to something else to avoid worry and rumination about the anxiety-provoking situation (for an example, see Rimm & Masters, 1974). This technique can be useful in the hospital, generally in combination with other techniques that involve addressing the feared stimulus more directly.

Induction of Anxiety Symptoms

One useful procedure in the outpatient setting involves allowing patients to experience the physiological symptoms of anxiety, and perhaps enhancing them, to allow patients to realize the symptoms will not harm them and to allow the anxiety to peak and then decrease over time. This is generally not a useful strategy in the hospital setting. Regardless of the patient's medical issue, it is usually not helpful to stress her physiology to engage in an exercise like this. Besides the potential medical contraindications, interventions in the hospital are often interrupted by members of the medical staff, and then patients would not achieve the potential benefits of this intervention.

Distraction

Finally, for some patients, simple distraction strategies work best, either alone or in combination with the formal anxiety-management techniques described in the preceding text. Specifically, patients can be encouraged to generate tasks they can engage in to help to distract themselves from their worries and to promote relaxation. While in the hospital, common tasks include listening to soothing music, watching TV, reading, playing games, and socializing with family and friends. Patients are often aware of behaviors that have helped them to relax in the past, although they do not think to actively use them to help manage their anxiety while in the hospital. Once patients have generated some strategies that are likely to aid them in this endeavor, they can be encouraged to actively use these at specific times to help them manage their anxiety during the current hospital admission and after discharge.

Family Members With Anxiety

Family members may also experience significant anxiety regarding the health of their loved one. The patient may bring this to the psychologist's attention, or it may be readily apparent when the psychologist visits the patient and observes the family. At times, a referral for the family member to an outpatient therapist is appropriate. At other times, the health psychology consultant may intervene with the family member along with the patient because the anxiety management strategies appropriate to both parties may be similar. A joint treatment can also enhance the bond between the two parties, and they can support each other in their efforts to cope effectively. Exhibit 7.5 describes the case of a mother and daughter who were treated jointly for anxiety but then separated to address other issues.

EXHIBIT 7.5

A Patient With Recurrent Cancer and Her Daughter

Patient is a 54 y/o woman, treated for breast cancer 7 years ago and in remission until 6 months ago. Over the past few months, the patient received several rounds of chemotherapy and radiation, but the cancer did not remit and eventually metastasized to her lungs and liver. The patient was being seen by the health psychology consultant for anxiety management and to help her deal with end of life issues. She was divorced and lived with her 22 y/o daughter, who was also experiencing significant anxiety. At the patient's suggestion, the psychologist included the daughter in some of the patient's treatment visits that involved education about the disease, relaxation strategies, and distraction techniques. Both parties seemed to benefit from this joint work; they were able to practice their relaxation skills together and support each other in their efforts for self-care.

As the patient became more ill, however, the daughter became angry and expressed anger toward her mother for dying and leaving her behind. The patient was deteriorating physically and cognitively, and her daughter's reaction was overwhelming to her. Their treatment was then separated. The primary psychologist continued to see the patient, focusing on her immediate needs and concerns as she was dying. A second psychologist took on the treatment of the daughter, supporting her as her mother died, and then working with her to address her grief on an outpatient basis afterward.

Conclusion

In summary, there are many causes of anxiety symptoms in the inpatient medical setting, as well as a variety of available treatments. The best outcomes will be obtained when the health psychology consultant does a thorough evaluation and then chooses the intervention(s) most suited to the specific patient and the source of the anxiety.

Sample 7.1
Initial Health Psychology Consultation: Patient With Unexplained Gastrointestinal Pain

Pt referred by Dr. J for health psych evaluation. She is a 25 y/o woman admitted for work up of unexplained gastrointestinal pain. Pt with hx anxiety.

Pt lives with her mother, who provides emotional support. She attended school to 10th grade, reports being able to read and write, although she often requires help. No special classes or LD (*learning disabilities*). Pt worked at McDonald's for about 2 yrs in her teens and has been on disability for psych reasons for the past 3 yrs.

Pt reports long hx anxiety, with panic attacks that occur at particularly stressful times. She has had several inpatient psych admissions for extreme anxiety; most recent was 2 yrs ago. No suicide attempts. She is seen at XX Mental Health, where she sees a psychiatrist every 3 mths. She sees a counselor weekly, and attends day hospital 4 days/wk. Pt also has a case manager to help her organize her meds, medical apts, and transportation. Pt reports getting 2 psych meds from her psychiatrist, although she cannot name them; pt's mother will bring bottles in this afternoon. On admission last year, pt was taking sertraline (50 mg q day) and alprazolam (0.25 mg TID).

Pt today reports intense anxiety, with increased heart rate, significant worry, and hypervigilance. She denies feeling depressed, also denies problems with sleep, guilt, worthlessness, hopelessness. No suicidal ideation. No panic attacks past 2 wks. Pt denies manic sx, paranoia, hallucinations.

Pt denies subjective memory problems. On mental status exam she was alert and oriented × 3 (not day of week). Registration, short- and long-term memory were all intact. Judgment OK. Attention mildly impaired.

Impressions: Pt with chronic and severe anxiety, in intensive outpatient tx at XX Mental Health. (caseworker Sandra can be reached at xxx-xxx-xxxx). Today pt reports severe anxiety. Discussed diaphragmatic breathing (which she has used in the past) to help her cope with anxiety. Pt will need to be restarted on outpatient psych meds, as appropriate. Her mother will bring Rx bottles to pt's nurse this afternoon. Please consult Psychiatry if there are questions regarding med management this admission. We will follow to aid anxiety management and coping this admission.

(Note that this patient has a significant history of anxiety, suggested by her disability status and ongoing intensive outpatient treatment.)

SUMMARY OF HEALTH PSYCHOLOGY TREATMENT

The patient's mother brought in her medications; she was currently taking sertraline 40 mg and alprazolam 0.25 mg TID. Psychiatry evaluated the patient and then restarted these medications. The patient remained inpatient for 1 week. During this time, the psychologist saw her daily for brief visits and focused on specific issues that were increasing the patient's anxiety in the inpatient setting. The patient continued to use diaphragmatic breathing as needed, and she was receptive to the use of simple self-statements to calm herself. She remained anxious throughout the admission but was able to keep the anxiety at a manageable level. She was discharged back to her previous outpatient providers for ongoing treatment.

Sample 7.2
Initial Health Psychology Consultation: New Leukemia Diagnosis

Pt is a 33 y/o Caucasian woman, referred by Dr. G for health psych eval. Pt admitted with new dx acute leukemia; no significant past med hx. No substance use problems.

Pt completed college and works as an editor at a large newspaper. She lives alone, is unmarried, and has good family support.

Pt reports feeling fatigue over the past few months and scheduled a routine exam with her PCP. No obvious clinical problems were noted at that visit yesterday, and pt obtained routine blood work afterward and returned to work. By the time she arrived back at work, the MD's office had called and told her to go immediately to the hospital, that she had acute leukemia and needed to begin tx immediately. Pt was admitted to the hospital last night, had PICC (*peripherally inserted central catheter*) line placed, repeat blood work drawn, as well as other procedures to evaluate the functioning of other organs prior to beginning chemo.

Pt with no previous inpatient or outpt psych tx, no psych meds, no family hx. Pt reports being overwhelmed and anxious. She has been given basic education on acute leukemia and its tx (immediate chemo, later stem cell transplant). She is worried she will lose her job because she will need to be off work at least 6 mths to undergo treatment and is frightened that she may not live through this. She has contacted her parents, who are "freaking out" and coming to stay in the hospital with her.

Pt with very poor sleep last night, secondary to anxiety and rumination. She reports increased anxiety when medical personnel leave her room and she is alone. Anxiety is mostly worry and rumination, no significant physiological sx except for occasional increased heart rate. Pt feels out of control. She denies depressed mood, poor energy, appetite changes, poor sleep generally, suicidal ideation. No panic, hallucinations, paranoia.

Mental status exam deferred for now; no gross deficits noted during interview. Pt appears quite anxious, jittery, and hypervigilant.

Impressions: Pt with no formal psych hx. New dx acute leukemia has resulted in significant anxiety and worry. Discussed with pt the typical adjustment process and normalized her current reactions. Will follow and work with pt on relaxation, distraction, and cognitive strategies to help her to manage anxiety.

SUMMARY OF INTERVENTION

Patient was in the hospital this admission for 6 weeks and was seen by the psychologist for monitoring and intervention every 2–3 days. Patient learned and successfully used relaxation strategies, mostly to help her to relax and sleep at night. Her family brought her some activities to help her to pass the time, distract her from her worries, and decrease rumination. She played games with them, and read and played solitaire when on her own. Pt gained some feelings of control by educating herself regarding her treatment, and she was able to learn cognitive strategies to help her challenge her catastrophic thoughts and help her to develop reasonable expectations. Pt struggled with anxiety throughout this admission, although generally did well at coping with it. Before discharge her anxiety increased. Her oncologist prescribed alprazolam 0.25 mg prn, and the health psychology consultant made plans to continue to see the patient twice weekly when she came to the oncology clinic for outpatient follow-up appointments.

Sample 7.3 Initial Health Psychology Consultation: Chronic Obstructive Pulmonary Disease and Anxiety

Patient referred by Dr. B for health psych eval with concerns about anxiety. Pt is a 51 y/o AA woman, admitted with COPD exacerbation; pt on vent × 2 yrs. Pt lives alone, but she has 2 adult children who help out. She completed some college and worked as a receptionist until she became vent-dependent and went on disability 2 yrs ago. No hx substance abuse or psych tx.

Pt reports having COPD and managing it well most of the time. Even when it became necessary for her to use the ventilator continuously, she accepted that and coped with it well. She reports generally good quality of life, and she enjoys spending time with her grandkids.

Pt reports that she began experiencing anxiety about a year ago. Her son was preparing dinner, and his shirt caught on fire. At the time, patient was in her bedroom suctioning fluids from her system, so not on the ventilator. She heard her son screaming but knew if she went to his aid without the vent in place she would pass out herself and be unable to help him. Fortunately, a neighbor also heard his screams and called 911. Since that time, the pt has been experiencing anxiety, especially when she is briefly off the ventilator. She also now worries that the vent will malfunction. She has also begun to experience some depressive sx re: her medical situation, and she has begun to question her quality of life and to have passive thoughts of death.

Pt does not worry excessively in general, no panic. No problems with sleep, guilt, worthlessness, + hopelessness re: her medical issues at times. No suicidal ideation, plan, or intent. No mania, paranoia, hallucinations.

Pt denies subjective memory problems. On mental status exam she was alert and oriented × 3. Registration, judgment, long-term memory, concentration were all intact. Short-term memory mildly impaired (2/3).

Impressions: Pt with no significant psych hx or emotional problems. New anxiety for past year after frightening experience while off vent. Some mild depressive sx since then also. Will follow pt this admission to provide strategies to aid coping, and to address anxiety and depressive sx.

SUMMARY OF INTERVENTION

Pt remained inpatient for 5 days and was seen three times for health psych intervention during that period. At these visits, patient was reeducated about how the ventilator works and what she could do to get back on it quickly in case of an emergency. Next, cognitive strategies were introduced to help her to cope with new anticipatory anxiety about the brief times she is off the vent. Finally, a recommendation was made for patient to begin outpatient treatment with a health psychologist, who could continue to help her with the anxiety symptoms and also to monitor and address the new depressive symptoms. She was responsive to the interventions and agreeable to the referral for additional outpatient treatment to aid her coping with her medical situation.

Depression 8

Depression and concerns about mood are common referral questions for inpatient psychology consultation; one study reported that depressive disorders occurred in 26.9% of patients in internal medicine inpatient units, with only about half of those identified by their physicians (Rentsch et al., 2007). Depression has also been associated with longer hospital admissions (Aoki, Sato, & Hosaka, 2004) and also with decreased adherence (e.g., Turan, Yemez, & Itil, 2014; Wagner et al., 2011). Depressed mood is common in hospitalized medical patients, but new onset major depression that meets criteria for a *Diagnostic and Statistical Manual of Mental Disorders* (fifth ed.; American Psychiatric Association, 2013) diagnosis occurs less frequently on medical floors in the hospital. The intensity of the depressed mood can range from mild to severe, and patients may present with only depressed mood or with a constellation of other depressive symptoms, such as poor sleep and appetite, decreased concentration, apathy, withdrawal, decreased motivation, or loss of interest.

Sources of Depression

There are a variety of causes for depression and depressed mood in the hospital setting. Patients with premorbid depression (that may or may not be associated with a medical disorder) may be admitted to the hospital and referred for

http://dx.doi.org/10.1037/0000108-009
Health Psychology Consultation in the Inpatient Medical Setting, by S. M. Labott

help managing depressive symptoms. As with anxiety disorders, some medical illnesses result in symptoms of depression that can be confounded with a psychological disorder, and many medications cause symptoms of depression. Finally, there are psychological stressors associated with the hospital admission that could be associated with depressive symptoms in medical inpatients. All of these are described more fully here. As with anxiety, the etiology of the depressive symptoms will dictate the appropriate treatment.

PREMORBID DEPRESSION

Patients with ongoing problems with depression warrant special attention when they are admitted to medical floors of the hospital, especially if there is a history of severe depression with suicide attempts that has warranted psychiatric inpatient admission in the past. Depending on the severity of the depression, a consultation with Psychiatry may be warranted soon after admission so that the patient's outpatient medication can be continued or adjusted for the current situation. People with depression may have difficulty coping with the hospital milieu, tests and procedures, and bad news about medical issues, so regular follow-up from the psychologist is warranted. Sample 8.1 is a consultation report on a patient with premorbid depression that negatively impacted his hospital admission.

Many patients are admitted to the hospital with antidepressant medications as part of their outpatient drug regimen but without a clear rationale for the medication, and the patient may not be aware of the reason for it. The health psychology consultant will need to determine why the patient is taking the medication and then ensure it is continued during the hospital admission (if appropriate, given the current medical situation). As always, a thorough evaluation and history are warranted. Some patients have a long history of depression but may be symptom-free. Others may be taking the antidepressant for reasons other than severe depression (e.g., premenstrual syndrome symptoms).

For many patients on outpatient antidepressant medications, it is best to continue the antidepressant while the patient is in the hospital unless there is a medical contraindication. Because the inpatient hospital milieu can be stressful, discontinuing a medication that has presumably been helping to keep the patient symptom-free may result in a resurgence of depressive symptoms. In addition, because it may take several weeks for an antidepressant to take effect, discontinuing the medication may mean that the patient has to endure a resurgence of symptoms before again obtaining the benefits of the medication.

NEW-ONSET DEPRESSION SYMPTOMS WITH PSYCHOLOGICAL ETIOLOGY

Many people experience depressed mood when in the hospital, even if they have no past history of depression or other mental health problems. In fact, most patients referred for psychology consultations do not have a history of mental illness but are reacting to a new or difficult medical illness. The depressed mood and other symptoms that may be seen in the hospital may be a direct emotional result of the medical problem and associated with the patient's adjustment to the new medical situation.

In many cases, if the patient had not become sick, there would have been no need for a referral to a mental health professional, either in the hospital or as an outpatient. Consider a young woman who was recently diagnosed with breast cancer and admitted to the hospital for chemotherapy and radiation. She had no previous psychological history but had been experiencing depressed mood, poor sleep with rumination, anxiety, and poor appetite for the past week. While her symptoms do not qualify for a diagnosis of major depression, they are important and could negatively affect her medical situation if left untreated. If she had not been diagnosed with breast cancer, it is unlikely these psychological symptoms would have occurred at all.

Exhibit 8.1 lists additional causes of depressed mood for patients in the hospital. Patients may be concerned about the outcome of their treatment, and their mood might fluctuate over time, depending on how the medical treatment is progressing. Patients may have "good days" in which their mood is good because their treatment is progressing well and they are feeling better. These may be interspersed with "bad days" that occur if there are setbacks in the medical situation or increases in subjective symptoms.

Patients may also be experiencing other losses due to the hospital admission. There are often activities that they miss and significant social losses as they are unable to see and interact with people who are important to them. For patients with young children, it can be especially difficult because young children are usually not allowed to visit a parent in the hospital.

At times, the symptoms of depression and depressed mood can progress to a diagnosable major depression, especially if the patient has been in the hospital for a long time and with recurrent complications. A patient may have been admitted for a simple elective surgery with plans to go home 2 days later, but then gets an infection that delays discharge, then another medical problem is found that requires additional inpatient treatment, and this cycle goes on and on ("one thing after another"). This experience may result in a more intense depression with associated hopelessness that the situation will ever improve.

OVERLAP BETWEEN SYMPTOMS OF DEPRESSION AND THOSE OF OTHER MEDICAL DISORDERS

The diagnosis of depression shares symptoms with many medical diagnoses. For example, sleep apnea can present with poor sleep and low energy, and hypothyroidism may present with fatigue and memory problems. Cardiac problems can

EXHIBIT 8.1

Psychological Reasons for Depressed Mood in Hospitalized Medical Patients

Adjusting to a new diagnosis or to a change in a chronic medical problem
Uncertainty of treatment outcome
Loss of typical activities or relationships
Long length of stay
Recurrent medical problems

present with low energy, and gastrointestinal problems may be associated with poor appetite, weight loss, and fatigue. Mental status problems can also present with withdrawal, mood changes, and decreased concentration and can be confused with depression. Exhibit 8.2 provides a list of medical disorders that share symptoms with depression. A variety of neurological and endocrine disorders have been associated with depression, as well as cancer, infectious diseases, and metabolic imbalances. The diagnostic difficulty is in determining whether the patient has only a medical disorder that accounts for the symptoms, major depression alone, depression independent of a medical disorder, or depression and a medical disorder that interact with or exacerbate each other. Brief rating scales used to measure depression (e.g., Beck Depression Inventory—II; Beck, Steer, & Brown, 1996) often contain items that assess vegetative symptoms and so confound the psychological and medical issues. Although these scales can still be useful, they do not take the place of a thorough psychological evaluation, history, and medical record review when it comes to differentiating the psychological and medical contributions to the symptom picture.

Multiple sclerosis (MS) demonstrates the interplay between a disease and depression. There is some symptom overlap as fatigue and low energy are symptoms of both depression and MS. Further, research has consistently demonstrated that depression occurs more frequently in MS patients than in healthy subjects, with a prevalence of about 26% (e.g., Patten, Beck, Williams, Barbui, & Metz, 2003; Viner et al., 2014), and depression is associated with decreased quality of life, suicidal ideation, poor support, and poorer disease course in MS patients (Viner et al., 2014). The occurrence of depression in MS has been associated with functional limitations (Beal, Stuifbergen, & Brown, 2007; Dalton & Heinrichs, 2005) and also with relapse episodes

EXHIBIT 8.2

Medical Conditions Presenting With Depressive Constellations

Endocrine disorders: thyroid dysfunction (hypothyroidism or hyperthyroidism), adrenal dysfunction or syndrome (Cushing's disease or Addison's disease), diabetes mellitus, insulinoma, acromegaly, hypoparathyroidism, hypopituitarism

Neurological disorders: Parkinson's disease, Huntington's disease, multiple sclerosis, Alzheimer's disease, cerebrovascular diseases

Metabolic disorders: hypomagnesemia, hyponatremia, hypokalemia, hyperkalemia, uremia, Wilson's disease, pernicious anemia, pellagra, folic acid deficiency, pyridoxine deficiency

Neoplasias: oat cell carcinoma, pancreatic carcinoma, tumors of the central nervous system, lymphoma, leukemia

Collagen-vascular disease: systemic lupus erythematosus, giant cell arteritis, rheumatoid arthritis

Infectious disorders: infectious mononucleosis, hepatitis, influenza, syphilis, tuberculosis, acquired immune deficiency syndrome (AIDS), encephalitis

Note. From *Psycho-Oncology* (p. 531), by J. C. Holland (Ed.), 1998, New York, NY: Oxford University Press. Copyright 1998 by Oxford University Press. Reprinted with permission.

(Moore et al., 2012), but it has also been associated with neurodegeneration (Byatt, Rothschild, Riskind, Ionete, & Hunt, 2011; Hildebrandt & Eling, 2014) and with medications used to treat the MS symptoms (Arnett & Randolph, 2006; Fragoso et al., 2010). Depression symptoms may, in fact, appear before MS symptoms and can delay the diagnosis of MS (Byatt et al., 2011). Therefore, when a psychologist sees depressive symptoms in a MS patient, it may not be immediately clear whether these symptoms are due to psychological causes, organic causes, medication, or a combination of these factors.

Huntington's disease (HD) is a genetic disorder in which depression occurs in 33% to 76% of patients (Ossig & Storch, 2015). The symptoms of depression frequently occur before the onset of HD but can also occur as a reaction to the development of the HD symptoms (Ossig & Storch, 2015). Similarly, depression has been reported in 46% of acute stroke inpatients and appears to be associated with previous mood disorder (Caeiro, Ferro, Santos, & Figueira, 2006). Caeiro et al. (2006) noted that apathy and loss of interest differentiated the depression of the acute stroke patients from depression in cardiac patients and suggested that the apathy is caused by the brain lesion, whereas other symptoms of depression may be an emotional reaction to the illness.

Goldston and Baillie (2008) provided a good review of depression and coronary heart disease (CHD), noting the role of depression in the development of CHD, as an outcome after cardiac events, and as an indicator of poor prognosis. Specifically, depression is a risk factor for heart disease, with more severe depression creating greater risk. Further, 20% or more of patients who have myocardial infarction develop depression. The presence of depression in CHD patients is also associated with a greater number of cardiac events as well as patient mortality (Goldston & Baillie, 2008).

DEPRESSION CAUSED BY MEDICATIONS

Many medications and drugs can cause depression; Exhibit 8.3 lists examples. Several cancer drugs can cause depression, and some cause it with great frequency, e.g., vinblastine (used in the treatment of solid tumors) results in anxiety or depression in up to 80% of patients treated with it (Peterson & Popkin, 1980). Corticosteroids, often used as part of a chemotherapy regimen, can cause changes in mood and emotional lability, as well as anxiety and psychosis (see steroid section in anxiety chapter). Interferon, which is used to treat cancer, MS, and hepatitis C, has been associated with the development of depression in up to 45% of patients (Asnis & De La Garza, 2005) and creates additional risk for patients with a preexisting history of depression (M. Schaefer et al., 2005). It is also associated with poor sleep, weight loss, irritability, and cognitive changes. Tamoxifen, used in breast cancer or preventively for those at high risk of breast cancer, has been associated with depression, weight gain, and other menopausal-type symptoms (Chang, Chen, & Liu, 2015).

Even seemingly innocuous drugs have been associated with depression in medical patients, although perhaps only in specific circumstances; for example, taking two

EXHIBIT 8.3

Medications and Psychoactive Substances Associated With Depression

Antihypertensive medications	Cancer chemotherapeutic agents
Reserpine	Vincristine
Methyldopa	Vinblastine
β-blockers (in predisposed individuals)	Procarbazine
Contraceptives	L-Asparaginase
Corticosteroids	Amphotericin B
Benzodiazepines	Interferon
Histamine$_2$ receptor antagonists	Psychoactive substances
Cimetidine	Alcohol
Ranitidine	Opiates
	Amphetamine or cocaine (withdrawal)
	Anabolic steroids

Note. From *The American Psychiatric Publishing Textbook of Consultation-Liaison Psychiatry: Psychiatry in the Medically Ill* (2nd ed., p. 311), by M. G. Wise and J. R. Rundell (Eds.), 2002, Washington, DC: American Psychiatric Association. Copyright 2002 by the American Psychiatric Association. Reprinted with permission.

or more antihypertensive drugs has been associated with depression, whereas taking only one drug (regardless of the specific drug) was not (Johansen, Holmen, Stewart, & Bjerkeset, 2012). H_2-blockers (used to treat ulcers and gastroesophageal reflux disease) have also been implicated in the development of depression; for example, Stocky (1991) reported on three patients who demonstrated improvements in depression when ranitidine was discontinued.

However, not all or even most patients taking these medications experience symptoms of depression, and even if a patient does have symptoms of depression, it should not be assumed they are due to the medication. A cancer patient could be depressed due to the losses she will face if her treatment does not work, and the depressive symptoms may have little or nothing to do with the medication in that case. Again, a thorough psychological evaluation will delineate the cause or causes of the depressive symptoms.

Exhibit 8.3 contains a good list of some medications to be wary of, but it is not exhaustive, and new drugs and combinations continue to be developed. The psychologist will need to be aware of new developments in the medical specialty areas in which he works and remain attentive to researching new medications taken by his patients.

Suicide in Medical Patients

Active suicidal ideation occurs when someone is planning to take an active role in making his or her own death occur. Medical patients considering suicide will have thoughts about methods to bring about their own death; these thoughts are similar to those that can occur for any person who is contemplating suicide. For many patients, the suicidal ideation is associated with depression. In other cases, the patient may not be depressed, and the plans for suicide are a rational response to a terminal illness, to facing a poor quality of life, or overwhelming pain. (Assisted suicide is discussed in Chapter 14 of this volume.)

Suicidal ideation and suicide attempts are always a concern in depressed patients, and especially in patients with serious physical illnesses (with or without depression). It has long been known that medical illness is associated with suicide (Mackenzie & Popkin, 1987), and hospitalization for a medical illness is associated with an increased risk of suicide (Erlangsen, Vach, & Jeune, 2005; Voaklander et al., 2008). Some researchers have studied specific diagnoses to ascertain the relationship with suicide; Misono, Weiss, Fann, Redman, and Yueh (2008) reported that the risk of suicide in cancer patients is twice that of a healthy population, for example.

Although suicide is not uncommon in patients with physical illnesses, suicide attempts and completions are rarely made by patients admitted to the medical floors of a hospital (Mills, Watts, & Hemphill, 2014). Medical patients are more likely to be distressed because they are seriously ill; they want to live but are afraid they will die. Patients with medical illnesses are more likely to make a suicide attempt later, in the outpatient setting, when they are struggling to deal with chronic medical issues that have severely decreased their life quality. Therefore, even if a patient does not appear to be a high risk for a suicide attempt during the hospital admission, the health psychologist should be aware of the possible increase in risk that could occur after discharge.

The assessment of suicidality should be a part of every inpatient psychological evaluation. In many cases, patients can simply be asked if they have any thoughts or plans to kill or harm themselves. If they say no (convincingly), there is generally no need to discuss the issue further unless there is additional evidence that warrants further investigation. For those patients who are experiencing current suicidal ideation, a thorough evaluation of their thoughts and plans, mental status, social supports, and access to a means to attempt suicide is warranted. Following the evaluation, the consultant will need to document the findings thoroughly and accurately and also provide verbal notification of any risk of suicide to relevant providers (usually the patient's nurse and primary medical team).

Exhibit 8.4 lists risk factors for suicide that should be considered in medical patients. As with healthy patients, a history of past attempts, access to a means to kill oneself, and male gender are risk factors. Other factors, associated with the medical illness, such as pain, poor quality of life, loss of mobility, and the inability to communicate can also play a role. Depending on the specific medical illness, there may be additional risk factors to consider (e.g., the site of a cancer affects the risk of suicide; Wang, Chang, Weng, Yeh, & Lee, 2018).

In the inpatient setting, it is important to distinguish thoughts of death from suicidal ideation. Many hospitalized patients have good reason to be thinking about their death, either because they have been diagnosed with a terminal illness or have concerns that they will be. Patients in this situation may consider what their death will be like, as well as whether there is anything they can do to make their death more the way they would like it to be. They may consider their funeral (and often actively plan it),

EXHIBIT 8.4

Risk Factors for Suicide in Medical Inpatients

Severe psychiatric illness, chronic
History of past suicide attempts
Access to weapon, drugs for overdose, or other means
Lack of social support
No hope for improvement in medical illness
Significant pain
Sufficient physical stamina to successfully accomplish suicide
Poor quality of life and no hope for improvement
Mental status changes

and what the lives of their loved ones will be like without them. They may also try to wrap up loose ends in their lives (both emotional and financial) to make the death less complicated and stressful for themselves as well as their loved ones. These thoughts and plans for death can occur in someone who does not wish to die but realizes it is likely to happen, so they do their best to accept it and plan for it. Thoughts of death such as these may be completely unrelated to suicidal ideation and risk.

Delirious patients may be confused with suicidal patients in the medical setting. Delirious patients may be delusional and frightened. Although they may not be actively suicidal, they may accidentally hurt themselves as they react to their fears. For example, Mr. G was a 26-year-old AA man who was undergoing a stem cell transplant for sickle cell anemia. He had no past psychiatric history. The medical treatment had generally been going well, and the patient's mood was good with no significant symptoms of anxiety or depression. He then developed an infection with high fever, which progressed to sepsis. The patient became delirious and believed there were police in the hospital who were planning to kill him. He attempted to throw a chair through his 10th-floor window so that he could escape. The window cracked but did not break, but the patient sustained some serious cuts. Although the patient was not suicidal, he attempted to jump out the window to escape from those he feared would hurt him. Because his judgment was also impaired, he didn't realize that jumping from the 10th floor was likely to result in serious injury. The patient was moved to the intensive care unit (ICU), and the medical problem was successfully treated. The delirium cleared, and the remainder of his inpatient stay was uneventful.

Management of Depression and Suicide in the Inpatient Setting

The main goal in the management of a medical patient at risk for suicide is to keep the patient safe, using the minimal physical restraint possible, while removing opportunities for suicide attempts. If a patient is calm and not physically aggressive, often the use of a "sitter" is sufficient to ensure her safety. The sitter is generally a nursing student or aide who is hired by the hospital to simply be in the room to watch the patient and help with simple needs. (Although it is tempting to use a family member for this, if something goes wrong, it could result in legal liability issues.) Objects that a patient could use to harm herself should be removed from the room and attention paid to improving the patient's cognition as much as possible. No-suicide contracts can be made with the patient, and other interventions, such as cognitive strategies, can be used to help patients cope with the suicidal thoughts. Nursing staff should check on patients with suicidal ideation frequently and also carefully monitor medications.

As described earlier, there are several distinct etiologies for depressive symptoms in the hospital, although many cases of depression or depressed mood are multidetermined. The most effective treatment will be that which targets the specific cause(s) of the symptoms in a specific case. That is, a patient who has developed depressive symptoms that appear to be exclusively due to a chemotherapy agent will receive less benefit from a cognitive–behavioral intervention than a patient who is depressed due to the loss of her job and marriage since beginning treatment for cancer. Both patients, however, would likely benefit from education about the symptoms, causes, and treatments for depression. This education should be brief and user-friendly and can be helpful at providing patients with the background to understand their situation and to take an active role in their treatment.

The goals for any treatment of depression in the inpatient medical setting are to (a) address any issues that will affect the medical situation positively, that is, help the patient to change what she can; and (b) cope with what remains, including managing affect associated with the situation. Having a positive impact on the situation includes anything the patient can do to exert some control over the physical and psychological situation. Then, once all behavioral efforts have been made, the patient needs to deal with the emotional aspects of the situation. In the case of depression, this will involve using cognitive and behavioral strategies to cope with the difficult situation. Specific treatments for depression in medical inpatients are described next, including education, cognitive–behavioral interventions, the use of social support, and medication.

EDUCATION

Most laypeople feel they understand what depression is, but they rarely understand what would differentiate a severe major depression from the low mood that might be experienced due to daily life stressors. Because they do not know the specific symptoms associated with depression, patients often cannot say if they are depressed or not when they are asked. Therefore, one of the most useful educational interventions is to describe to patients the symptoms associated with depression, including down or low mood or feeling blue, changes in sleep and appetite, decreased motivation, apathy, withdrawal, decreased interest and energy, poor concentration, fatigue, worthlessness, guilt, hopelessness or helplessness, slowed cognition, irritability, agitation or retardation, and thoughts of death or suicide (some of this education may occur during the patient evaluation). Patients will need to understand that the number, intensity, and duration of the symptoms are relevant for the diagnosis and treatment. It is also helpful for patients to learn that depressed mood is not uncommon for patients in the hospital and that it does not always mean they are depressed in the clinical sense or that the depressed mood will turn into a more serious and ongoing major depression in the future. Normalizing the low mood will often help to decrease the patient's worry about the symptoms and improve his ability to cope.

Describing the etiology of the patient's depression can also aid his coping. For example, if a patient understands that depression is correlated with MS, he may be more open to ongoing treatment for depression that involves both medication and psychotherapy. Alternatively, if the depression is due to a specific medication that will only be taken briefly, the best course may be to educate the patient about cognitive strategies to help him to manage the symptoms until the medication can be discontinued.

Educating patients that the treatment will go better if they take an active role is another important part of the treatment. Inpatients have often learned to be passive and expect their doctors to make them better using various procedures and medications. Encouraging them to actively use specific strategies to manage their mood can provide a sense of purpose and efficacy that can also positively affect their mood.

COGNITIVE–BEHAVIORAL INTERVENTIONS

The major goal of cognitive–behavioral therapy for depression is to help patients change their thinking about their situation to alleviate the depression and to promote adaptive behavior. In the medical situation specifically, this will involve helping patients to think differently about their illness, to adjust expectations, and to become an active participant in improving their health.

One major area of intervention involves addressing a patient's expectations about the illness. A patient may be shaken and feel vulnerable if diagnosed with a serious illness. He may feel that his relationships and life plans have been completely disrupted and may not see how he can have a reasonable life in the context of the illness. These concerns can have a significant impact on mood, and some patients will allow the illness to take over and become the main focus in life. Alternatively, the patient could take a more adaptive stance in which he integrates the new illness as part of an otherwise good and varied life. Discussing the implications of the new illness as well as ways to integrate it appropriately into one's life can provide a more adaptive perspective and feelings of efficacy about managing the illness. The patient's expectations will also be influenced by the chronicity and seriousness of the illness; expectations and plans regarding a long-term chronic illness will be different from that for an acute terminal illness.

Once patients have adjusted to a bad diagnosis and prognosis, they are often optimistic about their chances of beating it (e.g., "I will be the one person in 10 who is successful with this treatment"). Over time, however, and especially with repeated treatments, bad news, and long hospital stays, the patient's optimism may decrease. The road to recovery may look hopeless, and patients may become depressed and even give up. Especially for patients with an uncertain future, it is helpful for them to keep their thinking in the present, without looking too far ahead into the future.

Depressed mood is often associated with the patient feeling there is nothing she can do to influence the current situation. Even in the face of devastating medical illness, however, there is typically *something* a patient can do to affect the situation, at least minimally. Actions a patient can take to improve her current situation may involve eating properly, adhering to occupational and physical therapy, working collaboratively with the medical team, or taking actions to improve her mood. Each of these provides a way for patients to exert some control and to play an active role in their medical care. Sample 8.2 describes a patient with a history of depression, with increased symptoms following a new cancer diagnosis.

Activity Scheduling

One of the main approaches to treating depression involves increasing activity, decreasing withdrawal and isolation, and increasing positive reinforcement. In the outpatient setting, this often takes the form of increasing social events, exercise, and hobbies, which will then provide additional positive reinforcement, decrease rumination, increase feelings of efficacy, and improve mood. The same idea applies to patients in the hospital, and an increase in activity can also serve to distract patients from their worries about medical issues and help them to pass the time.

Activity scheduling in the hospital, however, is more complicated than in the outpatient setting, and the activities available to a patient may be severely limited. When in the hospital, patients are generally limited to activities that can be done in a hospital room, and they are often physically unable to engage in many activities that involve physical exertion. Therefore, activity needs to be broadly defined to include physical, social, and intellectual activity. While in the hospital, focusing on a favorite television program could be considered "activity." Some patients may have an exercise bicycle in their room or on the hospital unit, or they may be able to walk the floors of the hospital. Others may not be able to exercise or to leave the room, but they can engage in intellectual activities, such as puzzles, games, or reading. When patients have both cognitive and physical limitations, the task of finding activities for them is more difficult, but may include listening to music or talking with friends on the telephone.

Pleasant Event Scheduling

In the outpatient setting, depression can be due to a lack of pleasant events or positive reinforcement, and clinicians often encourage their clients to engage in at least one pleasant event daily. In the hospital setting, it is common for patients to have few positive events in their day, and often for many days in a row. Because of the setting, selecting and engaging in positive events can be difficult, but patients usually understand the rationale for this and are willing to try it. There are published lists of events that can be used to improve mood (Lewinsohn & Graf, 1973), and hospitalized patients can use some of these (e.g., thinking about something good in the future, smiling at people). Often, however, patients in the hospital need to be creative. Some patients have been successful at asking for privacy for a short time or asking a family member to bring in a favorite food, special music, a movie, or their favorite soft blanket. Although seemingly simple, these objects and activities can positively affect a patient's mood and quality of life while in the hospital.

SOCIAL SUPPORT

Social support is an important component in a patient's ability to cope with a hospital admission, as well as his ability to manage a chronic or terminal illness. Much research has documented the beneficial effects of social support in medical patients; it is associated with emotional adjustment (Curtis, Groarke, Coughlan, & Gsel, 2004), illness self-management (Gallant, 2003), and also self-efficacy and adjustment to illness (Yohannes, 2013).

Many patients have family and friends who are willing to be either emotionally or instrumentally supportive, or both. In many cases, however, the family does not know what to do to be helpful to the patient and requires some direction regarding what the patient wants or needs. Patients often do not independently think of this and need to be reminded that their loved ones are not mind readers. Yet they are generally open to the idea of specifically asking family and friends for what they want. At times, patients would like friends and family to bring an object or activity to the hospital for them; most often, however, the patient wants time from the family, and asking for it clearly will often have good results. Many family members will go out of their way to visit more often, spend a night with the patient in the hospital, or spend more time with the patient on the telephone. Patients need to be aware that family members may refuse their request, but most understand that they have little hope of getting what they want if they don't ask for it.

Some unfortunate patients have family members who will not be responsive to their requests, however; patients can often predict this ahead of time, based on their past history with them. One 10-year-old boy was dying in the ICU and desperately wanted his mother to be with him. When the mother was contacted by the health psychology consultant and asked to come in to spend some time with her son, she refused, stating that she did not want to see him this way and that it was too distressing for her. She would not be convinced to come to the hospital to be with her son. In this situation, the boy's aunt visited to provide support, and the psychologist spent additional time with him also. Yet although these surrogates were helpful to the patient, they could not take the place of his mother.

MEDICATION

It may seem obvious that antidepressants would be the treatment of choice for depressed medical inpatients, but traditional antidepressants may create unwanted side effects that are especially problematic for medical inpatients, such as orthostatic hypotension, confusion, urinary retention, sedation, and cardiac toxicity (Barreira,

1994). In addition, a positive response to the medication often does not occur for several weeks, and many patients are no longer in the hospital at that time. Many patients will not have an outpatient provider to monitor the effects of the medication, and (depending on the cause of the depressive symptoms) they may not need long-term treatment with antidepressant medications.

The selective serotonin reuptake inhibitors (SSRIs) such as fluoxetine (Prozac), sertraline (Zoloft), and paroxetine (Paxil) are associated with fewer and less severe side effects, but patients can develop agitation or sedation, insomnia, gastrointestinal problems, and sexual dysfunction (Rush & Nierenberg, 2009) when taking SSRIs. Yet the SSRIs are generally well tolerated by most people, making them popular with patients and physicians. Rush and Nierenberg (2009) summarized available antidepressant medications, possible side effects, and dosing information.

Psychostimulants, such as methylphenidate (Ritalin), can quickly—within a few days—improve a patient's energy, decrease fatigue, and provide an increased sense of well-being. This is useful in the inpatient setting when a boost in energy and mood can help patients to participate in physical therapy, eat better, and engage with visitors, facilitating the patient's recovery. Kerr et al. (2012) documented improvements in fatigue and depression with methylphenidate, and it has also been shown to decrease the vegetative symptoms of depression induced by interferon treatment (Camacho & Ng, 2006).

The patient's attending physician often has the required expertise and feels comfortable prescribing antidepressants or psychostimulants; the medical specialist will likely also be aware of dosing adjustments that need to be made in the context of the specific physical illness that the patient is dealing with. Otherwise, a psychiatry consult should be requested to evaluate the patient for these medications.

In summary, symptoms of depression occur commonly in medical inpatients and may be due to psychological stressors, associated with specific illnesses, or due to medications used to treat medical diseases. Treatment may include education, cognitive–behavioral interventions, social support, or psychotropic medication and will be most successful when tailored to the specific etiology of the patient's symptoms.

Sample 8.1 Premorbid Depression

Patient is a 64 y/o Caucasian man with hip fracture 2 weeks ago, s/p surgical repair, now admitted to acute rehab unit. Consult requested by Dr. S with concerns about noncompliance and pt's inability to work well with nurses, OT, and PT. Pt is a retired factory worker, divorced, and with 2 grown children who live >5 hrs away. He lives alone and was able to manage at home alone prior to hip fx. He completed h.s. and reports minimal social support.

Pt with hx depression × 8 yrs, treated by his PCP. Pt has taken a variety of psych meds over the years (e.g., Paxil, Zoloft), but has been on no psych meds for the past 2 yrs. (Records indicate PCP noted increased sx past year and recommended restarting Zoloft but pt refused.) No hx suicide attempts, no psychotherapy, no psych inpt admissions.

Pt today reports + depressed mood, + hopelessness, poor sleep and motivation, + irritability, no suicidal ideation, appetite OK. He feels these sx have been ongoing for a while but that they are worse since hip fx. Pt complains that nurses do not understand the pain he experiences, and so he is not willing to do what they request of him. He also feels therapists from PT and OT push him too hard, and he is now considering leaving the hospital bec he feels he needs more rest and less activity.

On mental status exam pt was alert and O × 3. Registration, attention, judgment, short- and long-term memory, abstract thinking all intact. Mood slightly irritable.

Impressions: 1) Pt with depression. He is aware of his symptoms, and also willing to restart meds. 2) Educated pt re: recovery process, needing to push himself in his therapies, also discussed how to communicate effectively with providers when he has problems. 3) Discussed pain issue with nurses, PT, and OT. Pt will be given pain meds 30 min before therapy sessions. Will also ask MDs to reeval pain meds and dosing. 4) Will follow to monitor mood and coping.

Sample 8.2
Depression When Coping With New Cancer Diagnosis

Patient is a 46 y/o man, diagnosed with liver cancer 3 days ago. Patient has a history of depression, has been taking Zoloft (sertraline) 50 mg for 10 years and feels this has been working well for him. Since the diagnosis, patient reports increased hopelessness about the future, with serious concerns about his ability to continue to work and provide for his family, as well as concerns for their future if he dies. Sleep is poor; no suicidal ideation or past attempts. Patient is also reporting anxiety about the results of ongoing testing regarding the extent of his illness, also anxiety about upcoming chemotherapy.

Discussed with patient the adjustment process as he comes to terms with his new medical situation, as well as supports he can enlist to help him deal with this. Patient is aware of symptoms of depression, and feels he is generally doing OK, but with some increase in symptoms since diagnosis. Patient is unsure about his prognosis and should know more later in the week as test results become available. Encouraged patient to avoid thinking of the worst outcomes and to withhold judgment on these issues until he knows more. He will use distraction from TV and reading to help with this. Taught patient diaphragmatic breathing to help him relax, as well as cognitive strategies to help decrease anxiety. Will plan to follow up with him daily to help him to cope with the new diagnosis and its implications.

9 Delirium and Acute Cognitive Changes

Delirium is a clinical emergency in which a medical problem causes impairment in cognition, psychotic symptoms, behavioral changes, or a combination of these. The fifth edition of the *Diagnostic and Statistical Manual of Mental Disorders* defines delirium as involving disturbances in attention and cognition with a rapid onset and fluctuating course that represents a change from the patient's baseline functioning and is due to a medical condition, medication, or substance intoxication or withdrawal, and not to a preexisting neurocognitive disorder (American Psychiatric Association, 2013). The presentation may be dramatic, as in the case of an agitated and aggressive patient, or it may be subtle, as seen in a calm patient who is disoriented and quietly hallucinating. Delirium is an emergency because it represents the failure of brain function, which is serious. The brain is resistant to insult, and if it is not functioning properly, the issue must be remedied as quickly as possible. Prompt and correct diagnosis and treatment are paramount because untreated delirium can result in death. Delirium may be referred to in the medical record as acute confusional state, encephalopathy, intensive care unit (ICU) psychosis, or altered mental status.

Delirium occurs most frequently in older adults (Inouye, Westendorp, & Saczynski, 2014), in those with serious or terminal medical problems (Hsieh, Ely, & Gong, 2013), and in the context of dementia (Leonard et al., 2014). It

http://dx.doi.org/10.1037/0000108-010
Health Psychology Consultation in the Inpatient Medical Setting, by S. M. Labott

is fairly common in the inpatient medical setting, but it is rarely seen in healthy outpatient populations. The occurrence of delirium in elderly people living at home is low (1%–2%), but its development at home often prompts the presentation of the patient to the emergency department where the prevalence is higher (8%–17%; Inouye et al., 2014). Delirium occurs most commonly in the intensive care setting where patients are the sickest (hence, the term *ICU psychosis*). On the basis of a review of previous reports, Inouye et al. (2014) reported that 7% to 50% of patients admitted to the ICU have delirium, and new-onset cases after admission to the ICU range from 19% to 82%. However, delirium occurs throughout the inpatient setting, with an incidence of 21% to 63% after hip replacement and 13% to 48% poststroke (Maldonado, 2008).

Delirium has consequences for patients beyond the specific symptoms of the delirium itself because it places them at risk for other medical issues, such as aspiration, pressure ulcers, and decreased food intake (Fong, Tulebaev, & Inouye, 2009). Delirium is associated with longer hospital stays and increased mortality, longer term cognitive problems, and also posttraumatic stress disorder (Flaherty, 2011; Hipp & Ely, 2012). Therefore, timely diagnosis and treatment are paramount to minimize both the duration of the acute episode and the longer term sequelae.

Clinical Features of Delirium

The clinical features of delirium can include changes in behavior, personality, and cognition, as described in this section.

CHANGES IN ATTENTION AND AWARENESS

Patients experiencing delirium may have difficulty maintaining attention to a specific task, or even to an interview question. They may be distractible or unable to shift attention to a second task when asked to do so. This may be demonstrated by perseveration on a topic, even after they have been asked repeatedly to shift focus. Patients with delirium may be somnolent (unable to maintain wakefulness) or simply unfocused and nonresponsive to stimuli. It is not uncommon for a patient with delirium to fall asleep repeatedly during an interview. Some patients will doze off midsentence and after a few seconds will wake and continue speaking, only to doze off again a few seconds later. In other cases, patients may physically orient to the interviewer but not respond verbally.

COGNITIVE CHANGES

Delirium usually involves acute cognitive changes that are a notable change from the patient's baseline cognitive functioning. These cognitive changes can take a variety of forms, and there is no consistent pattern to the cognitive deficits that a patient will demonstrate. Patients with delirium may evidence problems with orientation, memory, perception, language, visuospatial deficits, poor judgment, executive functioning, or other aspects of cognition. A patient may demonstrate a host of acute cognitive changes or may demonstrate one cognitive change in an otherwise intact cognitive picture. For example, one patient with no history of cognitive problems was able to provide a completely correct mental status examination, except that she believed it was 1984 (in 2015). Alternatively, a patient may provide a mental status examination that shows deficits in orientation, short- and long-term memory, and also attention.

RAPID ONSET

Delirium typically develops over hours. That is, an initial symptom may be noted and then other symptoms continue to unfold until significant impairment is evident. These symptoms are a notable change from the patient's baseline (e.g., disorientation in a patient who has never had problems with orientation previously or a patient who believes he saw cats running around in the hospital room late last night in the context of no history of psychopathology or dementia). Because the delirium results from a medical problem, as the medical issue intensifies, the symptoms of delirium intensify as well (e.g., as an infection takes hold in the patient's body, the symptoms of delirium begin to appear and may increase in severity as the infection does). Similarly, as the infection is treated, the symptoms of delirium will gradually decrease until the patient returns to his cognitive and emotional baseline.

FLUCTUATING COURSE

It can be difficult to diagnose delirium because the symptoms can fluctuate, called *waxing and waning*. It is not uncommon for one provider to assess a patient and diagnose delirium based on the symptoms described here. When another provider reevaluates the patient a few hours later, the patient may present a different picture (e.g., he is aware that there were no cats in the hospital last night and is correctly oriented to time). For this reason, the symptoms need to be tracked carefully over time, or it could be incorrectly determined that a delirium has cleared when, in fact, the symptoms have simply fluctuated.

PSYCHOTIC SYMPTOMS

For psychologists, it is natural to think about schizophrenia or some other psychopathology with psychotic symptoms when a patient demonstrates hallucinations, delusions, or paranoia. Hallucinations are not uncommon in delirium, and these hallucinations are likely to be visual hallucinations, rather than auditory hallucinations, which are found more commonly in schizophrenia (Slooter, Van De Leur, & Zaal, 2017; Wise, Hilty, Cerda, & Trzepacz, 2002). The hallucinations may be frightening to the individual (e.g., people coming through the walls who intend to harm the patient; soldiers running through the hospital hallway with guns). In these cases, patients may try to climb out of bed and run away and can hurt themselves in the process. This scenario is often responsible for a patient's fall out of the bed, an attempt to jump out a window, or a patient who is roaming the stairwell looking for a way to escape. Alternately, the hallucinations may not be frightening at all and could be comforting to the patient; one patient reported that Superman was hovering outside her hospital window to keep her safe; another patient was happy about the puppies that she saw in a basket in the corner of her hospital room.

Paranoia is a common accompaniment to delirium and may be focused on medical staff or family members. Patients with delirium may be fearful that nurses and doctors are trying to harm or kill them, rather than help them. This can result in patients being uncooperative, combative, or feeling they need to leave the hospital to protect themselves. This presentation is clearly paranoid and needs to be distinguished from the more normal discomfort of an elderly patient who is alone at the hospital, slightly hard of hearing, and worried that the nurses are talking about her (which they are, in the course of managing the patient's medical care). This experience is uncomfortable for the patient but would not be a sign of delirium if the patient does not feel the staff is plotting to harm her and she remains intact cognitively and psychologically.

Delusions may be associated with the paranoia (e.g., the patient may describe how and why a nurse is planning to hurt him) or can occur independently. One patient described in great detail how she was taken from the hospital in the middle of the night to go shopping for a new dress and some flowers for an upcoming family event. She described the experience as pleasant for her. Another patient described being taken on a harrowing car ride with bank robbers who were being chased by the police. Patients who describe situations like these are usually unable to explain how they got out of and back into the hospital. Although many descriptions of events such as these are clearly delusional, others are not so clear. One female patient described inappropriate fondling and sexual activity with a male nurse the previous night. In this case, there were no other signs of delirium at the time, so more data needed to be gathered to determine whether the sexual activity had actually occurred or if this was a delusion as part of a delirium (more detail on this case is in Chapter 16 of this volume).

IRRATIONAL THINKING

Patients who are delirious are often not thinking clearly, and this can be evidenced by poor insight and judgment. For example, one patient believed that nurses were trying to hurt him, so he decided to sneak out of the hospital to drive home where he would be safe. This occurred after an abdominal surgery that made it impossible for him to ambulate independently, his car was not at the hospital, and he wouldn't have been able to drive it anyway. The patient lived alone and would have been unable to care for himself even if he did get home safely. Despite all these reasons why going home by himself was not a good plan, the patient was certain it was a good idea to try to escape the hospital to save himself from the nurses. Because delirium may decrease a patient's ability to make rational decisions and use good judgment, it can affect their ability to make rational decisions about their medical care. Especially if a patient is making decisions about refusing a lifesaving treatment, the psychologist needs to be sure that the patient is thinking rationally and has the capacity to make his own decisions. (Decisional capacity is discussed further in Chapter 11.)

UNCHARACTERISTIC BEHAVIORAL AND EMOTIONAL REACTIONS

Family members or medical personnel who know the patient well may first notice changes in the patient's behavior. This typically involves irritability, uncooperativeness, or emotional lability in a patient who is typically calm and polite. Although all patients have bad days and may react strongly to problems with the hospital admission or a bad diagnosis, the personality changes associated with delirium are often dramatic and more intense than emotional reactions that would be expected when patients get bad news or have other problems in the hospital. (Some patients tend to be more characterologically oppositional and irritable; for them, the irritable and uncooperative behavior would not suggest delirium as it would in the person who is always friendly and cooperative.) One patient's daughter tearfully explained that her father had always been supportive of her, but today he has been swearing at her—which had never happened before—and berating her for a variety of issues. He was also uncooperative with requests to take medications, allow blood draws, and shower, and he threw his lunch tray at a nurse. All of this was completely atypical for him. Similarly, a patient might refuse to call a nurse for pain medication or help getting to the bathroom because of anger at some mistreatment they feel a nurse has committed against them.

HYPERACTIVITY OR HYPOACTIVITY

Patients can experience either increased or decreased psychomotor activity during an episode of delirium, or a mixed presentation. Hyperactivity or agitation can involve aggressive behavior toward providers, physically running to escape from perceived threats, picking at bedding and hair, or pulling out IV lines or other medical equipment. Often referred to as *excited delirium*, this type of delirium is also associated with violent encounters with police outside the hospital setting, often due to drug toxicity (Gill, 2014). Patients with hyperactivity are easiest to diagnose because their symptoms are observable, but they can be dangerous to manage because they may be frightened and trying to protect themselves while not thinking clearly.

In contrast, a hypoactive delirium is often more difficult to diagnose because the patient may be calm and appear comfortable, without dramatic behavioral changes or overt psychotic symptoms. The delirium diagnosis is often missed or may be mistaken for depression. Hypoactive presentations of delirium are commonly seen in palliative care settings (Friedlander, Brayman, & Breitbart, 2004; Leonard et al., 2014), but are seen in hospitals as well. A patient with a hypoactive delirium will be able to provide little help in making the diagnosis because she may be only minimally verbal, so most data will need to be gathered from other sources.

As mentioned earlier, patients who are agitated may pull out IV lines, feeding tubes, or catheters and may extubate themselves. Either physical or chemical restraints may be necessary to keep them from unintentionally harming themselves. However, hypoactive patients may also be at risk for these same issues. Often hypoactive patients will continue to touch and play with lines, ultimately pulling them out, although without the overt intent that may be seen in hyperactive patients. With quietly delirious patients, it is tempting to explain repeatedly what the line or tube is for, reminding them to leave it alone. They will acknowledge what was said and may even stop for the moment, but they are soon back to manipulating the line, either because they do not remember what they were just told or because they are unable to tolerate the discomfort that would be manageable if they were cognitively and psychologically intact.

Some causes of delirium are associated with specific presentations. Hepatic encephalopathy, for example, is a type of delirium caused by decreased functioning of the liver and occurs commonly in patients with chronic liver disease who are waiting for a liver transplant. These patients may have repeated episodes of hepatic encephalopathy that are associated with changes in liver functioning over time. The patient's speech, thinking, and behavior are all slowed, and the patient may have difficulty staying awake. If not treated, the liver function will continue to deteriorate, and the patient's behavior and cognition will slow more and more, resulting ultimately in coma and death.

Patients with hypo- and hyperactive delirium may demonstrate similar problems with cognition and other symptoms, and the main difference may be only in terms of activity. Further, a patient may evidence a mixed picture in which he is active and combative at times but hypoactive and lethargic at others. Liptzin and Levkoff (1992) initially described the characteristics of the three subtypes (i.e., hyperactive, hypoactive, mixed). Current research is inconsistent on the association between the etiology of the delirium and the demonstrated motoric subtype (e.g., Meagher et al., 2011; Meagher, O'Hanlon, O'Mahony, Casey, & Trzepacz, 2000), although the subtype does seem to be related to outcome, with those demonstrating a hypoactive delirium having the poorest survival (Meagher et al., 2011).

REVERSIBILITY

Delirium is a temporary state that resolves when its cause is treated. Delirium symptoms then resolve, restoring the patient to her baseline cognitive and emotional state. As the patient is being treated for the cause of the delirium, the psychologist can often observe the symptoms improve, until the patient is back to baseline. One exception, however, occurs in patients who are nearing death and in whom the causes of the delirium cannot be adequately treated and resolved, such as in the case of a patient with organ failure that cannot be repaired. In these cases, although theoretically reversible, the delirium cannot be reversed. This is sometimes referred to as a *terminal delirium*.

THE DELIRIUM EXPERIENCE

In a review of qualitative studies of the delirium experience, Bélanger and Ducharme (2011) reported on several studies in which patients felt distressed due to confusion and feeling they had no control over the situation. Patients described frightening experiences in which they were in danger or held against their will. They felt disoriented and confused and experienced hallucinations and illusions. Some patients described feeling suspicious of others and felt that their lives were at risk. Some reported a need to escape to save their lives, while others distanced themselves from family members or behaved aggressively to medical staff. They also reported difficulty communicating their concerns to others.

Misak (2004) presented an excellent description of a patient's experience of psychotic symptoms while in the ICU, noting that the experience is particularly frightening because the delusions and hallucinations mix with reality so that it is difficult to sort out what is true and what is not. This is further complicated if the patient is intubated and unable to discuss the experiences with others. Misak also noted the problems created in the patient–physician relationship if the patient believes the medical staff are conspiring against her.

Sample 9.1 presents the evaluation of a patient with a hypoactive delirium, who is unable to maintain wakefulness and demonstrates problems with orientation and memory. Note the brevity of the report—the patient was a poor reporter, and there was little additional history available. The initial evaluation was done by a trainee, with a follow-up visit a few hours later by the faculty supervisor.

Causes of Delirium

Delirium involves psychological, cognitive, and behavioral changes that occur due to a medical problem or a drug. It may also occur in the context of multiple causes in which each issue itself is not sufficient to cause the delirium but the combination of factors results in symptoms. Unless the specific cause or causes are properly diagnosed and treated, the delirium will not clear, and the patient will have ongoing symptoms. Exhibit 9.1 lists some of the major causes of delirium. Although each of these factors has been associated with the development of delirium, it is not the case that every individual who experiences one of these problems will have an episode of delirium. Delirium occurs most frequently in those who are physically or cognitively vulnerable: people with serious medical problems and the elderly. Delirium often occurs when a precipitating factor or factors (such as those in Exhibit 9.1) occur in a patient with preexisting risk factors (e.g., dementia, hearing or vision impairment, old age; Inouye et al., 2014).

The most common cause of delirium is infections, specifically urinary tract infections (UTIs) and respiratory infections or pneumonia in older adults (Arinzon, Peisakh, Schrire, & Berner, 2011; Eriksson, Gustafson, Fagerström, & Olofsson, 2011). Infections in a generally healthy adult will not typically result in delirium, but in an elderly patient with multiple medical problems or mild dementia, a seemingly simple infection can result in visual hallucinations, disorientation, agitation, and other symptoms of delirium. Almost any infection can result in or contribute to the development of delirium in a patient with risk factors such as old age or serious medical illness.

Drugs and medications account for a large portion of delirium diagnoses. It may be obvious that abuse, intoxication, and withdrawal from street drugs or alcohol can result in delirium, but many prescription medications can also cause delirium (Flaherty, 2011; Maldonado, 2008). Medications with anticholinergic effects are especially likely to cause cognitive and behavioral changes (including tricyclic antidepressants and

EXHIBIT 9.1
Etiologies of Delirium

Infections: urinary tract infection, respiratory infections/pneumonia, sepsis, HIV, meningitis, encephalitis
Medications/drugs
- Use: chemotherapy drugs (e.g., methotrexate, cisplatin, prednisone, bleomycin, vincristine); H2 antagonists (Pepcid, Tagamet, Zantac); narcotic pain meds (codeine, morphine, meperidine); steroids (e.g., prednisone, cortisone, dexamethasone); anticholinergic drugs (tricyclic antidepressants, antihistamines)
- Abuse/intoxication: antidepressants, lithium, antihypertensive drugs, digoxin, street drugs (amphetamines, cocaine, PCP), alcohol
- Withdrawal: benzodiazepines, barbiturates, alcohol

Metabolic: electrolyte imbalances (hyponatremia; hypo- and hypercalcemia), hypoxia, dehydration, liver or renal failure
Neurologic: hemorrhage, epilepsy, concussion, stroke
Cardiac: congestive heart failure, myocardial infarction
Endocrine: hyper/hypothyroid, hypo/hyperglycemia
Deficiencies: vitamin B_{12}, folate, thiamine
Other toxins: heavy metals, carbon monoxide, pesticides

antihistamines; Krishnan, Leung, & Caplan, 2014), and many chemotherapy drugs can result in delirium (e.g., Breitbart & Cohen, 1998). Narcotic pain medications can cause hallucinations, vivid and upsetting dreams, and confusion. For all of these medications, decreasing the dose of the medication may help to decrease the symptoms of delirium, or switching to another medication may resolve the problem; for example, in the case of pain medications, a nonnarcotic pain medication may accomplish the same pain relief without the narcotic side effects. Especially if the delirium is severe, discontinuing the medication or replacing it with something else should result in improvement or disappearance of the symptoms. In some cases, however, the specific medication that seems to be causing the delirium is required for adequate treatment of the medical issue. In these cases, the medication must be continued, and the symptoms of delirium must be managed for the duration of the medication use.

When corticosteroids are a cause, the delirium may be referred to as a *steroid psychosis*. Chapter 7 describes some of the common side effects of steroids; some of these, although creating a challenge for the patient to manage (e.g., poor sleep, weight gain, nervousness), would not qualify as delirium. These symptoms may be disruptive and upsetting to the patient, but they would not be diagnosed as delirium unless additional symptoms typical of delirium are present.

Other side effects of steroids, such as psychotic symptoms and cognitive changes, could result in a diagnosis of delirium. A steroid psychosis most commonly occurs with high doses of corticosteroids (generally more than 40 mg prednisone equivalent per day; West & Kenedi, 2014) with symptom onset during the first week or two of treatment (Kenna, Poon, de los Angeles, & Koran, 2011). The occurrence of a steroid psychosis is not correlated with a previous negative reaction to corticosteroids or a past history of psychosis (Kenna et al., 2011). The usual presentation of a steroid-induced psychosis includes restlessness and agitation, hallucinations, delusions, emotional lability, and, at times, suicidal ideation. Making the correct diagnosis is important; if these symptoms were misdiagnosed as generalized anxiety disorder and treated with cognitive strategies, the treatment would have little effect.

Another scenario for delirium occurs when a medication becomes toxic, either because too much has been administered or because the medication isn't clearing properly from the patient's body and builds up. One example of a medication that can become toxic is digoxin, a medication commonly used to treat cardiac problems. If the digoxin level in the blood becomes too high, the patient can become delirious. Delirium has also occurred secondary to lithium toxicity (Wilkinson, Gavine, & Black, 2009) and discontinuation of lithium (Lin & Mao, 2010).

The H2 antagonists (blockers) are used to treat gastroesophageal reflux disease. Several, such as Pepcid, Tagamet, and Zantac, are sold over the counter. These are commonly used and tolerated by most people but can result in delirium in those who are vulnerable, usually the elderly (Tawadrous et al., 2014). Symptoms may include confusion, agitation, and hallucinations. One patient had multiple medical problems and took a variety of narcotics for pain without any problems. When an H2 blocker was started to protect her stomach from irritation caused by other medications, she developed hallucinations of people coming through the hospital room walls. These hallucinations were frightening to her and occurred consistently until the H2 blocker was discontinued. The hallucinations did not recur.

Finally, a patient may tolerate individual drugs, but as additional medications are added, the interactions may cause side effects that cause delirium. For example, even if a patient tolerates lithium on its own, if it is combined with other medications, the interaction effects can result in delirium (e.g., Faaij, Ziere, Zietse, & Van der Cammen, 2009; Miodownik, Alkatnany, Frolova, & Lerner, 2008). Because many medical inpatients take numerous medications, one important aspect of the delirium workup includes an assessment of the specific medications being taken as well as the potential interactions among them.

Electrolyte abnormalities are common in medical inpatients and can result in the cognitive or behavioral changes of delirium. Specifically, hyponatremia (low sodium), hypercalcemia (high calcium), hyper- or hypomagnesemia, and hypophosphatemia are some of the more common electrolyte problems that can result in delirium (Frontera, 2012).

Hypoxia occurs when the patient does not have enough oxygen, and the brain is unable to function properly. This is typically remedied by the administration of supplemental oxygen to the patient. Liver and kidney failure result in the toxins that are typically removed by these organs remaining in the system, resulting in cognitive and behavioral changes. Kidney patients on dialysis can often correlate changes in cognition with their dialysis schedule; if dialysis does not occur, the symptoms worsen, ultimately increasing to a clinical delirium and death if the situation is not remedied with transplant or dialysis.

Strokes, hemorrhage, and myocardial infarction are a few of the neurological and cardiovascular insults that can cause delirium. Often these medical issues are acute in nature, and the resultant delirium may improve slowly after the acute issue is remedied. Thyroid problems can result in a variety of psychological symptoms, including anxiety, depression, and delirium. Similarly, significant changes in blood sugar can result in delirium, coma, and death if the problem is not promptly diagnosed and treated. Nutritional deficiencies, such as thiamine, B_{12}, niacin, and folate can also be causes of delirium (Frontera, 2012), as can dehydration.

Uncommon causes of delirium in medical inpatients include toxins, such as pesticides, carbon monoxide, and heavy metals. These causes are generally only explored if all of the more common causes of delirium have already been ruled out but symptoms remain.

Assessment and Diagnosis

The assessment of a delirious patient may be different from a typical evaluation. Many delirious patients are unable to provide accurate data, so other sources of information may need to be relied on.

THE REFERRAL

It is rare that patients are referred with a diagnosis of delirium; more common is a referral for uncooperativeness or changes in behavior. Physicians may see a patient who is angry or refusing medications and procedures and become concerned that there is a psychiatric or personality issue that will interfere with the medical treatment. It is often helpful to ask the referral source what it is that she saw that prompted the referral. Uncooperativeness, excessive reactions to pain, suspiciousness, mutism, somnolence, poor understanding of the medical situation, wandering, and aggressive behavior might all be symptoms of delirium. Knowing what specific behaviors have prompted the referral can aid the consultant with the evaluation and diagnosis of the patient. With thorough evaluation, the psychologist can determine whether these symptoms signify a delirium or some other psychological problem. Because the incorrect diagnosis will result in the incorrect treatment, it is vital to establish the correct diagnosis for each patient.

The overall approach to the assessment of delirium is similar to the general biopsychosocial evaluation described previously. The main difference is that patients with delirium may be unable to participate in a long interview, due to somnolence, irritability, or paranoia. These symptoms may mean it is necessary to keep the interview with the patient brief and to rely on other data to make the diagnosis.

MEDICAL RECORD REVIEW

When there is a question of delirium, the medical chart should be thoroughly reviewed for evidence of acute changes in behavior and cognition, current medical issues, medications that are associated with delirium, and any history that could account for cognitive or psychotic symptoms. For example, in an emergency department note, a newly admitted patient with multiple chronic medical problems was described as agitated, uncooperative, and disoriented when arriving at the hospital, and the patient's daughter said that he might have taken his multiple medications twice today (instead of once as prescribed). Another patient, recently discharged from the hospital after a cycle of chemotherapy, was unable to stay awake at home for several days. She stopped answering the telephone because she felt the FBI was listening in and trying to trap her, and she had never demonstrated symptoms like this before. In each of these cases, the symptoms had an acute onset, seemed to be associated with a change in the patient's medical situation, and there was no previous history of psychiatric problems, suggesting the possibility of delirium.

A review of the patient's history and current medical issues will provide clues to the presence of a delirium. Exhibit 9.2 summarizes specific information in the medical record that can aid the psychology consultant when dealing with a potential delirium. For example, a patient who had a recent stroke or a new infection, or a patient who recently started high-dose steroids or a new chemotherapy medication, would raise questions about the possibility of delirium in response to these medical issues. A review of vital signs could show that the patient has developed a fever over the past few hours that might reflect a new infection that has not yet been diagnosed. Further, current laboratory results may demonstrate that a patient has new metabolic abnormalities (e.g., hyponatremia [low sodium] or hypercalcemia [high calcium]) that could explain a delirium.

Past notes in the medical record should be reviewed to determine whether the patient has a history of problems that could present with symptoms similar to those of delirium. A patient with a history of schizophrenia may have psychotic symptoms that indicate psychiatric decompensation rather than delirium. However, both possibilities need to be evaluated thoroughly because people with a history of psychosis can also develop delirium due to an underlying medical problem and the current symptoms may have nothing to do with the premorbid psychiatric issue.

A history of dementia is especially important when considering a diagnosis of delirium. The symptoms of delirium and dementia overlap to some extent (see Leonard et al., 2014, for a comparison of the features of delirium and dementia in palliative care), but it will be important to obtain the correct diagnosis because the course and treatment of these disorders are different. Delirium is temporary and

EXHIBIT 9.2

Specific Issues to Attend to in the Medical Record When Assessing for Delirium

Admit and other current notes that contain data about the patient's current behavior and cognitive status, family reports of changes in cognition or behavior

Older notes that could include baseline information on mental status and psychological history and functioning (e.g., notes from neurology, family medicine, or psychiatry)

Results of tests and procedures that could show abnormalities associated with delirium

Medications associated with delirium

Vital signs, especially fevers

reversible, whereas dementia is chronic and progressive. Delirium is a medical emergency that warrants aggressive and immediate treatment; dementia is typically less of a medical emergency. However, individuals with dementia are more vulnerable to a delirium (e.g., Fick, Agostini, & Inouye, 2002; Leonard et al., 2014); one study of ICU patients reported that those with dementia were 40% more likely to be delirious, even after controlling for illness variables (McNicoll et al., 2003). Therefore, a patient's current presentation may reflect a delirium superimposed on a more chronic dementia. A delirium that is not treated (i.e., the underlying medical issue is not corrected) will certainly result in decreased quality of life for the patient and can result in injury and ultimately death. Knowing the patient's baseline cognitive and psychological status will help the psychologist evaluate the current symptoms, make the correct diagnosis, and then deliver the appropriate treatment. Sample 9.2 describes the case of a patient with a delirium superimposed on dementia who was admitted with infection.

THE PATIENT INTERVIEW

As noted earlier, the interview with the patient may need to be abbreviated and should focus on an assessment of the patient's cognitive status, as well as other symptoms of delirium. In addition to the standard assessment of cognition that would occur with any inpatient, additional assessment may be useful in patients for whom there are concerns about delirium. Drawings are often used (with both delirium and dementia patients) to evaluate a patient's constructional ability. Patients are simply asked to draw pictures—of a clock face designating a particular time, of a daisy in a flowerpot, or of a house, for example (see Strub & Black, 2000, for details on the administration and scoring of these and other drawings). A clock face is most commonly used and can demonstrate problems with fine motor behaviors, visual perception, and organization; patients may also provide additional information as they do the task, indicating that they don't understand the concept of time, for example. Wise et al. (2002) and Strub and Black (2000) all provide sample drawings and interpretations for patients with delirium or dementia.

Much of the standard biopsychosocial interview, and especially that dealing with psychological symptoms, will need to wait because delirious patients are unable to accurately report on psychological issues such as depression and anxiety (although they may be willing to provide information they think is accurate at the time). Yet the psychologist can learn much from observing the patient's behavior. For example, a patient with delirium may pick at the bedding or his clothing, may be distracted by visual hallucinations, and may be unable to stay awake or sit still. A constellation of behavioral and cognitive symptoms that are a change from the patient's baseline would suggest delirium.

Some patients with delirium are unable to articulate what is wrong or the symptoms they are experiencing, and others will not discuss their experience because they feel unsafe. It is often useful for the psychologist to ask whether the patient feels safe and, if not, then to attempt to make the patient more comfortable before proceeding with the evaluation. In many cases, patients are aware that something is wrong and that they are not themselves, although they may be unable to explain it any more than that. The psychologist can ask the patient if he does not feel like himself, is not right in his own body, or is not behaving as he typically would. Similarly, some patients can report that their memory and thinking are not as good as usual. They may also be able to acknowledge that they are having "strange" or "weird" experiences (e.g., seeing things that aren't really there). Patients often agree with the idea that they are unable to cope and feeling out of control, and that they are frightened and overwhelmed by their current experience. Patients can also be asked to notify their nurse if any "strange" experiences reoccur, although they may not do so because of poor memory or paranoia.

MEASURES TO ASSESS DELIRIUM

Many scales have been developed to assess the presence and severity of delirium (Grover & Kate, 2012, and Wong, Holroyd-Leduc, Simel, & Straus, 2010, provided good reviews). Some measures were developed as checklists for medical professionals to rate a patient's symptoms on the basis of their observations or interactions with the patient (e.g., Breitbart et al., 1997; Trzepacz, Baker, & Greenhouse, 1988). Other delirium assessment measures have been developed for a particular setting, such as the ICU (Confusion Assessment Method [CAM]–ICU; Ely et al., 2001) or the emergency department (CAM–ED; Lewis, Miller, Morley, Nork, & Lasater, 1995). Standardized cognitive screening measures are also useful in the evaluation of delirium (Mitchell, Shukla, Ajumal, Stubbs, & Tahir, 2014) but should be used in conjunction with other measures or data that address the noncognitive symptoms. Many of the scales developed to assess delirium have been used more frequently for research, but they can also be useful clinically.

Clinicians experienced with delirious patients become experts at noting even subtle changes in behavior and cognition and can then interview more thoroughly to elicit additional information to establish the correct diagnosis. For those new to working with delirious patients, it can be difficult to recognize subtle symptoms or to make the diagnosis for a patient who is largely rational. Structured measures can be useful in any case and may serve to draw the clinician's attention to relevant symptoms, as well as symptom severity. Outside of the research context, many delirium measures may be more useful qualitatively, that is, to focus attention on the relevant clinical symptoms, rather than to generate a specific score used to determine the diagnosis. At other times, especially if the clinician wishes to track changes in symptoms over time, a quantitative score is useful.

The CAM (Inouye et al., 1990), the Delirium Rating Scale—Revised (DRS–R–98; Trzepacz et al., 2001), and the Memorial Delirium Assessment Scale (MDAS; Breitbart et al., 1997) are three of the most popular quantitative measures to aid in the diagnosis of delirium. The CAM takes about 5 minutes to administer and involves rating symptoms of delirium such as attention, thinking, and agitation. It is likely the most commonly used screening measure for delirium. It does not require psychiatric training to administer, and it demonstrates good sensitivity and specificity (Inouye et al., 1990).

The DRS–R–98 is a revision of the original DRS (Trzepacz et al., 1988). It includes 16 items that address symptom presence and severity. It can be used as a brief screener for delirium and is useful for repeat evaluations over time. Proper use of the DRS–R–98 requires clinical expertise. Interrater reliability, internal consistency, sensitivity, and specificity are good, and cutoff scores for the diagnosis of delirium are provided (Trzepacz et al., 2001).

Finally, the MDAS is a 10-item rating scale in which clinicians rate symptoms of delirium based on the patient's recent behavior, using both cognitive and behavioral items (Breitbart et al., 1997). The MDAS demonstrates good interrater reliability and internal consistency, is correlated with other measures of delirium, and can differentiate delirious patients from other groups. It is designed for repeated use to track change over time (Grover & Kate, 2012).

COLLATERAL INFORMATION

When evaluating a potentially delirious patient, collateral information from someone who knows the patient well can provide the necessary baseline data from which to evaluate the current symptoms. This is especially important if there are no data regarding the patient's baseline functioning in the medical record and if a patient is unable to provide adequate information on his baseline functioning. Family members are often the first to notice changes in behavior and are able to provide detailed information on these changes. However, family members may also miss subtle changes, so the psychologist needs to ask appropriate questions to elicit the relevant information. When interviewing family members for information to aid in the diagnosis of delirium, it is useful to ask whether there is anything different about the patient over the past few days, in terms of behavior, thinking, and attention. Asking about confusion and the ability to remain awake is useful. Historic information can also be obtained from the family to help establish a baseline, specifically regarding a history of past cognitive problems or psychopathology. When asked specific questions, family members can often provide relevant data that they had not considered until they were asked pointed questions by the psychologist.

Even if family members are aware of and able to articulate information about acute changes in the patient's presentation, they often do not understand what the symptoms mean and may interpret changes in behavior as a personality issue that is under the patient's control, rather than the result of a medical problem. Family members often chide patients for uncooperativeness and other "bad" behavior and expect the patient to be able to control such behavior (which is unlikely). Educating the family of a delirious patient regarding what delirium is, what to expect from the patient, the expected course of the disorder, as well as what they can do to help, will be important in the overall management of the situation.

Treatment and Management

Once diagnosed, the first step in the treatment of the delirium involves treating the underlying medical issue (e.g., the UTI, kidney failure, or hyponatremia). The health psychology consultant is responsible for managing the patient's behavior and keeping him safe and comfortable as the medical treatment progresses. It is often the case that the medical issue causing the delirium is the same problem that brought the patient to the hospital, and this is often already being treated by the time the health psychologist has been consulted. For example, an elderly man diagnosed with delirium had been admitted to the hospital with a UTI and dehydration. He was being treated with antibiotics and fluids to address those medical issues, and some improvement, reflected in laboratory tests, had already occurred. As a result, the symptoms of delirium also began to subside.

While the patient is delirious, the psychologist should assess and monitor the patient's cognition and behavior daily to be sure the symptoms are decreasing as the medical treatment progresses, until the delirium clears completely. During this time, however, the patient needs to be kept safe and as comfortable as possible. Many delirious patients are frightened and may fear for their lives or those of family members, especially if they are paranoid, delusional, or hallucinating. These patients are at risk for hurting themselves in their efforts to protect themselves during this time. Further, they perceive a lack of understanding from others, and that may result in aggression or irritation (Fagerberg & Jonhagen, 2002). Even frail patients with IVs have been known to try to climb over the bed rails in an effort to escape, resulting in falls with broken bones and concussions, which place them at additional risk for further medical problems. Even if patients do not demonstrate psychotic symptoms, they may evidence poor judgment that puts them at risk (e.g., a patient attempts to leave the hospital because she feels she is doing OK and can manage at home on her own). Physical restraints may need to be used at times, but these should be avoided as much as possible because it frightens patients even more, reinforces the belief that others are out to hurt them and does nothing to help the symptoms of delirium.

It is critical to help the patient feel safe and comfortable for the duration of the delirium. The best strategy is to have a support person (a close family member or friend) stay with the patient—all day and all night, if possible. This support person may be the only person in the hospital that the patient trusts while in this state. A family member who has been educated about delirium and what she can do to help the patient cope with the experience can reassure the patient and help him to stay calm. The support person can also be an ally when the patient is dealing with nurses that he doesn't trust and can explain medical issues and plans for the patient's medical treatment, procedures, and tests. If a family member or friend is not available, many hospitals have "sitters"; these are typically off-duty nurses, certified nursing assistants, or students who simply stay with the patient to monitor his safety and to keep him physically and emotionally comfortable. Because sitters are initially unfamiliar to the patient, they are less good at comforting and reassuring the patient, but they can observe the patient to ensure that he doesn't do anything to inadvertently hurt himself.

Exhibit 9.3 lists general strategies for managing the delirious patient while waiting for the causative medical issues to resolve (see also Irwin, Pirrello, Hirst, Buckholz, & Ferris, 2013; Mittal et al., 2011; and Slooter et al., 2017). It is important to provide delirious patients with ongoing information to help with their perception

EXHIBIT 9.3
Management of Delirious Patients

Enlist a support person to stay with the patient to promote comfort.
Reorient the patient frequently.
Educate the patient and family regarding delirium symptoms, causes, expectations.
Avoid restraining the patient if possible.
Use familiar medical providers.
Use pharmacological management of symptoms as needed.
Improve communication as much as possible (e.g., make sure patient has glasses, hearing aids).
Promote sleep.
Ensure physical safety.

and cognition. Leaving lights on makes the hospital room less frightening and may enable patients to remain oriented, relax, and sleep. Similarly, open blinds, clocks in the room, and familiar nurses who make eye contact and continue to reorient the patient can be helpful. Patients should also be given any relevant aids to improve their perception and communication, such as glasses and hearing aids. In addition, it is important to promote appropriate sleep and to put plans in place to avoid falls.

Educating the patient may also help him to deal with the delirium. This education will be very basic, but would (a) empathize with the patient that he is "not himself" right now (because of the medical problem or medication) and that (b) medical staff will help him to get through this and he should be back to his baseline behavior and cognition soon. Delirious patients may forget this information, but it may temporarily comfort them to understand that their providers are aware of what they are experiencing and trying to help. Once the delirium has cleared, most people do not remember it. Some do, however, and may have difficulty coming to terms with the experience of being out of control. They may also experience fears that it will reoccur. Education about what has happened and why it resolved may provide some comfort.

The best approach is to facilitate the patient's comfort and safety using nonpharmacological measures while the medical issue responsible for the delirium is being treated. However, in many cases, pharmacotherapy is needed to manage the patient's behavior, especially if the patient is hyperactive, psychotic, and aggressive, because these factors place them at risk for additional harm. Several authors have described specific dosing requirements and the efficacy of various psychotropic medications that can be used for this purpose (e.g., Hipp & Ely, 2012; Mittal et al., 2011; Zaal & Slooter, 2012). The first line of treatment for delirium is haloperidol, especially for patients who are agitated; other medications commonly used to treat the symptoms of delirium include atypical antipsychotics such as olanzapine, quetiapine, risperidone, and ziprasidone (e.g., Irwin et al., 2013). Consultation-liaison psychiatrists in the inpatient medical setting are experts in the use of these medications to control the symptoms of delirium and should always be consulted when medical management is warranted in addition to the nonpharmacological management strategies.

Because of the high incidence of delirium in the inpatient setting, especially in the elderly population, recent work has been focused on interventions designed to prevent the development of delirium in the first place. Early assessment for delirium symptoms, creating an environment that provides lighting and signs to improve orientation, attention to specific medical issues that are frequently associated with delirium, medication and nutrition reviews, promoting sleep, and an educated medical team are all important components of delirium-prevention programs (e.g., Kalish, Gillham, & Unwin, 2014; O'Mahony, Murthy, Akunne, & Young, 2011). The Hospital Elder Life Program, a comprehensive plan to prevent delirium and optimize functioning in elderly hospitalized patients, has shown success in improving outcomes for patients (Reuben et al., 2000).

In summary, delirium is often an unknown entity for psychologists without experience in the inpatient medical setting. Careful assessment is important to obtain the correct diagnosis and etiology of the delirium. Then, while the medical issues are being treated, the psychologist can help manage the patient's behavior and comfort.

Sample 9.1 Report—Hypoactive Delirium

Pt referred by Dr. S for health psych eval; concern is that pt has been tired and sad past few days. She is a 64 y/o AA woman with CABG at outside hospital last year, L AKA 2 mts ago, admitted now with wound infection, on dialysis.

Pt was somnolent. She reports that she has 3 children and was living with her daughters PTA. She denies any previous inpt or outpt psych tx, no hx of emotional problems. Pt today denies feelings of depression, sadness, anxiety, worry, suicidal ideation, hallucinations, paranoia. She says there is nothing bothering her.

Pt also denies any problems with her thinking or her memory, although this is inconsistent with her performance on mental status exam. Pt oriented to person, but not to place—although she was able to select hospital from a list of possible places. She thinks it is 2/19/83 (it is 6/5/2016). Registration and long-term memory intact; short-term memory moderately impaired (1/3).

Impressions:

Pt is somnolent, dozed off many times during this interview. Her thinking is very slow. She is disoriented to time, and her short-term memory is poor. She denies psych sx, but her report is questionable due to cognitive impairments.

d/w Dr. S who indicated that this presentation is not pt's baseline. Please seek and treat reversible causes of delirium. We will follow to monitor cognition and to evaluate mood when pt is able. Thanks. Pager xxx.

Follow-up note:

Pt was asleep on approach but was easily awakened. Her speech was slowed and quiet. She was disoriented to both date (3/24/93) and place (she was able to say she was in a hospital but did not know the name of the hospital, the city, or the state). She correctly reported her birthdate and her current age, but this information was provided in response to an unrelated question ("how is your mood today"). We will continue to follow to monitor mental status. Should pt's cognition improve, we will assess for mood and coping. Please page with questions, # xxxx

Sample 9.2
Report—Delirium and Dementia

Pt referred by Dr. S with concerns about being able to manage at home alone. Chart reviewed; pt interviewed as well as daughter, landlady, and pt's nurse.

Pt with aortic aneurysm, glaucoma, HTN. Admitted with UTI. Inpatient meds are Bactrim, Tagamet, Colace, slo mag, Tylenol. No hx substance abuse.

Pt is 84 y/o WF. She lives alone, in same apartment × 46 yrs. Landlady reports pt's apartment is filthy and animal-infested, stove does not work, windows do not open. Landlady has been trying to remedy these issues, but pt resists. Pt was briefly married once, raised one daughter on her own. Daughter and son-in-law live about 1,200 miles away. Pt completed 3 yrs h.s. and worked at various jobs until retirement.

Pt reports that she doesn't cook but can care for herself, and spends her days downtown with friends. No previous psych hx. She denies depression, suicidal/homicidal ideation, hallucinations, appetite/sleep problems, panic. Pt reports decreased energy and high anxiety most of her life. Pt friendly and cooperative during eval today.

Pt was agitated and hostile last week in ICU; she does not recall that now. She has had several head injuries due to falls and mugging. She denies subjective memory problems. On exam today, pt was alert and oriented × 3. Immediate memory 3/3, recent memory impaired (0/3 after 5 min). Pt refused serial 7's, could spell WORLD, refused backwards. Pt can name common objects, follow 3-stage command, name 2 presidents and mayor, knows own address, not phone number.

Impression: Delirium—cleared; Dementia.

Recommendations: Pt was most likely delirious on admission, due to anemia, UTI, decreased Mg, and these factors accounted for her behavior and confusion. These issues are now corrected or improved, and pt has returned to baseline. Impairments suggest dementia. 1) Pt can live independently and care for herself ONLY with significant input from others, e.g., social services, family, friends. 2) Due to poor memory, judgment, and understanding of medical condition, pt cannot function totally on her own, without help. She cannot take care of daily meds and medical issues. 3) Consider further dementia w/u.

Thanks, please call with questions, pager # xxxx

d/w Dr. S

Substance Use and Abuse

10

Substance use and abuse play significant roles in the medical issues of many hospitalized patients. Estimates of alcohol misuse range from 16% to 30% (Kouimtsidis et al., 2003), and 34% of patients referred for psychiatric consultations have substance use problems (Specker, Meller, & Thurber, 2009). Usually patients who are acutely intoxicated or high are seen in the emergency department, and most or all of the effects of the substance have worn off by the time they are admitted to the hospital floor, so these patients are rarely seen by inpatient psychology consultants. Patients are most often referred because a substance is having a negative impact on a medical problem. Although treatment typically takes longer than an inpatient medical admission, the psychologist has an opportunity to provide a positive beginning to treatment while the patient is admitted.

Hospital Admissions Associated With Alcohol

Inpatient referrals to psychology may be made for the management of patients who are (a) actively withdrawing from alcohol, (b) admitted for treatment of a medical issue directly caused by alcohol, or (c) being treated for an unrelated

http://dx.doi.org/10.1037/0000108-011
Health Psychology Consultation in the Inpatient Medical Setting, by S. M. Labott

medical problem that has been affected by alcohol use. Each of these scenarios is discussed in the following sections.

WITHDRAWAL

Alcohol withdrawal may be the reason for a patient's hospital admission because medical management may be necessary to ensure the patient is safe medically and physically. Withdrawal from alcohol can present with mild to quite severe symptoms, with the most severe symptoms related to greater alcohol use. Symptoms of alcohol withdrawal can begin a few hours or up to 10 days after the patient's last drink or significant decrease in drinking. Initial symptoms of alcohol withdrawal can include nausea and vomiting, diaphoresis, tremor, anxiety, irritability, agitation, decreased concentration, distractibility, memory problems, and decreased judgment (Saitz, Ciraulo, Shader, & Ciraulo, 2003; Vale, 2008). Alcohol withdrawal seizures can occur, as well as hallucinations, which are most often auditory (Maldonado, 2010). Delirium tremens (DTs) can begin within a few days and is characterized by similar symptoms of increased severity, as well as by agitated confusion, sympathetic overactivity, mental status changes, combativeness, and tremor (Hyman, 1994; Maldonado, 2010; Schuckit, 2009). Without treatment, 15% of patients who experience DTs will die; in patients with certain medical illnesses, mortality increases to 20% (Maldonado, 2010).

Although withdrawal symptoms would be expected in a patient with a known alcohol problem, in the hospital setting, withdrawal can occur unexpectedly. Many people drink alcohol heavily, and daily, yet do not consider themselves to be alcoholics, and there may not be any social or medical problems associated with the heavy alcohol use. If a person with this history is admitted to the hospital with appendicitis, for an elective surgical procedure, or for many other issues not typically associated with alcohol, the patient's alcohol use would probably not be flagged as a problem. Yet a few days in to the hospital admission, this patient could begin to demonstrate withdrawal symptoms that warrant immediate treatment, as described in Exhibit 10.1.

The treatment for alcohol withdrawal involves management of any related medical issues, such as correcting electrolyte imbalances, improving nutrition, replenishing fluids, and managing seizures. Sedative-hypnotics are used to decrease withdrawal symptoms and to decrease the discomfort experienced by patients, and benzodiazepines are the treatment of choice for the prevention of seizures and delirium (e.g., Amato, Minozzi, Vecchi, & Davoli, 2010). Vale (2008) and Maldonado (2010) described recommended dosing regimens for a variety of sedative-hypnotics to manage alcohol withdrawal. Behavioral management components are also important aspects of the withdrawal protocol and may include frequent reorientation of the patient, maintenance of a typical sleep–wake cycle with proper lighting, and measures to keep patients physically safe (e.g., sitters or restraints; Maldonado, 2010).

MEDICAL PROBLEMS ASSOCIATED WITH ALCOHOL USE

Even if a patient is not actively withdrawing from alcohol, chronic and heavy use of alcohol is associated with a variety of medical problems. Cerebellar degeneration

EXHIBIT 10.1

Alcohol Withdrawal

Mrs. J is a 47 y/o Caucasian woman admitted with irregular heartbeat. She is married for 22 years and has two children in high school. She has a master's degree and works as the principal of an elementary school. She has good family support.

Mrs. J had no history of psychotherapy or inpatient psych admissions. She took an antidepressant for about 4 months after the death of her mother about 10 years ago. No history of drug or alcohol treatment or problems.

The patient was admitted to the cardiac unit for heart monitoring and for workup of likely atrial fibrillation. About 30 hours into the admission, she became confused and agitated and reported tactile hallucinations (something crawling on her skin). She could acknowledge that she was not feeling like herself. Workup for delirium revealed no medical problems that could account for these symptoms, but interviews with the patient and her husband revealed that she drank about four glasses of wine each evening and that she had not had any alcohol for the past 2 days. The withdrawal symptoms were a surprise to the patient and also to the medical team.

The patient was treated with diazepam to help calm her and to manage the withdrawal symptoms. Within several hours, she was calm and comfortable.

Atrial fibrillation was conclusively diagnosed, and she was started on prophylactic medications (rivaroxaban) to decrease the likelihood of stroke if these episodes were ongoing. She was also encouraged to decrease alcohol intake, and she was willing to make plans to do so. These plans included strategies for her to use at home to decrease alcohol use, as well as a referral for outpatient substance use treatment.

(resulting in poor balance and gait problems), peripheral neuropathy, gastrointestinal problems (such as inflammation of the esophagus, cirrhosis, or pancreatitis), cardiovascular problems (hypertension and hypercholesterolemia), decreased white blood cell count, cancer, and sleep problems are all associated with heavy alcohol use (Schuckit, 2009). Patients may be admitted to the hospital for treatment of a medical issue for which alcohol abuse is the likely cause (e.g., liver failure associated with cirrhosis). In other cases, alcohol may contribute to the medical problem but is not a clear sole cause (e.g., hypertension). Alcohol can also affect the metabolism of some drugs, decreasing their positive impacts on the medical disease or increasing their effects to a level potentially harmful to the patient.

Patients admitted for a medical problem associated with alcohol are quite heterogeneous. Some individuals may be newly diagnosed with the medical problem and are still actively drinking or working toward abstinence. Others may have been diagnosed long ago and have been abstinent from alcohol for years; many others fall between those extremes of the continuum. The health psychology consultant will need to evaluate the patient to determine where he or she is on this continuum and will then be able to determine the appropriate intervention(s).

SEEMINGLY UNRELATED MEDICAL ISSUES

Many patients are admitted to the hospital for issues seemingly unrelated to alcohol, although alcohol use (perhaps not even abuse) plays a role in the patient's medical problem, often because it influences compliance with a medical regimen. For example, even if a patient does not drink alcohol frequently or excessively, there may be occasions during which she drinks minimally and then forgets to take her medication or to order refills of her prescriptions. Depending on the medical situation, even a few missed doses of her medications could have significant implications and result in a hospital admission. Alcohol use can also decrease motivation, resulting in missed doses of medication or missed medical appointments. Overall, excessive use of alcohol tends to decrease the patient's ability to manage the medical issues, and the greater the alcohol use and the more complicated the medical issues, the worse is the problem.

In many cases, doctors and nurses are well aware that the patient has an alcohol problem, either because the patient is actively demonstrating symptoms of abuse or withdrawal or because the patient is admitted with a diagnosis that has been documented previously as due to alcohol. In those cases, medical professionals are aware of and dealing with the role of alcohol in the patient's illness. In the case of the patient without clear medical issues related to alcohol, no one may suspect that alcohol is a problem until the psychologist interviews the patient and finds evidence that it plays a role in the patient's medical situation.

Illicit Drug Use

In 2014, 27 million Americans over age 12 (slightly more than 10% of the population) reported using illicit drugs (Center for Behavioral Health Statistics and Quality, 2015). Marijuana was the most frequently used illicit drug; others used were opioids, sedatives, stimulants, and hallucinogens.

OPIOIDS AND HEROIN

When used medically and in proper doses, opioids have few medical complications, but significant medical problems can occur when these drugs are used nonmedically or prescription drugs are overused or abused (as described later in this chapter). About 435,000 Americans use heroin; although it is used less often than many other illicit drugs, its use has recently increased dramatically (Center for Behavioral Health Statistics and Quality, 2015). Heroin is highly addictive, and its use is associated with increased mortality due to overdose, infections, and suicide (Strain, Lofwall, & Jaffe, 2009). In 2014, more than 11,000 hospital admissions were associated with heroin poisoning (Centers for Disease Control and Prevention [CDC], 2017).

Strain et al. (2009) described a variety of medical problems (e.g., skin infections, pulmonary emboli, staphylococcal pneumonitis, endocarditis, and septicemia) that occur when people do not use sterile procedures for injecting the drug. Other problems occur due to the injection process itself (e.g., edema, lymphadenopathy, skin popping) or due to contaminants from filters or injection materials that were intended for oral use. Heroin use also plays a role in the development of cardiac problems, HIV, tuberculosis, liver disease, chronic pain, and immune system dysfunction.

People using opioids for illicit purposes also have higher rates of comorbid psychiatric disorders, including mood and anxiety disorders and antisocial personality disorder (Strain et al., 2009).

Opioid withdrawal symptoms depend on the half-life of the drug and the chronicity of use; these begin about 10 hours after the last dose (Franklin, Leamon, & Frances, 2002). Opioid withdrawal symptoms include anxiety, cravings, and flulike symptoms (Franklin et al., 2002; Maldonado, 2010) that can last for several weeks. Methadone maintenance is the most common treatment for opioid addiction because it decreases the "high" and also the need to seek more drug to maintain a high. Buprenorphine is also used to treat opioid dependence (Franklin et al., 2002).

SEDATIVE-HYPNOTICS

About 330,000 people used sedatives for nonmedical reasons in 2014 (Center for Behavioral Health Statistics and Quality, 2015); benzodiazepines and barbiturates are those most commonly abused. Diazepam and alprazolam are the most commonly abused benzodiazepines, and they are often mixed with alcohol (Maldonado, 2010). Withdrawal symptoms generally begin a week to 10 days after stopping or reducing intake of the drug; withdrawal symptoms may occur also in patients using sedative-hypnotics appropriately for medical reasons but who abruptly stop the drug (e.g., if they run out of the medication). Symptoms of withdrawal from benzodiazepines include anxiety, psychosis, cognitive changes, agitation, and cardiovascular collapse (Franklin et al., 2002). Barbiturate withdrawal symptoms are similar and include uneasiness and anxiety, insomnia, anorexia, tremor, orthostatic hypotension, electroencephalographic changes, seizures, delirium, and hypothermia (Ciraulo & Sarid-Segal, 2009). Withdrawal symptoms are managed by a slow taper of the drug, typically using diazepam (for benzodiazepines) or pentobarbital (for barbiturates); Ciraulo and Sarid-Segal (2009) presented guidelines for discontinuing benzodiazepines and barbiturates and for managing withdrawal pharmacologically.

STIMULANTS

Amphetamines, methamphetamine, and cocaine are commonly abused central nervous system (CNS) stimulants. Amphetamines and methamphetamine are used by 1.6 million people over age 12, and cocaine is used by an additional 1.5 million (Center for Behavioral Health Statistics and Quality, 2015). In 2014, hospitalizations associated with cocaine and methamphetamine poisoning were 13,265 and 8,290, respectively (CDC, 2017).

Amphetamine toxicity can occur in individuals who take a large dose but use the drug infrequently; it can result in anxiety, restlessness, irritability, lability, headache, vomiting, hallucinations, and seizures that may last a week (Weiss, Greenfield, & Mirin, 1994). Serious cardiovascular and CNS effects can also occur (McCann & Ricaurte, 2009). Amphetamine psychosis is not uncommon and presents with symptoms similar to paranoid schizophrenia (Franklin et al., 2002; McCann & Ricaurte,

2009). Amphetamine withdrawal symptoms include depressed mood, decreased energy, fatigue, hypersomnolence, cravings, and decreased concentration (McCann & Ricaurte, 2009).

Cocaine use is also associated with a variety of medical complications, including dental problems, malnutrition and dehydration, endocarditis, HIV, emphysema, pulmonary emboli, and other cardiovascular, neurological, and respiratory problems (Franklin et al., 2002; Weiss & Iannucci, 2009). It can also result in paranoia, which worsens over time (Weiss & Iannucci, 2009). Comorbid alcohol use is a significant problem in cocaine users (Carroll, Rounsaville, & Bryant, 1993) and can complicate treatment. Cocaine withdrawal is associated with agitation, anxiety, depression, irritability, decreased concentration, insomnia, and cravings; these symptoms usually last for several weeks (Weiss & Iannucci, 2009). Medical treatment for withdrawal involves administering benzodiazepines for anxiety and haloperidol for psychosis (Franklin et al., 2002); individuals should also be monitored for suicidal ideation because suicide attempts have been reported in 43.5% of cocaine dependent patients (Roy, 2009).

HALLUCINOGENS

Used by about 1.2 million people over age 12 (Center for Behavioral Health Statistics and Quality, 2015), hallucinogens include LSD, PCP, MDMA ("ecstasy"), and others. Use of these drugs commonly results in perceptual changes and can also result in anxiety, mood, and psychotic disorders. Episodes of severe anxiety and paranoia can occur, and individuals may experience flashbacks that continue even after the drug is stopped (Franklin et al., 2002; Jones, 2009).

A few studies have demonstrated success at treating flashbacks using clonidine, naltrexone, and sertraline (Franklin et al., 2002). Otherwise, the main treatment for the symptoms is reassurance, with diazepam sometimes used for panic or psychotic symptoms (Weiss et al., 1994).

MARIJUANA

THC (delta-9-tetrahydrocannabinol) is the active ingredient found in marijuana and hashish. In 2014, 22.2 million Americans over age 12 (8.4% of the population) reported current use of marijuana, the most commonly used illicit drug. It is typically smoked in cigars, pipes, and blunts but can also be ingested in foods or brewed in tea (Volkow, Baler, Compton, & Weiss, 2014).

Individuals under the influence of THC demonstrate cognitive and motor problems that are associated with an increased likelihood of motor vehicle accidents. Chronic use may also cause subtle changes in higher cognitive functions (W. D. Hall & Degenhardt, 2009). THC causes increased heart rate (problematic for patients with cardiovascular disease) and symptoms of chronic bronchitis (such as coughing and wheezing); it is also associated with the development of chronic obstructive pulmonary disease, pulmonary and other cancers, and decreased immunity (Hall & Degenhardt, 2009). However, THC also has several therapeutic medical uses. Medical marijuana has been approved by the U.S. Food and Drug Administration for the relief of nausea and vomiting and to improve appetite in medical patients; it has also been used for muscle spasticity and chronic pain (Hill, 2014).

Withdrawal from THC can result in anxiety, irritability, cravings, and decreased sleep and appetite (Haney, 2005). Few medications have been useful at alleviating these symptoms, but oral THC has shown some promise at decreasing withdrawal symptoms (Haney, 2005).

Due to decriminalization of marijuana in some areas, there has been an increase in calls to poison centers due to overdose from edible marijuana products (Cao, Srisuma, Bronstein, & Hoyte, 2016). Over a 3-year period (2013–2015), 430 calls were reported. Most at risk were children under age 5. There were no deaths, but 3% of the patients were admitted to the hospital for treatment in intensive care.

Prescription Drug Abuse

In 2015, 119 million Americans over age 12 (44.5% of the population) used prescription drugs, and 18.9 million of them misused prescription drugs (Substance Abuse and Mental Health Services Administration [SAMHSA], 2016). This misuse involved taking an increased dose, taking the medication longer than the time for which it was prescribed, or using someone else's medication. Unintentional misuse can also occur; the elderly may be most vulnerable, due to memory problems that can affect their ability to comply with a complicated prescription regimen. The most commonly misused prescription drugs are opioids (for pain), stimulants (to increase energy and alertness), and CNS depressants (for anxiety and sleep; National Institute on Drug Abuse [NIDA], 2015).

Physicians become concerned about patients abusing prescription drugs if they run out of medication before their refill date, report losing drugs and request more, have several doctors prescribing similar medications, go to the emergency department for additional medication, forge prescriptions, increase the dose despite the physician warning them not to do so, steal or "borrow" drugs, or abuse illicit drugs (see Portenoy, 1994, for more information on these and other variables that are more and less predictive of addiction). In the inpatient setting, patients may be referred because they are "drug-seeking," which means the patient is requesting medications (often pain medications) before the time they are due or repeatedly requesting additional medication. Although it is true that individuals abusing pain medications may demonstrate these behaviors, patients who have pain that is undertreated and those who have developed tolerance for the medication may also demonstrate these same behaviors (Schnoll & Weaver, 2003). Therefore, without proper evaluation, it is incorrect to assume that patients who repeatedly request pain medications are abusing prescription medications.

Evaluation of Drug and Alcohol Use

A review of the medical record, screening questionnaires, and patient interviews can all provide important information when evaluating a patient's substance use.

MEDICAL RECORDS AND TOXICOLOGY SCREENS

Medical records can often provide history regarding a drug or alcohol abuse problem. Previous providers may have documented excessive use and/or problems associated with substance use, such as falls or physical fights. Medical records should also be reviewed for past and current toxicology screening results.

Toxicology (tox) screens are typically run using blood samples, but some can also be performed with saliva or urine. There are tox screens for many drugs, both illicit drugs and prescription medications. Tox screens can be used to detect the presence of illicit drugs, but they can also detect if either too much or too little of a prescription drug is in the patient's system. These are generally ordered by the patient's medical team when the patient is admitted to the hospital if they seem warranted at that time. These tests, however, are not infallible and can be influenced by extraneous factors (e.g., ingesting poppy seeds in a muffin can result in a tox screen that is positive for opiates). Nonetheless, tox screen results can be helpful to the psychologist because they provide objective evidence of drug use that can be important in the case of a patient who denies any drug use.

SCREENING QUESTIONNAIRES

A variety of screening questionnaires are available to help determine the patient's level of risk for alcoholism, alcohol-related problems, or drug abuse. Several of the most common screening measures for alcoholism are described in this section. Cooney et al. (2008) and Haller, Acosta, Newville, and Herron (2015) have provided information on many additional formal assessment measures pertaining to drug and alcohol use.

The simplest and easiest screening measure is the CAGE questionnaire (Ewing, 1984), which consists of four items that ask the patient if he has ever felt (a) the need to cut down on drinking, (b) annoyed by others criticizing his drinking, (c) guilty about drinking, or (d) if he has ever taken a morning eye-opener. Patients with alcoholism generally respond positively to three or four items, while those without alcohol problems rarely score above two.

The Alcohol Use Disorders Identification Test (AUDIT; Saunders, Aasland, Babor, de la Fuente, & Grant, 1993) is a 10-item screening questionnaire for alcohol problems. It measures the domains of alcohol consumption, drinking behavior, and alcohol-related problems. Scores on the AUDIT can range from 0 to 40; 92% of patients with harmful alcohol use score above 8.

The Michigan Alcoholism Screening Test (MAST; Selzer, 1971) is another brief method that can be used to detect alcohol problems. Consisting of 25 items, it assesses feeling bad about drinking, job loss, hospitalizations, arrests, and other issues related to alcohol abuse and takes about 15 minutes to administer. Many of the items can be useful clinically, even if the MAST is not formally scored.

SCREENING, BRIEF INTERVENTION, AND REFERRAL TO TREATMENT

Screening, Brief Intervention, and Referral to Treatment (SBIRT) is a program developed and disseminated by SAMHSA (2011) that describes specific items a clinician can use to screen for substance use, provide brief intervention, and refer for more comprehensive treatment. The program was developed for use in hospital and community settings in which intensive ongoing treatment is not possible and lends itself to the health psychology inpatient consultation setting.

SBIRT begins with a brief NIDA (n.d.) screening questionnaire to assess drug and alcohol use and to identify patients who need more intensive treatment. Instructions and resources to use SBIRT are available online (SAMHSA, 2015). The screener begins with items that assess for the frequency of alcohol, tobacco, prescription drug, and illegal drug use. On the basis of the patient's answers, the clinician is directed to ask additional screening questions (e.g., regarding specific drugs used) or to deliver a brief intervention. For example, if the patient acknowledges heavy alcohol use, the clinician is directed to assess for alcohol use disorders and is then provided with instructions to explain the results to the patient and intervene by setting goals and considering referral to other providers for those who need more intervention than the brief SBIRT program already provides.

Several reviews and meta-analyses have demonstrated the effectiveness of the SBIRT and other brief interventions for reducing alcohol use (Kaner et al., 2009; SAMHSA, 2011). However, it has not yet been established that these brief interventions increase a patient's receipt of more intensive, ongoing treatment for alcohol use (Glass et al., 2015; Simioni, Cottencin, & Rolland, 2015).

The evidence on the effectiveness of brief interventions intended to decrease illicit drug use is contradictory. Saitz (2014) and Saitz et al. (2014) have reported that there is little evidence for the efficacy of brief interventions for illegal and prescription drug abuse, except for those individuals who are seeking help. Others, however, have reported improvements in drug use with brief interventions such as SBIRT (Madras et al., 2009) or Project QUIT (Quit Using Drugs Intervention Trial; Gelberg et al., 2015).

DETAILED SUBSTANCE USE INTERVIEW

A brief evaluation of alcohol and drug use should be performed with all patients, even those with no known drug or alcohol problems. The brief interview should include information on drug and alcohol history, any past drug or alcohol treatment, and current use of alcohol and drugs. Generally, tobacco use is also included. If the patient denies problems with substance use during screening, and if the initial interview uncovers no issues with substance use, there may be no need to pursue substance use further, at least at the present time. If, however, problems are discovered in the patient's management of the medical issue or if there is suspicion that alcohol has an impact on the medical situation, an expanded interview will be needed.

An interview about substance use should be performed in a matter-of-fact, nonjudgmental, and collaborative manner. Frequently other providers have already discussed substance overuse with the patient. Patients often perceive these discussions as judgmental and condescending and may be defensive and uneasy discussing the issue further with another provider.

Hospital personnel often believe that substance abusers are difficult to deal with interpersonally, and some patients demonstrate comorbid personality disorders that may make it difficult to build rapport. Yet substance use (especially alcohol) is pervasive, and many users have no other significant psychological or personality problems. Psychiatric disorders and negative affect are associated with relapse (Douaihy, Daley, Stowell, & Park, 2007; Witkiewitz & Marlatt, 2009); treatment of these additional psychiatric issues will ultimately make them less of a complication when addressing the substance use.

Presenting the interview as a collaborative effort to find ways to improve the patient's health is useful because patients are often motivated to make changes in their behaviors when in the hospital and actively dealing with a medical problem. The clinician should take the perspective that most people drink alcohol, and the goal is to determine patterns of use. Patients should not be asked "if" they drink alcohol, but rather "how much" they drink. Many patients without an alcohol problem have reported feeling guilty and put off by a question about "if" they drink because it may imply that even minimal alcohol use is morally wrong and warrants intervention. (People who do not drink alcohol at all do not seem to be offended by a question that implies that they do.) Drug use is somewhat different because in most settings, drug use is not the norm. Asking patients "if" they use drugs seems acceptable to most patients. If a patient reports using one type of substance, they should also be asked about the use of others. People often use more than one substance, and that pattern can complicate both the medical and the psychological treatment.

Even if the interview questions are phrased in the most nonjudgmental manner, almost everyone, even those who do not abuse substances, tend to underreport their use of alcohol and drugs. The clinician can keep this in mind and does not need to overtly challenge most patients on their reports (i.e., if the patient reports drinking eight beers daily, it makes little practical difference if he really drinks 10). If family members are present, their nonverbal reactions to the patient's report of substance use will often provide important cues about the veracity of the patient's report. However, many patients with a clear history of substance abuse will either completely deny any current use or will deny the history of abuse. If there is objective evidence of substance abuse (i.e., repeat positive toxicology screens), the inconsistency will need to be addressed with the patient because intervention is unlikely to be effective if the clinician accepts the patient's denial of substance use. Some patients may want to avoid using terms such as *substance abuse* or *alcoholism*; if the patient is willing to acknowledge the behavior and the problem that needs to be addressed, the terminology can be flexible. Some patients, however, will choose terminology that enables them to deny that there is a problem; for example, "OK so I drink a lot, but I'm not really an alcoholic, so I don't need any treatment."

There are several good resources available to health psychology consultants for use in a detailed assessment of alcohol and drug use. Glidden-Tracey (2005) presented an outline and specific questions for use in a detailed assessment of substance use. The evaluation includes information on the patient's substance use history, to include specific substances used, as well as patterns of use. Physical and psychological symptoms of substance use are assessed, including medical issues that may be relevant to the substance use. Detailed information about past inpatient and outpatient treatment for substance use and mental health issues is also obtained, as well as information on contextual factors associated with substance use (e.g., social support, family history, legal problems). Finally, the patient's motivation for treatment is assessed, to include his feelings about the need for treatment and his perceptions of his own ability to decrease or stop using the alcohol or drugs. Cooney, Kadden, and Steinberg (2008) also described the importance of a thorough assessment of substance use that includes factors such as readiness to change, self-efficacy, coping skills, drinking expectations, spirituality, cravings, and comorbid psychopathology, and provided information on questionnaires available to help with the assessment of these factors.

Determining a specific reason for the drug or alcohol abuse is helpful, although not always possible. For many patients, the issue that prompted the start of overuse or abuse is in the distant past, and currently there may be no specific trigger that can be delineated. The current drug or alcohol use is now simply part of the patient's daily life and no longer connected to the initial cause. Common reasons for current abuse include habit, poor coping or self-medication, and attempts to manage anxiety or depression. In the case of prescription drug abuse, causes may also include poor attention to the details of the regimen, cognitive problems that interfere with adequate management, symptoms that are not well managed on the current regimen, or other medical needs that are not met.

Psychological Treatment of Substance Use and Abuse

In the inpatient setting, psychologists can use concepts of relapse prevention, motivational interviewing, and other strategies to begin the process of substance use treatment. These and other interventions are described in this section.

EDUCATION

Everyone knows that drug and alcohol abuse and misuse are harmful, in a general sense. Yet patients rarely have specific knowledge about the implications of substance abuse, given their particular medical situation. For example, many people with diabetes do not understand that drinks with alcohol contain a significant amount of sugar. People also do not commonly understand that drinking alcohol before bed can interfere with sleep (even though it initially may relax them and enable them to fall sleep), nor do they understand that it can suppress their respiration, making sleep apnea more dangerous. Education about the specific implications of alcohol or drug use, given the patient's specific medical issues, can help them to see the rationale for decreasing or discontinuing the use of alcohol and drugs.

Patients who are misusing prescription drugs may not understand the proper use of the medications. This should be reviewed with them, and barriers to adherence should be addressed (see Chapter 12, this volume). If patients continue to misuse prescription medications after they understand the proper use of the medication and also the implications of misuse, then other issues will need to be addressed.

COMMUNICATION

Improving the patient's ability and willingness to communicate openly with the treatment team about the substance use will improve the likelihood of success of any intervention. Often patients are ashamed of the drug or alcohol use, and they may have spent years trying to hide it from family and medical providers. Patients are often responsive to a discussion about how the drug use is not a moral issue but rather a medical one, and that, as with any medical issue, treatment is more successful if all members of the team collaborate in treating the problem. Especially with treatment of prescription medication abuse, it will be important to include the patient's doctors in the development of a treatment plan that the patient is able to adhere to and that also appropriately addresses the medical issue.

FIND ANOTHER WAY TO MEET THE NEEDS

What needs are being met by the drug or alcohol abuse? If those needs can be met in other ways, it will be easier to decrease substance use. For example, young adults who are socially anxious may overuse alcohol to decrease anxiety and self-consciousness and to help them relax in social situations. People may overuse benzodiazepines to manage anxiety or take pain medications to help with insomnia. Others use alcohol to numb feelings of depression. Interventions can be developed to address each of these issues, decreasing the patient's motivation to use the drug to cope with the issue.

RELAPSE PREVENTION

Relapse prevention (RP) is a term used to describe a set of cognitive–behavioral strategies and procedures that are designed to identify situations in which an individual is at risk of relapse, and then to generate strategies to help the patient to prevent the relapse. The RP model proposes that relapse is due to a variety of factors and interactions that can occur when individuals are faced with high-risk situations. Specifically, background factors, physiological states, cognitive processes, and coping all interact to predict relapse. (See Witkiewitz & Marlatt, 2004, for more detail on the model, as well as empirical evidence in support of it.)

When using the RP model clinically, patients are initially taught to recognize high-risk situations in which they are most vulnerable to relapse, as well as potential triggers for relapse. Patients then learn strategies to allow them to cope effectively with these threats. Interventions are designed to improve the patient's self-efficacy and management of negative emotional states. Patients are also helped to recognize cravings and cues to cravings, and they learn to manage cognitive errors that can lead to relapse. Douaihy et al. (2007) described these clinical strategies for treating patients with substance use problems and provided case examples.

Motivation is also an important aspect of this model and includes both motivation to change the behavior and motivation to use the substance (Marlatt & Witkiewitz, 2005). Motivation to change can be assessed using the five stages of readiness to change proposed by the transtheoretical model: precontemplation, contemplation, preparation, action, and maintenance (Prochaska, DiClemente, & Norcross, 1992). Motivational interviewing (Anstiss & Passmore, 2012; W. R. Miller & Rollnick, 2013) can then be used to improve a patient's readiness to change.

Motivational interviewing interventions are designed to decrease ambivalence about change and to increase the patient's motivation to change. One strategy is to ask the patient to consider the pros and cons of changing the behavior; another is to help the patient see discrepancies between his goal of decreased use or abstinence and his current behavior. Generally, a patient is asked to consider the specific impacts that using or not using substances will have on her health and other aspects of her life. She is asked to consider changes that would need to happen for any positive impacts to occur, as well as the likelihood that she would actually make the required changes. The first steps to get started on making the required changes can then be generated. (W. R. Miller and Rollnick [2013] presented detailed instructions on how to use motivational interviewing.) Much evidence supports the use of motivational interviewing in the treatment of substance abuse (Wilbourne & Miller, 2002). It has commonly been combined with cognitive behavior therapy and other approaches (including relapse prevention) with good outcomes (e.g., Moyers & Houck, 2011; Stein & Lebeau-Craven, 2002; Turner, Welches, & Conti, 2013).

When hospitalized, people are often motivated to change their behavior because they can clearly see how the substance use has become problematic. Further, they have already quit the substance for the duration of their hospital admission. The health psychology consultant can reinforce that they have already taken a significant step and can then help the patient develop strategies to keep the momentum going after discharge.

Motivation to use the substance (i.e., positive expectancies about the effects of the substance) is associated with relapse (Witkiewitz & Marlatt, 2004) and can be addressed by challenging the patient's expectations. Douaihy et al. (2007) also suggested the use of medications, such as disulfiram (Antabuse) or methadone, to help patients with initial abstinence and RP. A plan for thorough assessment of the factors involved in RP is found in Donovan (2008). Many studies have supported the effectiveness of RP in the treatment of alcohol and illicit drugs (Douaihy et al., 2007; Witkiewitz & Marlatt, 2009).

BASIC COGNITIVE–BEHAVIORAL STRATEGIES AND SOCIAL SUPPORT

Although it is not possible to do a significant amount of substance abuse treatment while the patient is in the hospital being treated for a medical problem, the process of intervention and education can begin. Because there is often a delay in starting outpatient treatment, intervention that begins during the hospital admission is warranted.

There is evidence that brief inpatient substance use consultations can be useful. Alaja and Seppä (2003) reported that at 6 months after discharge, 37% of patients who had inpatient substance use consultations reported either decreased substance use or abstinence, with more improvement in women and in patients who had not received previous treatment for substance use. That is, inpatients without comorbid psychiatric problems and chronic substance use problems benefited most from a brief hospital consultation. However, only 19% of patients returned for follow-up treatment. These results are relevant for inpatient health psychology consultation because they provide evidence that even a brief consultation can be helpful to certain patients.

On the basis of the treatments described here, there are some simple interventions that can be used in the inpatient setting to provide patients with basic tools to get started on their goal of decreasing or discontinuing substances. Although many patients will need additional outpatient treatment, brief inpatient interventions can have a profound impact. Exhibit 10.2 provides a list of basic interventions that can be used in the inpatient setting to help the patient begin a program to manage substance use problems. The interventions described are consistent with the RP model and can enable patients to begin to develop awareness and generate adaptive strategies to help them address the substance use problem.

EXHIBIT 10.2

Basic Interventions for Substance Use in the Inpatient Setting

Increase motivation: What are the benefits of making the effort to change, especially in the context of the current medical problem?

Increase awareness of triggers for substance use: When is the patient most at risk for use or abuse? How can the patient make changes to those situations to decrease risk? Are there situations a patient should avoid altogether?

Make plans to manage high-risk situations: Help the patient develop coping strategies to deal with specific events, such as parties, as well as any anticipated social pressure to use substances.

Consider changes to routines: How can the patient make changes to avoid habitual use of substances (e.g., meet friends for dinner rather than happy hour)?

Cognitive strategies: Patient reminds himself or herself that this can be mastered over time and of the positive medical, social, or legal results of decreasing or discontinuing substance use.

Enlist family support: Are there ways families can support the individual (e.g., removing alcohol from the home)?

Begin treatment for comorbid disorders, such as anxiety and depression.

Social support is also an important factor because it influences a patient's abstinence from substances and can have either a positive or negative impact. Positive social support is associated with abstinence, but many patients have experienced family members nagging at them for years to decrease their substance use. In some situations, it will be useful to educate the family about the treatment plan and their role in it, so that they can support the patient appropriately. Negative social support (which can take the form of social pressure to use substances) is associated with relapse (Marlatt & Witkiewitz, 2005).

REFERRAL FOR ADDITIONAL TREATMENT

There are many options available for treatment of substance abuse, including intensive inpatient treatment, day hospital, halfway house, traditional outpatient individual or group therapy, and support groups such as Alcoholics Anonymous. When making referrals for ongoing treatment after discharge from the hospital, it is important to consider the level of care the patient's problem warrants, the availability of the necessary services, and the likelihood the patient will attend those services. A large part of a successful referral for substance abuse involves helping the patient see that the treatment is warranted and that it will be of benefit.

In summary, the health psychology consultant will frequently encounter patients with medical issues in which substance use or abuse is operative. A thorough evaluation can delineate the specifics of the patient's situation; treatment can begin in the inpatient setting with ongoing outpatient treatment recommended as needed.

SPECIAL ISSUES IN THE HOSPITAL SETTING

IV

Decisional Capacity

11

A health psychology consultation may be requested to provide documentation that will allow the medical team to follow (or not follow) a patient's wishes regarding treatment. That is, patients are allowed to refuse any treatment if they have capacity to make their own decisions. Likewise, patients are not allowed to make their own decisions if they do not have capacity. In those cases, someone else makes decisions for them.

Competence Versus Capacity

Those who do not work in medical or forensic settings may use the terms *competence* and *capacity* interchangeably, although they mean different things. *Competence* is a legal term; a competent individual is an adult who is "of sound mind" and has legal rights to manage his own affairs and to make his own decisions (e.g., to sign a contract, to stand trial, to execute a will, to make medical decisions; Leo, 1999). For a normal adult, competence is generally assumed, unless there is reason to doubt it. If that occurs, the decision about competence is made by a judge, and the court's decision about competency refers to all aspects of the individual's legal life. If the individual is found not to be competent, a guardian is appointed to handle his affairs for him.

http://dx.doi.org/10.1037/0000108-012
Health Psychology Consultation in the Inpatient Medical Setting, by S. M. Labott

Decisional capacity refers to the individual's ability to make an informed decision and is determined by a clinician with expertise in this area (a psychiatrist, psychologist, or other qualified physician). In the hospital, clinicians are asked to provide an opinion of the patient's decisional capacity for a specific medical decision (e.g., to consent to a treatment, to manage medical issues independently, or to refuse medication). The capacity assessment is with respect to a specific decision and is typically not a global assessment of the individual's functioning. (See American Bar Association [ABA] Commission on Law and Aging & American Psychological Association [APA], 2008, for extensive information on capacity in a variety of contexts.) Medical problems can influence decisional capacity at any age, and patients may experience either a permanent or a temporary loss of decisional capacity. In some cases, the patient's ability to make decisions may fluctuate as her medical status changes.

Capacity Assessment Referrals

Decisional capacity assessments are requested when the primary medical service is concerned that the patient may be unable to make an informed medical decision. In practice, capacity assessments are likely to be requested if the patient seems to be making the "wrong" decision, that is, refusing a treatment that is recommended by the doctor. Logically, it is difficult to understand why a person would refuse treatment after they presented to the hospital requesting treatment, especially if the recommended action is expected to prolong the patient's life or improve life quality. The converse is also true: A capacity assessment is often not requested if the patient is making the "correct" decision, regardless of how impaired the patient is. Especially with family support for the decision, the patient's capacity is practically less relevant if she is making the "correct" decision; even if the patient doesn't fully understand, if she was deemed incapable of deciding for herself, the family would make the same decision.

In practice, there are many decisions made each day regarding a patient's care in the hospital. Minor decisions about the patient's care are unlikely to result in capacity referrals because it is relatively easy to comply with the patient's wishes regarding small matters. For example, venipuncture technicians frequently make their rounds to perform blood draws at 4 to 5 a.m. (so that the physicians have results when they start their treatment of patients a few hours later). Patients frequently complain about being awakened for blood draws and may refuse. At that point, a capacity evaluation could be requested to determine whether the patient retains capacity to refuse, but this generally does not happen. The technician can usually find a way to accommodate the patient and also get the blood drawn. In practice, the venipuncture technician will ask the patient if it is acceptable that she return later for the blood draw, and usually a patient will agree. The blood draw can be accomplished later, without putting the patient through a comprehensive capacity evaluation. A similar strategy can also work for a health psychology consultation: A consultant can negotiate with a patient to return to complete the evaluation later in the day if it is not a good time for the patient when the consultant initially arrives.

Kahn, Bourgeois, Klein, and Iosif (2009) reported on 88 capacity referrals from a psychosomatic consultation service at an academic medical center. Decisional capacity referrals most frequently occurred for patients who wished to leave the hospital against medical advice (AMA), when there was a question of a patient's capacity to accept or refuse medical and surgical procedures, or when there were concerns about a patient's capacity to participate in discharge planning (i.e., to decide on placement after leaving the hospital). Individuals referred for capacity assessments were slightly more likely to be male (64%). The average age of the patient was 60 years, but the range was 22 to 92 years, demonstrating that decisional capacity can also be a concern in younger people in the hospital. The consultants in this setting had determined that 88% of the patients (77 of 88) who were referred for decisional capacity evaluations did not have capacity to make their own decisions.

LEAVING AGAINST MEDICAL ADVICE

In the United States, only about 1% of hospitalized patients leave the hospital against medical advice (Ibrahim, Kwoh, & Krishnan, 2007; Tawk, Freels, & Mullner, 2013). Patients leave the hospital AMA for many reasons, including social or personal, financial or legal reasons, or problems with their hospital care. Personal reasons are most common and include such things as the need to attend an important event (a child's graduation or a father's funeral), the need to provide child care for one's children, or family emergencies. Financial factors can motivate someone to leave the hospital AMA; examples of these include when a patient needs to return to work to continue to support his family, or when a patient leaves the hospital because she has no insurance and is fearful of generating high medical bills that she will not be able to pay. People may also leave the hospital AMA to attend court dates or other legal proceedings. Finally, patients may leave the hospital because of a perceived problem with their medical care; a patient may disagree with the doctor who says he needs additional treatment or may feel he is not receiving proper care, for example. Patients may also leave AMA because they are tired of waiting for discharge paperwork to be completed. Although some of these problems can be resolved, others cannot, and then patients leave the hospital AMA.

People who wish to leave the hospital AMA are required to sign a document that states they are leaving against the advice of their doctor. They are often told by their resident or attending physician that if they leave the hospital against the doctor's advice, their insurance company will not cover the cost of the admission. This is often done to encourage the patient to remain in the hospital and is widely believed by physicians, although the evidence does not bear this out (G. R. Schaefer et al., 2012).

A health psychology consultant may be asked to assess decisional capacity to determine whether the patient is able to rationally decide about leaving AMA or may be asked to reason with a patient who has capacity to convince her to stay in the hospital for additional testing or treatment. Often patients are angry by the time the psychologist is called because they feel the medical team is not listening to their wishes—and now the doctor has even called a "shrink" to see if they are crazy! These are challenging consultations, but they provide an opportunity for the psychologist to empathize with the patient's frustration and then enlist her collaboration to try to resolve the issue.

If it is determined that a patient has decisional capacity, it is his decision to leave AMA if he wishes to do so. Patients who exercise this right and leave the hospital AMA tend to be male and have Medicaid or no insurance (Ibrahim et al., 2007; Kraut et al., 2013; Tawk et al., 2013). They demonstrate a wide variety of medical problems. Alcohol or drug abuse seems to be a frequent problem in those who leave the hospital AMA (12%; Kraut et al., 2013), whereas those with cancer are among the least likely to leave AMA (0.5%; Ibrahim et al., 2007).

DECISIONS ABOUT MEDICAL TREATMENT

The most common referral for decisional capacity assessment in the inpatient medical setting involves the case of a patient who needs lifesaving treatment but refuses it. Consider a 55-year-old woman with a long history of diabetes and end-stage renal disease who has been on dialysis for several years and hates it. She has developed gangrene in a toe. An amputation will likely remove the infection completely and will allow her to continue to live her life, although she may need to walk with a cane to aid her balance after the amputation. If she does not have the surgery, the infection will continue to spread and will probably kill her within a few months. The patient refuses the lifesaving amputation, stating that she has lived a good and long life and that she is tired of spending all her time dealing with medical problems. Similarly, a 40-year-old woman, diagnosed with breast cancer about 8 years ago, was successfully treated with a mastectomy, chemotherapy, and radiation. She has now developed leukemia, likely as a secondary effect of the chemotherapy that was used to treat the cancer previously. She is now facing more chemotherapy and a possible stem cell transplant. These treatments would be expected to prolong her life, perhaps for several years. She refuses them, saying that she has had enough treatment and will live out her time without any additional chemotherapy or any other intervention to treat the leukemia.

Although it appears that in both of these cases, it is in the patient's best interest to agree to undergo the recommended treatment, it is the patient's right to refuse if she has decisional capacity. Either of these patients might have provided the medical team with some data indicating they may not have capacity (e.g., acute cognitive changes this hospital admission), or she may be referred for an evaluation because it does not seem reasonable for a patient to refuse a treatment that has a good likelihood of prolonging her life.

Alternatively, consider a patient with severe dementia who has lung cancer and multiple other medical problems, but no understanding of the medical issues. She is taken to surgery to remove part of her lung because she agrees with the doctors (and her daughter) who feel the surgery is necessary to prolong her life. In this case, her capacity to make her own decisions is likely poor, but it was not questioned because she seemed to be making the "correct" decision. If she had refused the surgery, it is likely that a capacity evaluation would have been requested. If her capacity for decision-making was then found to be impaired, her daughter would have made the decision for her, and she would have had the surgery anyway. Therefore, although the patient perhaps did not have decisional capacity, questioning it would have resulted in more evaluation and would probably not have changed the outcome. Because the doctors, the patient, and her daughter all agreed that the surgery was warranted, raising a question of her capacity was not practically relevant.

PLACEMENT DECISIONS

Most patients are eager to return home after a hospital admission, but in some cases, patients need additional care, perhaps in an acute rehabilitation facility or a nursing home, either briefly or permanently. Most patients can be convinced to agree to a short stay in a rehabilitation facility—for example, after a hip replacement or a long illness in which they have become weak and deconditioned—but some people are adamant that they want to go home and do not want to go to a rehabilitation program or nursing facility, even briefly. If the patient lives alone, has a history of difficulty managing at home alone, and also demonstrates cognitive impairments, discharging him home on his own may not be safe. A case like this is slightly different from the other decisional capacity questions, in that this is not a question of the capacity to make one specific medical decision but involves a decision that will then result in a host of other decisions that the patient will need to make to be safe and healthy at home. Decisions involving placement will involve a focus on the patient's judgment, both past and present, as well as her physical ability to manage at home. Neuropsychological testing may provide a more thorough picture of the patient's cognitive functioning, and an assessment of the safety of the patient's home and other available resources (e.g., family support) may also be used to help determine whether the patient will be safe if discharged to home alone.

Issues That Impact Decisional Capacity

Decisional capacity can be impaired in patients with delirium and dementia, as well as those with other psychopathology, such as psychosis, depression, and personality disorders. In the Kahn et al. (2009) study, cognitive disorders (including delirium, dementia, and cognitive disorder not otherwise specified [NOS]) accounted for the greatest proportion of patients who lacked capacity (64%). Other, less frequent diagnoses that resulted in a lack of capacity were psychotic disorder NOS, mood disorders, and alcohol dependence or abuse.

Any of these factors can affect an individual's ability to make a rational decision, but simply because a patient has been diagnosed with one of these disorders does not automatically mean he lacks the capacity to make his own decisions. Certainly a person with active command hallucinations in which voices tell him to kill himself would not have capacity to decide about undergoing surgery for a bowel obstruction. However, if the patient has been diagnosed with schizophrenia but is stable on medication and in treatment, it is likely that she would retain the capacity to make her own medical decisions.

Similarly, delirium and dementia may influence an individual's ability to make informed decisions, but not all patients with cognitive diagnoses have decisional impairments. People with mild dementias often retain decisional capacity, and people with delirium may have capacity that fluctuates with their symptoms. (Decisional capacity can also fluctuate in patients with certain types of dementia; see Trachsel, Hermann, & Biller-Andorno, 2015.)

Kim, Karlawish, and Caine (2002) reviewed studies of decisional capacity in people with cognitive impairments. They concluded that people with dementia or other cognitive problems were more likely to lack capacity than those without the diagnosis of a cognitive problem. However, those with mild-to-moderate Alzheimer's disease can often perform adequately on measures of decisional capacity. So although dementia is correlated with a lack of capacity, a diagnosis of dementia (or any other cognitive problem) does not indicate that the patient automatically lacks decisional capacity. Therefore, regardless of a patient's diagnosis (be it dementia, schizophrenia, or something else), the patient needs to be evaluated to determine exactly what her capabilities are and whether she retains capacity.

Criteria for Decisional Capacity

The President's Commission for the Study of Ethical Problems in Medicine and Biomedical and Behavioral Research (1982) indicated that the necessary elements for decisional capacity include the following: (a) the possession of a set of values, (b) the ability to communicate and understand information, and (c) the ability to reason and deliberate about one's choices. In practice, these criteria have been expanded to encompass four domains to be evaluated in a decisional capacity assessment: communicating a choice, understanding relevant information, appreciating the situation and the decision's consequences, and the ability to rationally manipulate relevant information (Appelbaum & Grisso, 1988; Leo, 1999; Searight, 1992).

COMMUNICATING A CHOICE

To have decisional capacity, a person needs to have an opinion or to have made a choice about the decision in question. Although there is some room for adjustments in the decision if the medical situation changes, the patient must generally make a choice and be consistent in this choice over time. If a patient is unable to make a decision, or if his decision changes every few hours, he would not meet this most minimal requirement for decisional capacity.

People also need to be able to express their choice. This does not mean that they need to state it verbally, but they need to be able to communicate it clearly, perhaps by writing it down, by nodding their head in response to relevant questions, or in some other way. However it is communicated, the patient's choice must be clearly understood by others. Many patients meet this most minimal requirement for decisional capacity, in that they have an opinion and are able to express it to others. Yet decisional capacity also requires that they meet the following additional criteria.

UNDERSTANDING INFORMATION RELEVANT TO THE DECISION

The choice the person expresses is irrelevant if they don't understand what they are talking about. Patients should be able to describe the medical illness they are being treated for, as well as its anticipated course. They should also be able to describe relevant treatment options that have been presented by their doctors. Typically physicians have recommended one option as the preferred treatment, and that is the decision for which the patient's decisional capacity is being evaluated.

Patients also need to be able to describe the risks and benefits of the treatment in question. Even the most educated patients don't necessarily have the medical knowledge to articulate this well. It is most important that they understand and explain the main points, even if they don't understand the details and nuances of the medical issues. For example, a patient should be able to say that he has gangrene, an infection, or a "problem" with his foot. He should be able to describe what treatments have been discussed (e.g., amputation, antibiotics, or no treatment) and the risks and benefits of each. He should know that there are risks of undergoing surgery but that amputation could save his life. If the administration of antibiotics is another option, he should know that this option is associated with less risk than surgery, but the antibiotic treatment is also likely to be less successful at completely resolving the infection (and then perhaps the surgery will need to be reconsidered later). The patient should also be able to explain that if no treatment is provided, he will likely die from this infection in a few weeks or months. The patient does not need to know the name of the antibiotics that could be given or exactly how the surgery would be done, but he needs to have a general sense of the potential risks and benefits of the treatment options he is being asked to consider.

All of the information about the proposed treatment (as well as the other options) will have been discussed with the patient beforehand by the medical team, but that does not mean the patient will recall or be able to articulate that information when asked to do so by the health psychology consultant. It is sufficient if he "knows" all this information after the consultant discusses it with him again, providing repeat education as needed. Patients may not understand all of the medical issues a priori, but additional education (from the psychologist, a nurse, or doctor) may improve their understanding and enhance their decision-making. This criterion is more stringent than the previous one, in that individuals need to be able to articulate relevant information. To meet this criterion, they need to understand the facts about the proposed treatment.

APPRECIATION OF THE DECISION'S CONSEQUENCES

The third aspect of decisional capacity relates to the patient's ability to weigh the options and to understand the consequences of the decision—both immediately and for the future. This is more than simply knowledge of the objective facts about the illness and the proposed treatment; it also includes an understanding of how these facts will subjectively affect the individual's life. It involves the ability to look into the future and anticipate the potential risks and benefits associated with the treatment or procedure and what those will mean to the patient. It is not about what the likely outcomes would mean to most people, but it is an individualized focus on the meaning of the events to this specific patient.

Consider a person making a decision about the removal of part of a finger after an accident with a lawn mower. Many people would agree that if they remained generally healthy overall, the loss of a fingertip could be managed; not so for a pianist who feels she will have no quality of life remaining if she loses her career and also her major passion in life. Similarly, for some, undergoing a neurosurgical procedure that could result in paralysis is preferable over death, while others would prefer to die than to live with quadriplegia. The patient's individual values regarding the potential outcomes and the implications of them are paramount here: The patient needs to understand the potential consequences of the decision and evaluate how that will affect *her* life.

On occasion a patient will make a decision that is consistent with his values, such as deciding to refuse the neurosurgery, but then as he comes closer to death, he begins to reconsider and imagines that there could be some quality of life available for him even if he was paralyzed after the surgery. Sometimes the initial decision can be reversed later and the surgery can then be performed, but many times the appropriate window of time for the recommended treatment is past (e.g., if the disease has progressed, and the treatment would no longer be useful), and then the treatment is no longer appropriate.

ABILITY TO RATIONALLY MANIPULATE RELEVANT INFORMATION (REASONING)

Patients need to be able to think logically, weighing the pros and cons of the treatment options, and then come to a conclusion based on that. They should be able to describe their thought process and how they came to their decision. A mental status examination may be useful here to provide a measure of the patient's ability to think clearly, but it cannot be the only piece of data used to evaluate rationality and the ability to think about the information. Delusions or other problems with thought processes might not be evident if the patient is given only a brief mental status examination.

It is important to realize that even if a patient is able to think clearly and manipulate information, she may not come to the "correct" or preferred decision (from a medical standpoint). That is, rational manipulation of information does not mean the patient will make the "right" decision—it simply means he has the capacity to make the decision, and then the decision he makes is up to him, even if the medical providers do not agree with it. Consider again the patient with gangrene for whom an amputation has been recommended. She is aware that she has diabetes and says she does not want an amputation (articulates a choice). She can explain that she has been told she needs an amputation to treat the infection (understanding of the facts), and she can acknowledge that she understands the amputation would save her life (understands likely consequences). She then weighs the implications of her decision for her future life and decides she will not have the amputation because she feels that her quality of life will be poor afterward and she doesn't want to live that way (manipulates relevant information). The patient can also explain that her mother had diabetes and became depressed after an amputation, then died shortly afterward anyway. The differences between the patient's and her mother's situations had been discussed with her, and she understood that her mother had a history of depression even before her illness (which the patient did not). Yet she still did not wish to undergo the surgery. Because this patient had demonstrated capacity to make her own decision, her decision was respected and followed, even though her doctors felt it was best for her to have the amputation.

The Decisional Capacity Evaluation

The decisional capacity evaluation may include content from the general biopsychosocial evaluation presented earlier, or it may be almost exclusively focused on the specific data necessary to make the decisional capacity determination. If the patient is able, the thorough evaluation is preferable, although often patients are not able to participate in extended evaluations. When assessing capacity, the psychologist will want to review the medical record and collect information specific to the capacity issues, such as living wills and advance directives. The patient should be "prepared," that is, by adjusting medications and providing aids (e.g., glasses, hearing aids), so the patient is at his best for the interview. Mental status should be assessed, and other standardized measures for capacity assessment may also be useful. Collateral information from those who know the patient well should also be obtained. These aspects of the decisional capacity evaluation are discussed in more detail next.

COLLECT RELEVANT INFORMATION

As with any inpatient consultation, the psychologist needs to review the patient's medical record to obtain background information on the patient's medical history and current status. For a decisional capacity evaluation, a review of a living will or advance directive can provide background on the patient's values and wishes for treatment before the current medical problem (which is especially useful if the patient is currently unable to communicate). It is also usually necessary to have a discussion with the referring physician about the patient's situation because the psychologist needs some specific information that may not be found in the patient's medical record. To evaluate capacity, the psychologist needs to understand what decision is being made, the expected course of the disease (with and without treatment), risks and benefits of the potential treatments, and other information relevant to the specific patient and decision. Although some of this information will be in the medical record, it will likely not all be there, or will not be there in sufficient detail for the consultant's needs. The psychologist will need to know the answers to all the interview questions that she will be asking the patient. In addition, it will be important to know what information the patient has been given on all of these issues, and the discussions he has had regarding the treatment with his medical team. The decisional capacity evaluation is similar to an academic test, and the test will be "graded" by the psychologist, so it is critical that he knows the correct answers to the test questions.

PREPARE THE PATIENT

Patients referred for decisional capacity evaluations are often quite sick and not at their best to complete an evaluation. One possible outcome of the capacity evaluation is that the patient loses her right to make her own decision; therefore, it is critical that the patient is enabled to perform at her best, so that if she has capacity to make informed choices, she is able to demonstrate that. Part of the psychologist's responsibility is to see that the patient is provided with her best chance at demonstrating clear thinking and understanding.

A variety of steps can be taken to ensure that the patient has an opportunity to perform at her best during the evaluation. Those patients who have hearing or vision impairments may be unable to understand the consultant and are at a disadvantage when it comes to demonstrating their ability to understand and think rationally. Patients will need to have glasses, hearing aids, or any other aids that will help them to see and hear what is occurring around them. These items may not be in the hospital, and family members will need to bring them from home.

The patient's nurse can typically provide valuable input on other issues that can improve the patient's ability to perform in the decisional capacity evaluation. Often a patient is most lucid at a certain time of day; if this is the case, the consultant should plan the evaluation for that time. If a patient is less cognitively intact or somnolent after taking a certain medication, perhaps that medication can be held until the capacity evaluation is finished. If the patient would be in too much pain without the medication, perhaps the dose can be decreased temporarily. The goal is to have the patient be as alert as possible, but also as comfortable as possible.

There may also be additional issues that, if treated, would improve the patient's thinking and performance (e.g., depression, sleep apnea). In practice, there may not be time to fully treat all of the issues that could potentially affect the capacity evaluation, especially if a decision needs to be made quickly to maximize the benefit a patient will receive from the treatment. If so, the determination of a patient's decisional capacity will be made based on the patient's current functioning, even if it is likely that his functioning will improve in the future. That is, on the basis of how the patient is functioning today, she does (or does not) have capacity for the decision. If the situation changes over time, because the patient's cognitive ability either improves or worsens, capacity may need to be evaluated again. Consider a delirious patient who should theoretically be able to make her own decisions, but today she cannot because of the delirium. If the delirium clears in a few days and there are remaining decisions about her treatment to be made at that point, capacity could be reevaluated, and perhaps she will be capable at that time. Except for the case of a patient with severe and permanent cognitive damage, such as an intellectual disability or a severe brain injury, it is expected that capacity may change over time and may need to be reevaluated as the patient's cognitive status changes.

INTERVIEW THE PATIENT

Exhibit 11.1 provides a list of questions that a psychologist can ask to assess the four criteria for decisional capacity discussed earlier (see also Etchells et al., 1999, and Searight, 1992); note that these may not be asked in the order presented, for example, asking why the patient is in the hospital is often the first question. As always, good interviewing skills are necessary. If a patient is verbal, open-ended questions should be used. In cases in which a patient cannot communicate well, the psychologist will need to ask very simple questions that the patient can respond to with yes–no answers, nods, or gestures.

To demonstrate decisional capacity, patients are expected to describe the current medical problem, the expected course of the illness without treatment, the recommended treatment (and other options), and the risks and benefits associated with each treatment option. They will need to state their choice and also describe the potential consequences of this choice. It is not acceptable for patients to simply say that they will "get worse"; they need to be able to articulate specific facts about what

EXHIBIT 11.1

Interview Questions to Assess Decisional Capacity

Communicating a choice

What do you think about what your doctors are recommending? What do you think you want to do?

Understanding information relevant to the decision

What brings you to the hospital? What is the name of the medical problem?

What are your doctors recommending that you do? What would this involve (e.g., procedures, injections, medication, surgery, length of treatment, other interventions)?

Are there other alternative treatments for this condition? What would those involve?

What are the possible risks of each of these treatments?

What are the potential benefits?

If not treated, what will likely happen?

Appreciating the decision's consequences

What could happen to you if you do this? Or if you don't do this? How could the recommended treatment help you?

Do you have concerns about the treatment?

What are the likely consequences of your decision—now and also in the longer term? Do you see possible benefits of this decision for you? What about risks?

How does this decision fit with your values about your life and medical care? (As needed: Do you understand that you will die if you don't have this treatment?)

What if you decide not to do this now? What if you change your mind later?

Ability to manipulate information

How did you come to your decision? What are the pros and cons?

Have you discussed this with your family? What do they think? How would you explain your decision to your family?

will happen if they refuse treatment. They also need to demonstrate that they can weigh information and come to a conclusion based on careful thought. Beware that some patients will jump to an impulsive decision and state it adamantly, loudly, and repeatedly, but they are unable to demonstrate that any careful and rational thought has gone into the decision. As noted earlier, patients may not be able to provide sophisticated answers to these questions, but they need to understand the basic ideas.

Beyond the specific questions to assess decisional capacity, the patient needs to be asked about other issues that could be influencing his decision (e.g., depressive symptoms, financial worries, family conflicts). These will often be raised by the patient in the course of the capacity evaluation (e.g., "I don't want to have chemo because it is expensive and my wife will need to care for me now and then pay for it after I am gone"). Each of these issues will not be relevant to all patients, but sufficient background knowledge will enable the consultant to decide which additional issues should be addressed.

As with any other inpatient interview, the patient's mood and behavior will need to be observed or assessed. The consultant will want to note any issues that could affect the patient's ability to make rational decisions, such as agitation, severe pain, hallucinations, or suicidal ideation. Any such issues will then need to be evaluated further to determine their relevance to the patient's decisional capacity.

It is not uncommon for information to be uncovered during a capacity evaluation that puts a variety of other issues into perspective and obviates the need for the capacity evaluation. Consider a patient admitted to the hospital with severe stomach pain. He has a fourth-grade education. Since his admission 2 days ago, he has been refusing blood draws and all other medical procedures. He is now planning to leave AMA, and the referral is to determine whether he retains capacity to make that decision for himself. During the course of the capacity evaluation, the patient continued to complain about not getting enough pain medication to adequately manage his pain and asserted that all the doctors wanted was to run tests to increase his hospital bill so they could make money. The doctors were, in fact, trying to minimize his pain medication use to avoid masking any further symptoms, and they were unable to diagnose the problem without the laboratory tests and procedures that the patient was refusing. Without the proper diagnosis, they were unable to recommend a course of action to treat the problem. During the discussion that occurred as part of the decisional capacity evaluation, the patient began to understand the purpose of the testing and also the reason for minimizing the pain medication. Once that occurred, he was willing to comply with the diagnostic testing, understanding now that this would result in a diagnosis and then treatment that would include adequate pain management in the short term as well as a solution to the problem in the longer term.

MENTAL STATUS TESTING

Because the ability to attend to and process information is relevant to a decisional capacity evaluation, using a brief mental status screener, such as the Mini-Mental Status Examination (MMSE; Folstein, Folstein, & McHugh, 1975) can be helpful. In a review of articles using the MMSE to assess decisional capacity, Sessums, Zembrzuska, and Jackson (2011) reported that scores less than 20 were associated with incapacity, scores greater than 24 were associated with capacity, and scores 20 to 24 showed no consistent pattern. The mental status examination should be viewed as one component of the comprehensive capacity evaluation, not used *instead of* the comprehensive evaluation, because a high score on a mental status exam can occur in a patient who lacks capacity, and a low score can be seen in a patient who retains capacity. Therefore, although the mental status examination is a useful component of the overall capacity evaluation, it is not sufficient in and of itself to determine a patient's capacity to make decisions.

STANDARDIZED CAPACITY ASSESSMENT MEASURES

Many formal measures are available to help a clinician to assess the capacity of a patient to make a treatment decision. At least 15 of these are currently available for clinical purposes (as well as many others designed to assess capacity for research decisions). The clinical measures tend to either use vignettes to elicit the patient's thinking about a specific decision (i.e., to provide a demonstration of the patient's thinking process, albeit not specifically regarding the current decision) or the vignettes are specifically related to the current decision. Overall, the available measures differ in terms of the training needed to administer them properly, as well as the time needed to administer them to the patient. Good reviews and comparisons of the most commonly used instruments are provided by the ABA Commission on Law and Aging and APA (2008) and by Dunn, Nowrangi, Palmer, Jeste, and Saks (2006). Although many of these measures can provide useful data to aid the health psychology consultant's thinking about the patient's decisional capacity, none of them provide a single score to answer the capacity question without a thorough evaluation.

Three of the most useful instruments for decisional capacity assessment in the hospital are the MacArthur Competence Assessment Tool for Treatment (MacCAT–T; Grisso, Appelbaum, & Hill-Fotouhi, 1997), the Hopemont Capacity Assessment Interview (HCAI; Edelstein, 2000), and the Capacity to Consent to Treatment Instrument (CCTI; Marson, Ingram, Cody, & Harrell, 1995). All three of these measures evaluate a patient's understanding, appreciation, reasoning, and the expression of a choice. Administration times range from 15 to 60 minutes, with the MacCAT–T being the shortest. All three of these measures use vignettes to assess capacity, and all have good interrater reliability. One benefit of the MacCAT–T is that the vignette is relevant to the *actual* decision that people are dealing with, so it is more immediately relevant than the other measures, which use hypothetical scenarios. The MacCAT–T does not determine global capacity, but it identifies the patient's strengths and weaknesses with respect to the major criteria (i.e., understanding, appreciation, reasoning, expressing a choice), and it is intended to be interpreted in the context of other clinical information. Good training materials (manual and video) are available.

Moye, Karel, Azar, and Gurrera (2004) compared the CCTI, MacCAT–T, and the HCAI in a group of mild-to-moderate dementia patients versus matched control participants. The dementia patients demonstrated impaired reasoning on all three measures compared with the control participants. However, most adults with dementia scored within the normal range on each of the four aspects of decisional capacity, highlighting the importance of using these in conjunction with other information to assess the patient's decisional capacity.

COLLATERAL INFORMATION

There may be a role for family members to play in the capacity evaluation, especially if they can provide background on the patient's personality and values that can help the health psychology consultant determine whether the wishes the patient is currently embracing are consistent with his beliefs and personality. Family members may also have access to living wills or other documents that describe the patient's values about medical treatment and end-of-life issues. Finally, family members can also provide background information on the patient's cognitive baseline that can help the psychologist determine whether the patient's current presentation is typical.

Most family members are well intentioned, and they know the patient much better than the psychologist does, but they may also have their own ideas about what is best for the patient that can interfere with their ability to objectively report on the patient's values. They are also more likely to be paternalistic, and they are more likely than physicians to view the patient as incompetent (Vellinga, Smit, Van Leeuwen, Van Tilburg, & Jonker, 2004). The consultant would do well to obtain information from family and friends and then attempt to engage them in a collaborative effort to determine what the patient would want in this situation.

Patients Lacking Decisional Capacity

If, after a thorough evaluation, the patient has not demonstrated capacity to make her own decisions, the clinician should review the situation once more before making the formal determination that the patient is unable to make the decision. This review should include another look at the information the patient was provided about the decision, that is, were they given complete information? Unfortunately, physicians sometimes present information to patients and think they have been clear in their presentation, but the patient did not understand it. If that is a possibility, the information should be reexplained, and the patient should be allowed to ask questions, and then her capacity to make the decision should be reevaluated.

If it is clear that the patient does not have capacity and that presenting additional information will not change that, then consider whether this is likely to be a temporary or permanent situation. If the patient is delirious due to an infection but the infection is being treated and is improving, then the patient's cognition may improve in the near future. In this case, if the decision needs to be made quickly, the patient will not have capacity to make it today, but if the decision can be safely delayed, it should be delayed; the patient's capacity can then be reevaluated in a few days. Perhaps by that time, the patient will have regained his capacity to make his own decisions.

If the patient does not have capacity for a decision that needs to be made, then someone else has to be designated to make the decision on the patient's behalf. Patients may have planned for this previously by designating someone as their POA (power of attorney) for health care. If not, a surrogate decision-maker needs to be appointed to make decisions for the patient while she does not have capacity to do so herself. Individual states have legislation that outlines who can make surrogate decisions for a patient and provides for advance directives and instructions for designation of surrogates. There are limitations specific to each state regarding what decisions can be made by surrogates, as well as rules for what is to be done if the patient is "unbefriended" (has no family or friends to act as a surrogate for them). In 1993, the Uniform Health Care Decisions Act (Sabatino, 1994) was proposed in an effort to standardize the approach taken to decision-making across states if a patient lacked capacity. This act has been adopted by several states but is not yet a consistent standard.

In a majority of states, a spouse is the most likely person to be appointed as a surrogate, followed by other family members, and some states also allow friends to serve as surrogates. In Illinois, for example, the Health Care Surrogate Act (Office of State Guardian, 1998) allows for a surrogate to be appointed to make decisions about most medical treatment (not only terminal illness or a vegetative state) without judicial involvement, if the patient lacks decisional capacity. The individuals who can serve as a surrogate include a guardian, the patient's spouse, an adult child, a parent, adult sibling, adult grandchild, a close friend, and the estate guardian (in that order). Generally, capacity is assessed by a qualified professional, and the appropriate surrogate is selected to make decisions if the patient is unable, without involving the courts. If no surrogate is available, then the court needs to appoint a guardian.

Surrogates are expected to make decisions according to a "substituted judgment" standard in which they consider the patient's wishes when making a decision. Some states require evidence of the patient's values or preferences regarding medical decisions. In other states, if the patient's wishes are unknown, the surrogate is allowed to make decisions based on what is expected to be in the patient's "best interests."

These cases may be complicated if, for example, a patient demonstrates fluctuating capacity, changes her mind frequently, has ongoing conflicts with the medical team, or has no family or friends to help with decision-making. Many large medical centers have ethics committees that will evaluate the patient's situation and provide recommendations if it is unclear how to proceed in a specific case. (See Chapter 14 for more on proxy decision-making.) If it appears that an ethics consultation is warranted, the psychologist should make this recommendation to the medical team and discuss the rationale for it with them before proceeding.

Concluding the Decisional Capacity Evaluation

The psychologist's conclusions should be discussed with the referring physician and also, perhaps, with the patient, the patient's family, or both, depending on the patient's awareness and the family's involvement. Conclusions should also be clearly documented in the medical record, along with data to support the psychologist's conclusions. Recommendations for further evaluation, especially if the patient's medical situation changes, may also be warranted as part of that report. Sample 11.1 is a consultation report that demonstrates these issues.

Note that in this case, the patient was cognitively intact and had capacity to make her own decision. There was no reason to expect her cognition to fluctuate now (although it would be expected to deteriorate as time goes on if she does not have hemodialysis). Another case, described in Exhibit 11.2, features a patient who did not have decisional capacity at the time of the initial evaluation. This case demonstrates some of the complicated issues involved in evaluating patients with acute cognitive

EXHIBIT 11.2

A Patient With Impaired Decisional Capacity

Mrs. S was admitted to the intensive care unit with pneumonia and respiratory distress. She had received bilateral lung transplants previously and was now in chronic rejection and was relisted for transplant. She was well known to the health psychology consultant. She had no formal psychological history before the medical issues. While dealing with ongoing lung problems and transplant issues, she experienced anxiety at times but coped well using cognitive techniques and distraction.

At the initial evaluation this admission, the patient was on a ventilator, communicating with head nods. She was somnolent, tearful, confused, and oriented to person and place only. She reported frightening hallucinations and that she felt like giving up. (A complete evaluation could not be done at this point.) This presentation was notably different from her cognitive and emotional baseline.

The next day, the patient was able to communicate some understanding of her medical situation, but her presentation was similar to that at the first visit. She tried to write her thoughts down, but she was unable to do so (because it was too complicated cognitively). She was interested in trying to spell some words when given the alphabet, and she spelled the words "want" and "die." It was not clear whether the patient was asking for the withdrawal of life support.

At this point, a decisional capacity evaluation could have been requested, but it was not. The patient's doctors understood that she was delirious and continued to treat her based on their understanding of her previous values, that is, that she wanted any and all measures that would help her to live and regain the quality of life she had previously. Her family supported this plan.

Over the next few weeks the patient's pneumonia improved, and she was extubated (removed from the ventilator) and she was able to talk about what she meant when she communicated that she wanted to die. She reported that she had not been asking for the medical staff to remove her from life support but that she was communicating her upset at certain aspects of her personal life.

changes that influence their decisional capacity, as well as the importance of evaluating a patient over time, if possible. There was also some conflict with the patient's family in this case; see Labott (2006) for a more detailed description of the entire case.

Sample 11.1 Decisional Capacity Evaluation

Patient referred by Dr. S for decisional capacity eval. She is a 48 y/o AA (*African American*) woman with MMP (*multiple medical problems*), admitted currently for worsening ESRD (*end-stage renal disease*). Pt refusing dialysis (*hemodialysis; HD*).

Pt is divorced, lives with her 31 y/o daughter and 3 y/o grandson. She is on medical disability, worked previously as a clerk until about 5 yrs ago. She attended school through 11th grade.

Pt saw a counselor for about 4 mts in 1995, after she divorced and was feeling anxious and depressed. No inpt psych admissions, no psych meds, no family hx.

Today, pt denies feeling depressed; she also denies problems with sleep, guilt, worthlessness, hopelessness. Appetite poor. No suicidal ideation. She reports some "stress" re: her current medical problems, but denies anxiety, significant worry, panic, manic sx, hallucinations, paranoia.

On mental status exam pt was alert and oriented × 2 (knew year and month, not date). Registration, attention, short- and long-term memory all intact. Thinking is concrete, linear, goal-directed. Judgment intact. Affect appropriate.

Pt is able to communicate that she does not want to start dialysis. She can explain that her doctors have told her that her kidneys are not functioning properly and that their functioning has been worsening over the past several years. They recommend that she begins HD now and also that she consider being listed for kidney transplant. She understands there is not really any other tx for this and that people who require HD and do not have it will die. She understands that HD will require her to attend apts 3× weekly for about 5 hrs each visit. Pt has a cousin who has had HD, so she is somewhat familiar with the procedures. Pt reports that she is a Christian and that she feels God will care for her. She sees HD as a procedure that is beyond what God would want her to do to preserve her life. She reports complying with meds and diet but sees HD as more extreme and unwarranted. Pt understands that refusing HD may result in her death, and she sees nothing that would make her change her mind as she gets sicker. She has met with her minister and also her daughter, and has clarified her values with both of them; they support her decision (even though pt's daughter would prefer that pt agrees to HD).

Impressions: Pt with ESRD, refusing HD. Mental status is WNL; no significant psych sx or hx. Pt is able to communicate her choice to refuse HD, and she understands what HD involves, as well as relevant risks and benefits. Her decision to refuse is based on her religious beliefs, and she feels HD is too extreme a measure for her. She understands that this decision means she will likely have only a few weeks or months left to live. Pt is comfortable with this, as is her social support system.

Conclusion: Pt retains capacity to make her own decision re: HD.

Nonadherence 12

Adherence refers to the degree to which a patient follows the recommendations for medication, diet, exercise, and other aspects of the treatment regimen that is prescribed by the medical providers. *Nonadherence*, or *noncompliance*, refers to the situation in which the patient does not follow all or part of the provider's instructions. At times, the term *noncompliance* seems to imply a more negative or judgmental attitude, that is, that the patient is behaving badly. However, in the field it is also commonly used in the broader sense of the patient not fulfilling his or her responsibilities in the treatment plan. In this chapter, as with this entire book, the term *nonadherence* is used to describe the situation in which a patient does not follow treatment recommendations.

Adherence Rates

Adherence may not be an all-or-none phenomenon; patients may follow certain aspects of the regimen (take medication as directed) but not others (avoid exercise). Nonadherence occurs frequently in the outpatient medical setting but also occurs in the inpatient setting, even though medical personnel have more control over a patient's behavior in the hospital than they do

http://dx.doi.org/10.1037/0000108-013
Health Psychology Consultation in the Inpatient Medical Setting, by S. M. Labott

in the outpatient setting. Nonadherence in the hospital creates a crisis in the patient's treatment and is often the impetus for a health psychology consult.

In the outpatient setting, individual studies, typically of specific diseases, report nonadherence rates with medications of 8% to 71% (Unni & Farris, 2011). Studies evaluating adherence to medications designed to manage chronic illnesses have reported adherence rates of about 50% and have also noted that adherence decreases over time (Leventhal, McCarthy, Leventhal, & Bold, 2015). Solid organ transplant patients should be highly motivated to adhere to their medication regimen because nonadherence can result in graft failure and death, but nonadherence in organ transplant recipients ranges from 20% to 50% (Laederach-Hofmann & Bunzel, 2000). Medications most associated with nonadherence include diuretics, hypnotics, analgesics, and bronchodilators (Barat, Andreasen, & Damsgaard, 2001), although patients may be noncompliant with any or all of their medications. In the inpatient setting, adherence is better because patients are monitored by nurses who dispense medications, and the patients are not personally responsible for taking them on their own. Any refusals of medication or other aspects of treatment in the hospital are obvious and generally result in actions by hospital staff to remedy the situation.

Nonadherence with dietary changes is also a major problem in the outpatient setting and has been studied most in the context of diabetes and heart disease; Broadbent, Donkin, and Stroh (2011) reported that only 22% of their sample of diabetic patients reported complete dietary adherence. In the hospital, medical staff can order a particular diet for a patient (e.g., low salt, soft, or renal diet). Although this provides some control over the foods and liquids that a patient ingests, it is common for patients to avoid eating or drinking items on their meal tray, and family members may (knowingly or unknowingly) bring foods for patients that are not part of their prescribed diet.

Exercise may be recommended as part of the patient's treatment plan, usually to decrease risk (e.g., in the case of heart disease) or to improve mobility (e.g., after hip replacement). Several studies have reported that prescribed exercise is associated with improved medical outcomes, such as decreased symptoms and relapse prevention (Dunbar-Jacob & Schlenk, 1996). Exercise program adherence is more difficult for patients than medication adherence because it takes more time, may require adjustments to a patient's routine, and may be associated with pain or discomfort. As a result, adherence to both risk reduction and rehabilitation exercise programs is about 50%, with dropout rates for on-site programs at 50% (L. E. Burke, Dunbar-Jacob, & Hill, 1997). Adherence to both on-site and home-based exercise programs is initially higher in some populations (such as cancer patients) but may then decrease over time (Pinto, Rabin, & Dunsiger, 2009). In the hospital, the prescribed exercise may take the form of physical therapy sessions up to several times daily. Adherence is high in the hospital, when the physical therapist comes directly to the room, but many patients still refuse to participate.

Patients are often asked to quit smoking to improve their health, especially in the context of respiratory diseases. A variety of treatments (i.e., antidepressants, nicotine replacement, behavior therapy) are effective at helping people to quit smoking, which results in significant improvements in health and decreased mortality (Waldroup, Gifford, & Kalra, 2006). Yet adherence to these treatments also tends to decrease over time, jeopardizing outcomes, for example, one study of nicotine patch use reported 92% adherence initially, but only 61% adherence 3 months later (Stapleton et al., 1995).

In the hospital, patients are not allowed to smoke, and heavy smokers are provided with nicotine patches to avoid withdrawal and discomfort during the hospital admission. Although this gives patients a good start on a smoking abstinence plan, many return to smoking after discharge when they return to their home environment.

Consequences of Nonadherence

For patients, nonadherence can result in poorer management of the disease, affecting their quality of life in several ways. If patients do not follow recommendations for medication and exercise, they may experience increased physical limitations, pain, additional medical complications, and death. For example, an elderly man with a recent hip replacement who fails to do physical therapy activities may have limitations on his physical mobility. If this same patient refuses to take pain medication, he may be unable to participate in physical therapy at all. If he refuses heparin injections, he may develop a blood clot, which will result in additional treatment, slow his recovery, and increase the length of his hospital admission.

Prescribed medications may also slow the progression of a chronic disease, such as multiple sclerosis (MS) or cancer, or they may decrease the likelihood of secondary effects of a disease; for example, anticoagulants decrease the risk of stroke in patients with atrial fibrillation. Patients experience decreased benefits if they do not adhere to the medication regimen. If the disease progresses or if complications occur, the patient will spend more time in the hospital, experience decreased quality of life, and be at risk of additional medical problems. Lau and Nau (2004) reported that diabetic patients who were nonadherent to their medication schedule were 2.5 times more likely to have a hospital admission during the next year than those who followed the regimen greater than 80% of the time. Finally, although some patients are able to ignore all of these issues, others worry about nonadherence and the impacts it could have on their lives and their family, adding emotional distress to the negative physical impacts of nonadherence.

Nonadherence also has public health implications. To the extent that patients do not adequately follow a prescribed regimen, costs to society increase as more treatment, outpatient visits, or hospital admissions are needed. Osterberg and Blaschke (2005) reported that 33% to 69% of medication-related hospital admissions are due to nonadherence to medication recommendations. Further, the risk of serious illness for other members of society increases if individuals do not properly follow medication recommendations. Many drug-resistant organisms have developed, in part due to patients not taking medications long enough, allowing the organisms to strengthen and mutate and become resistant to current treatments. This problem has already been documented for antituberculosis medications, antibiotics, and antiretroviral medications (Dunbar-Jacob & Schlenk, 2001).

Nonadherence Patterns

Nonadherence is demonstrated by a variety of behaviors; Dunbar-Jacob, Schlenk, and McCall (2012) described several problematic adherence patterns, including failure to adopt the treatment regimen, stopping treatment too soon, alterations in dosing (too little or too much), variable adherence, and dosing interval errors. From a clinical perspective, an awareness of the specific type of adherence problem will aid the development of a proper intervention plan. For example, some patients do not begin the treatment at all; for example, Burns, Sneddon, Lovell, McLean, and Martin (1992) reported that 27% of elderly patients did not fill their prescriptions after hospital discharge. Others begin the treatment but stop it too soon. This is especially a problem with antibiotics: Patients feel better before the medication is gone, so stop taking the antibiotics, even though the medication needs to be taken for the full amount of time for the best outcomes.

Patients may not dose their medications properly; for example, it is common for patients to take antidepressants when they feel bad, rather than taking them consistently; as a result, these patients do not derive much benefit from the medication. Alternately, patients may take too much medication, as may occur with pain medication, especially if they feel pain is not well controlled on the prescribed dose. Patients may also take too much of a medication if they have missed doses and then take an extra dose later to catch up.

Variable adherence occurs when patients follow the regimen but not consistently. Often this occurs when the routine is not an integrated part of the patient's life, so they forget to take doses of medication; this can also occur when patients run out of medications and are unable to obtain orders for refills or are unable to afford them.

Finally, dosing interval errors occur when patients do not take the medications at the prescribed intervals or they do not develop a consistent exercise routine. Patients often try to avoid taking pain medications, so they hold the medication until the pain is intolerable, even though they would do better to take the medication as prescribed to avoid significant fluctuations in pain. Interval errors in dosing also occur when patients "spread out" their medications if they are unable to afford refills at the proper times.

Medical professionals often view nonadherence as unintended on the part of the patient and due to barriers that can be addressed, such as forgetfulness, financial problems, and poor social support. Yet many patients intentionally and knowingly decide not to adhere to a treatment recommendation. In these cases, the patient has thought through the decision and can articulate his rationale for nonadherence. For example, a patient who is already taking several medications for joint pain and hypertension is now prescribed a medication to decrease cholesterol. He is concerned about taking too many medications and so reviews the risks and benefits of all three and decides the new medication to decrease cholesterol is the one to skip. In another case, a recommendation to begin chemotherapy is made for a patient with cancer. The patient refuses it because she knows she will lose her hair and feels that will be so bad for her emotionally that the treatment is not worth doing, even if this decision shortens her life. A third scenario involves a patient adjusting doses of a medication to fit the requirements of his day, for example, holding a morning diuretic until he is home from work so that numerous trips to the bathroom do not disrupt meetings at work during the day.

Wroe (2002) reported that patients make nonadherence decisions based only on information the patient considers relevant, which makes the decision idiosyncratic and therefore not always logical from another's perspective. Gadkari and McHorney (2012) suggested that unintentional nonadherence may be predictive of later intentional nonadherence, as patients test the consequences of smaller lapses in adherence before they make a commitment to complete nonadherence.

Models of Adherence

A variety of theoretical models have been used to explain an individual's adherence (or lack of adherence) to medical recommendations. The health belief model (HBM) was developed to explain under what conditions people will make changes to their behavior in an attempt to improve their health. It postulates several important components, each of which play a role in determining whether the individual engages in the recommended behavior (Martin, Haskard-Zolnierek, & DiMatteo, 2010; Rosenstock, Strecher, & Becker, 1994):

1. Perceived susceptibility: The individual's perception of their personal risk of either developing a specific disease or of the risk of developing specific associated complications or disabilities from the disease.
2. Perceived severity: The patient's perception of how bad the consequences of the disease could be.
3. Perceived benefit: A patient's estimation of the usefulness of a recommended behavior in terms of managing the problem.
4. Perceived barriers: The patient's perception of potential negative consequences associated with undertaking the recommended action.
5. Self-efficacy: The patient's belief that he is able to successfully perform the recommended behavior.

The HBM predicts that the best adherence will occur in patients who feel at risk for a severe negative outcome and who believe that engaging in the recommended behavior could help to avoid that outcome. Further, the patient is more likely to follow a recommendation if he believes the potential negative consequences of engaging in the behavior are manageable and feels capable of successfully performing the behavior. Martin et al. (2010) reviewed the literature on these critical aspects of the HBM, and reported that each element has been associated with health behavior and change, with the relative importance of each factor depending upon the specific population and the recommended behavior. Because of the consistent evidence in support of the predictions from the HBM, it has become one of the most popular theories of behavior change for medical patients.

Another popular theory of health behavior change is the common sense model (CSM; Leventhal, Brissette, & Leventhal, 2003). The CSM postulates that patients behave as scientists as they assess illness threats; the patient's conceptualization of the threat then dictates behavior change goals. Information that people use to develop their assessment of the illness threat is based on their ideas about the symptom and name of the health threat, its consequences, cause, and controllability (Leventhal, Phillips, & Burns, 2016; Reynolds, Martin, Nanyonga, & Alonzo, 2012). Initial studies of the predicted relationships among cognitions, coping, and outcomes indicated support for the model (Hagger & Orbell, 2003), although a more recent meta-analysis reported that adherence was not predicted by the illness beliefs (Aujla et al., 2016).

Other models have also been used to explain health behavior change; two examples include social cognitive theory (Rosenstock, Strecher, & Becker, 1994) and the theory of planned behavior (Ajzen & Manstead, 2007). The transtheoretical model of change (Prochaska, DiClemente, & Norcross, 1992) has become popular in assessing a patient's readiness for change, which can then be addressed to move a patient to greater readiness and then action. These and other models of behavior change are reviewed by Martin et al. (2010).

The information–motivation–strategy model (IMS; DiMatteo, Haskard-Zolnierek, & Martin, 2012; Martin et al., 2010) has been developed to integrate and simplify some of the earlier models already described. The IMS model postulates three important components:

1. Information: Patients must be informed about what they are being asked to do.
2. Motivation: Patients need to believe the behavior will work.
3. Strategy: Patients know what to do and have resources to help them perform and maintain the behavior.

Nonadherence is then a result of a problem in one of these three areas (DiMatteo et al., 2012). These researchers have also described practical strategies to address any problems with information, motivation, or strategy to increase adherence (DiMatteo et al., 2012). This approach is consistent with the empirical literature on factors that influence adherence, which is discussed next.

Factors That Influence Adherence

Nonadherence makes no sense to medical providers—patients have come to them seeking treatment for a medical problem, are provided with recommendations to improve the problem, but then they do not follow the recommendations. Reasons why a patient would not adhere to provider recommendations have been studied extensively. Meichenbaum and Turk (1987) summarized the work in this area at the time and developed a list of 52 reasons why patients might not adhere to recommendations! Over the past 30 years, a significant amount of additional research has been done on adherence. Exhibit 12.1 lists some of the most important factors that have been demonstrated to influence adherence.

Several main categories of variables have been used to explain a patient's nonadherence to a medical regimen. Patient factors that have been studied include demographics, beliefs about illness and medications, and self-efficacy. Regimen and treatment factors comprise another major category, which includes variables such as the complexity of the regimen, inconvenience, and side effects. Disease factors include variables such as chronicity, fatigue, and cognitive changes associated with the illness. Finally, the relationship with the medical provider can impact adherence; for example, poor communication, provider unavailability, and dissatisfaction with the provider can all decrease patient adherence to recommendations.

PATIENT FACTORS

Demographic Variables

Gender, socioeconomic status, and race have not been consistently related to adherence (see Dunbar-Jacob et al., 2012). In the hospital setting, however, some patients

EXHIBIT 12.1

Factors That May Influence Adherence

Patient factors
- Demographics
- Emotions and personality
- Self-efficacy
- Social support
- Cognition and mental status
- Patient beliefs
- Adherence history

Regimen and treatment factors
- Complexity
- Side effects
- Immediate versus delayed consequences
- The hospital milieu
- Other issues associated with treatment

Disease characteristics
- Chronicity
- Severity
- Symptoms

Relationship with the medical provider
- Communication
- Satisfaction with provider
- Trust
- Provider availability

will report barriers to adherence that are related to socioeconomic status, such as being unable to exercise because they live in an unsafe neighborhood or can't afford a gym membership. Some studies have reported that older adults (generally over age 65) demonstrate better adherence to medication (e.g., Kripalani, Gatti, & Jacobson, 2010), continuous positive airway pressure (CPAP; e.g., Sawyer et al., 2011), and alcoholism treatment (Oslin, Pettinati, & Volpicelli, 2002), although others have reported no age effects on adherence in adults (e.g., Dunbar-Jacob et al., 2012; Young & Kahana, 1989).

Emotions and Personality

Much research has been done to explore emotional states that could influence adherence; studies of depression, anxiety, and hostility have produced mixed results (Dunbar-Jacob, Gemmell, & Schlenk, 2009). Personality factors, such as conscientiousness, neuroticism, extroversion, openness, agreeableness, and locus of control have also not consistently been associated with adherence (Dunbar-Jacob et al., 2009). Clinically, it is easy to find instances in which emotional states have had an impact on a patient's adherence in the hospital. Patients are less likely to follow a recommendation if they are overwhelmed and are unable to manage all the demands placed on them. They may also refuse to adhere to requests if they are frightened and trying to exert some control over the situation or if they are denying that they are sick at all (due to either personality or cognitive factors).

Self-Efficacy

Self-efficacy, the belief that one is able to adequately perform a required behavior, has also been studied as it relates to adherence. The literature generally shows a positive relationship between self-efficacy and adherence, in different diseases and with respect to different adherence behaviors (e.g., Chen et al., 2014; Colbert, Sereika, & Erlen, 2013; Dunbar-Jacob et al., 2009; McAuley et al., 2011). Self-efficacy has also been shown to mediate the effects of other variables on adherence; for example, Tovar, Rayens, Gokun, and Clark (2015) showed that self-efficacy can decrease the negative impact of depression on adherence.

Social Support

Adherence has been associated with social support in many studies (see reviews by DiMatteo, 2004, and Wheeler, Roberts, & Neiheisel, 2014), and in the context of many diseases, such as MS (Siegel, Turner, & Haselkorn, 2008), hypertension (Magrin et al., 2015), cardiovascular disease (Aggarwal, Liao, Allegrante, & Mosca, 2010), diabetes (Costa, Pereira, & Pedras, 2012), and HIV (Simoni, Frick, & Huang, 2006). Both practical and emotional support improve adherence, with practical support being most relevant (DiMatteo, 2004). Further, aspects of structural support (such as being married, living with someone else, and a stable home situation) are important in some contexts but not others (e.g., DiMatteo, 2004; Magrin et al., 2015; Wheeler et al., 2014).

In the hospital setting, the role of social support is abundantly clear as it relates to patient adherence (as well as other psychological variables, such as mood and coping). Family members have significant power when it comes to encouraging patients, explaining the medical issues, coaxing them to participate, obtaining additional information to aid the treatment team, and providing instrumental support to help patients compensate for physical and cognitive limitations.

Cognition and Mental Status

Cognitive deficits negatively affect adherence because patients with symptoms of dementia are less adherent to medications (Barat et al., 2001); delirious patients also perform poorly if allowed to manage medications independently. Further, normal forgetting in individuals without diagnosable cognitive problems is one of the main reasons patients provide to explain their nonadherence (Dunbar-Jacob et al., 2012). Similarly, a poor understanding of what is required is associated with nonadherence (Barat et al., 2001). Recent studies have also implicated poor health literacy as a cause of nonadherence, although the evidence so far is mixed (e.g., Chen et al., 2014; Dunbar-Jacob et al., 2009; T. A. Miller, 2016).

Patient Beliefs

When working with individual patients clinically, the role of patient beliefs is clear: If patients believe the behavior is important for their health, and they feel their health is important, they are likely to try to adhere and are also likely to succeed unless there are significant barriers that they have difficulty overcoming. They are less likely to follow a treatment recommendation if they do not believe their efforts will make a difference.

Some psychologists view the severity of the threat (i.e., a patient's diagnosis with a serious illness) as a wake-up call that has the potential to scare the patient and jolt her into adherence. There are certainly cases in which this occurs, although it can also backfire. That is, if a patient is too scared, she may become immobilized and give up. She may feel the situation is hopeless and that nothing she does will change the expected negative outcome, so she does nothing. For less serious illnesses, the patient may not be too concerned about the outcome and feels she doesn't need to exert much effort to influence it. This could occur with a patient who has no history of cardiac problems and doesn't feel sick, so she isn't motivated to take a statin to decrease cholesterol.

Patient beliefs often interfere with adherence, but they are generally not readily apparent to the clinician. Patients may also be unaware of or have difficulty articulating them, although these beliefs may be expressed incidentally when discussing other aspects of the treatment. For example, when asking a patient to explain the dosing schedule for a newly prescribed medication, she may preface her response with, "Well, many drugs don't agree with me so I don't like taking them." A statement like this provides a great deal of information that warrants more discussion and may explain a patient's nonadherence.

If the patient's beliefs do not become apparent through incidental comments, then the psychologist will need to elicit these beliefs during the interview. If they affect adherence, they will need to be addressed and so need to be clarified, discussed, and tactfully challenged. Perhaps the best way to begin this discussion is to ask the patient: "Do you have any concerns about the medication/diet changes/exercise that your doctors are recommending?" Any and all concerns should be addressed to the patient's satisfaction, or adherence is at risk.

Some research has begun to explore beliefs about medications as a factor in adherence. Unni and Farris (2011) reported that concerns about negative consequences of taking medications were associated with decreased adherence in older adults. Further, Schüz et al. (2011) studied a group of older adults with several medical problems and on several medications and reported that beliefs in the need for the prescribed medication to help control the illness were associated with increased intentional adherence. Patient beliefs that they were taking too many medications were associated with nonadherence in patients who forgot to take their medications. Patients also have ideas about the relative importance of various aspects of the regimen that influence adherence; diabetic patients rate medication as more important than diet and exercise in diabetes treatment, for example, and so adherence to medication is better (Broadbent et al., 2011).

Exhibit 12.2 lists common patient beliefs that can interfere with adherence to the regimen, followed by statements or questions that the psychologist can use to explore and begin to address them. The goal of these interventions is to move the patient toward more adaptive ideas and beliefs about themselves, the illness, and the prescribed treatment, ultimately to improve adherence. Although some of the clinician responses challenge the patient, the entire discussion should be done with empathy and in a nonjudgmental manner.

Adherence History

Previous adherence behavior often predicts future adherence behavior. That is, initial adherence to a specific health behavior (such as starting a new medication) is associated with later adherence to that same behavior (continuing the medication over time). However, previous adherence to one specific behavior, such as exercise, is not necessarily predictive of adherence to a different behavior, such as diet (Dunbar-Jacob et al., 2009).

REGIMEN AND TREATMENT FACTORS

Regimen Complexity

The complexity of the treatment regimen is the single most important factor that predicts nonadherence. Regimen complexity occurs when a patient has to take several doses of a medication daily, take multiple daily medications, or follow a combination of medication, diet, and exercise recommendations. In a review of medication dosing studies, Claxton, Cramer, and Pierce (2001) reported that adherence decreased as the

EXHIBIT 12.2

Patient Beliefs Associated With Nonadherence and Suggested Clinician Responses

"This medical issue is no big deal and so doesn't warrant much effort from me."

> What does your doctor say about the importance of doing this? Do you believe him? Does he have any reason to be dishonest with you? Do you expect this to take a huge amount of effort? Would you be more willing if we could find ways to make it easier?

"I know the doctor says that I need to take the medications and exercise to stay healthy, but I feel good, so I'm not worried."

> It's great that you feel good, and this isn't about making you worry. I think the idea is that he feels you won't continue to feel this good if you don't begin the regimen now. Do you see any benefits to doing this?

"I am a healthy person overall, so don't need medications. I'm not sick."

> It's good to be healthy—does taking this medication mean you are not? Many healthy people have medical issues to deal with and so take maintenance medications to stay healthy. Does taking medication, changing your diet, etc. mean you are sick?

"I'll wait until I'm not feeling good."

> Sometimes people do that, but by the time they decide to take action, the disease has progressed and you can't always reverse that, so it is usually better to start now before it gets bad.

"I don't like chemicals in my body, so I avoid taking any medications that I can."

> Avoiding unnecessary medications is always a good idea, but it sounds like there are times when medications are necessary. When in the past have you taken medication; under what conditions would you consider doing so again? Does this situation meet those conditions?

"I'm worried about side effects of the medication."

> What do you know about this medication? What side effects are expected—their frequency of occurrence? Severity? Let's weigh the possible side effects against the potential benefits.

"My uncle had this medical issue, never saw a doctor, took medication, or had any treatment, and he did OK."

> True that some people don't do treatment and seem to do OK, and back then we didn't have the options for treatment that we have now anyway. There is lots of data, though, that most people do better if they take the medication. I wonder if your uncle was just one of the lucky ones?

"I don't want to do this."

> Why not? Why wouldn't you make some changes to keep yourself as healthy as possible? What would you say to your wife if she said she didn't feel like taking her medication?

"It takes too much time"

> Let's talk about ways to make this easier.

number of daily doses of the medication increased, with adherence at 79% for one daily dose, decreasing with the number of doses until it was 51% for four doses daily. Ingersoll and Cohen (2008) reviewed 10 years of adherence research and noted that poor adherence is consistently associated with increased dose frequency and regimens that require several activities (e.g., multiple medications and diet).

It can be difficult for some people to learn to take one medication each morning with their breakfast, but if they need to take two oral medications at different times of the day, check their blood glucose and adjust a dose of insulin, use a CPAP machine at night, and institute a diabetic diet, the likelihood of adherence goes down dramatically. The more a person has to do, the more trouble she will have doing it. Not only does the patient have a lot to remember, but following the regimen takes significant time; she must buy and prepare the correct foods, clean CPAP equipment, check blood glucose, and calculate and deliver insulin. Further, certain aspects of the treatment may be inconvenient or may be difficult for the patient to integrate into her lifestyle (e.g., taking diuretics when working as a bus driver where there are few toilet options throughout the day).

Side Effects

Certain medications for HIV, MS, and cancer, as well as many others, are associated with side effects such as flulike symptoms that cause the patient to feel poorly much of the time. Nonadherence has been a serious problem with HIV medications and has been studied extensively (Bhatti, Usman, & Kandi, 2016). Especially if the patient feels no subjective benefit from taking the medication, these side effects can decrease adherence. In some cases, patients may adjust doses so that they are able to work or engage in other activities, but in other cases, they may stop the medications altogether because they interfere too dramatically with the patient's quality of life.

Immediate Versus Delayed Consequences

As with other behaviors, people are more likely to engage in the behavior (i.e., adhere to the regimen) if they receive immediate and positive consequences for doing so, and they are less likely to adhere if there are no consequences or the anticipated consequences are far in the future. For example, if a patient is experiencing pain but the pain lessens if he takes an oral pain medication or delivers IV medication using a patient-controlled analgesia pump, these behaviors will be reinforced by the pain relief and are likely to occur again. However, if a patient is asked to adhere to a schedule of twice daily Eliquis to decrease the likelihood of a stroke if she has an episode of atrial fibrillation, there is no immediate reinforcement for engaging in the behavior—the potential benefits are delayed, and the patient may not even know whether any benefit has ever occurred. Even if the problem that could occur (the stroke) could be life-changing and even life-threatening, there are no clear and immediate benefits, making it more difficult to gain adherence to the regimen now. This is an important issue because much of modern medical treatment is designed to prevent future problems, but patient motivation to adhere to the recommendations is more difficult to achieve and maintain for future prevention than for current symptoms.

The Hospital Milieu

When hospitalized, much of a patient's social support is less available to them, they have minimal privacy, and they lose control of their regular routine, creating significant stress for many people. Medical providers tend to believe that they ask little of hospitalized patients, but patients often see it differently. They are expected to eat food that is usually unappealing, participate in uncomfortable procedures, take many medications and other treatments, and shower when told to do so. They may also be expected to exercise and to learn lists of medications and their uses (if the patient is a candidate for transplant or some other special procedure). They also need to deal with a variety of medical providers who come and go throughout the day. All this may be overwhelming, and patients are expected to manage it all in the context of poor sleep and perhaps pain or other discomfort. Patients may refuse to follow some or all of the requests made by medical staff because they do not see requests as relevant or are trying to gain some control. Once discharged from the hospital, patients have more control over their lives, but then they are responsible for managing all aspects of their care by themselves (e.g., organizing medications, exercising, attending doctor appointments).

Other Issues Associated With Treatment

Tangential aspects of the treatment can also impact adherence. Patients are less likely to adhere to recommendations if they have difficulty getting timely appointments with the physician, have transportation problems, or experience financial or insurance issues that make adherence more difficult. It is not uncommon for patients to stop taking the medication that is the most expensive if they have financial problems.

DISEASE CHARACTERISTICS

As noted earlier, adherence to various aspects of a treatment regimen tends to decrease over time. Forissier (2011) reported on adherence rates for ongoing medications. Sixty-nine percent of the patients initially filled the prescription, but adherence decreased consistently over time, so that only 43% were refilling it after 6 months. Adherence to maintenance medications for chronic illnesses (e.g., high blood pressure, high cholesterol, diabetes) is often difficult for patients, and especially if they see no consequences of adherence versus nonadherence. Even if patients were initially motivated to follow the treatment recommendations, as they adjust to having the illness, and especially if it does not have much impact on their day-to-day lives, they can become complacent. However, there is also some evidence that severity and chronicity of the disease are associated with improved adherence (Wheeler et al., 2014). If patients experience ongoing problems and can see the benefit of consistently continuing their medication, adherence is better.

Some diseases (or treatments) are associated with symptoms that can influence adherence. A common symptom of MS is fatigue, which can make it more difficult for patients to motivate themselves to do the work associated with adherence to a medication or exercise regimen. MS may also result in cognitive deficits, such as slowing, memory problems, and decreased executive function; these can also make adherence more difficult for patients.

RELATIONSHIP WITH MEDICAL PROVIDER

Adherence to medical recommendations is affected by the patient's relationship with medical providers. Good communication, satisfaction, trust, and provider availability are all associated with improved patient adherence to the treatment plan.

Communication

Communication between patients and providers has been studied extensively. In a meta-analysis of more than 100 studies in varied populations, Haskard Zolnierek and DiMatteo (2009) reported that the research has consistently demonstrated that adherence is better in the context of good patient–provider communication; there is a 19% higher risk of nonadherence if communication is poor. Communication is therefore a pervasive factor in adherence and is operative among patients with different medical issues (e.g., Fox et al., 2009; Swain, Hariharan, Rana, Chivukula, & Thomas, 2015), and with patients of different ethnic backgrounds (e.g., Schoenthaler et al., 2009). Good communication with other medical providers, such as nurses and pharmacists, improves adherence similarly (e.g., Linn, van Weert, van Dijk, Horne, & Smit, 2016; Penn, Watermeyer, & Evans, 2011).

Satisfaction

Patient satisfaction with the treatment and providers is also related to communication and is associated with improved adherence. Specific provider behaviors associated with adherence and patient satisfaction include the provision of quality information that is tailored to the patient's specific situation, the provider listening and being willing to discuss issues with the patient, a collaborative approach to improving the patient's health, positive reinforcement, and friendliness (e.g., Linn et al., 2016; Wheeler et al., 2014). Certainly patients who have more information about their illness feel more in control and able to manage it. Provider support, over the long term, also serves to improve adherence.

Trust

Krueger, Berger, and Felkey (2005) reported on several studies in which "a trusting, supportive relationship" with the provider was associated with improved adherence. In a study of diabetes patients, trust was significantly correlated with adherence (Lee & Lin, 2009). Others have reported that adherence is 3 times higher among patients who trust their doctor and feel that she knows them; trust was also the best predictor of patient satisfaction (Safran et al., 1998).

Provider Availability

None of the relevant factors that influence communication, satisfaction, and ultimately adherence can occur if the provider is not accessible to the patient. Many patients admitted to the hospital have complained that they were unable to reach their doctor or nurse with a question about a new medication, so simply didn't take it. If the health psychology consultant points out that this is not an adaptive way to address the problem, they usually agree, but at the moment they were frustrated at being unable to talk with their provider about their problem, they did not consider other options.

Establishing Initial Adherence: Education

When patients are initially provided with recommendations for medication, diet, exercise, or any other health behaviors, the two most important goals are that they (a) understand what they are being asked to do and (b) know *why* they are being asked to do it. Exhibit 12.3 provides suggestions for patient education that can improve adherence. There is a significant amount of information that a patient needs to understand; with a new prescription, for example, the patient needs to know how, how often, and how long to take the medication; restrictions regarding food intake; handling of missed doses; and potential side effects.

The rationale for the recommendation provides the patient with a reason to exert the effort to follow the recommendation and should be presented clearly and in terms the patient can understand. For example, "The reason for taking this medication is that it will help your body to accept the transplanted kidney as part of you, so that the kidney will be able to function well and you can stay off dialysis" or "It is important for you to avoid sugar because your body is unable process it properly, and too much sugar in your system will cause you to feel lightheaded and faint, and can cause other medical issues such as skin problems, nerve pain, foot ulcers, and many others."

Providing the proper education initially can circumvent many of the adherence problems that can occur later; Barat et al. (2001), for example, reported that an understanding of the purpose of a medication and also the consequences of not taking it are associated with adherence. Initial education on medical recommendations will typically be presented by the physician, but the psychologist may review, reinforce, and expand on that information to enhance adherence.

Evaluation of Adherence Problems

Hospitalized patients are often referred to health psychology due to patient nonadherence to medical recommendations, both in the hospital and at home. The first step in improving a patient's adherence to a medical recommendation is to determine

EXHIBIT 12.3

Initial Patient Education to Enhance Adherence

1. Present the task explicitly and concretely.
   - Take a medication
     - How: orally, topically, etc.
     - How often
     - Take it with food or liquids? Avoid taking it with food/liquids or with certain food/liquids?
     - How to handle a missed dose
     - How long to take it (e.g., for a certain amount of time, until it is gone, until further notice)
     - Potential side effects to attend to
   - Dietary changes
     - What to eat and what not to eat—categories of foods/drinks and specific foods/drinks
     - Strategies to increase the amounts of foods that should be eaten and to decrease intake of those that should not
     - Portion sizes; number of meals/snacks daily
   - Begin exercise regimen
     - What type of exercise
     - How much
     - How often
     - How to start and then increase effort
     - How to monitor for safety, proper level of intensity
2. Present a clear rationale for the recommended behavior.
   - Avoid jargon; present the material in lay terms and at a proper educational and literacy level for the specific patient
   - Use interpreters as needed
   - Use diagrams or videos to reinforce the information; provide patients with written instructions to take home; encourage patients to take notes or have a family member present to help them to remember
   - Keep it simple: both the regimen itself and also the instructions; present the education in more than one visit if the material and regimen are complicated
3. Set up cues/reminders as needed (e.g., pill box, note on refrigerator).
4. Check on the patient's understanding of the regimen and rationale. Encourage questions and have the patient repeat the information back in their own words.
5. Be sure the patient agrees with the plan and knows what to do if problems develop; encourage patients to call or e-mail their provider with questions as needed.

the reason for the nonadherence. Consider a patient who is only sporadically taking a blood pressure medication. The patient may not take it because she does not like the side effects of the medication or because she does not believe the medication is necessary. She may be unable to afford the medication, or she may intend to but forgets to take it. The intervention for each of these issues is different; problem-solving ways for the patient to be able to afford the medication is irrelevant if the problem is that she forgets to take it when her grandchildren come over and distract her. Adherence is likely to improve only if the cause is accurately delineated and then addressed with the appropriate intervention.

The best source of information about a nonadherence problem is the patient. It is important to make this a collaborative and nonjudgmental interview because nonadherent patients often feel accused by medical staff and can be defensive when discussing the topic. The patient needs to understand that the goal of the interview is to obtain information to help him manage the medical issue as best he can so that he can be as healthy as possible and have the best quality of life possible. This discussion will usually begin with an assessment of the patient's understanding of the recommendations and of the rationale for them.

For hospitalized patients, a major reason for nonadherence is that patients do not fully understand what they are being asked to do and why. Even if patients are trying to follow medical recommendations, if they misunderstand the task, they have no chance at adequate adherence. In most cases, repeating or providing additional education about the disease and its expected course, the specific recommendations (e.g., exercising, taking medication), and the rationale for the recommendations will usually clarify misunderstandings as to the importance of what patients are being asked to do and why. During this conversation, patient beliefs about the disease and the recommended behavior will often surface and can be addressed. For many patients, resolving misunderstandings is sufficient to get their commitment to follow the recommendation. The next step, then, is to discover and remove any additional barriers that will keep them from following the recommendations.

A patient should be asked about anything that interferes with their performance of the recommended behavior. Financial issues, transportation, time constraints, social issues, side effects, and other nonmonetary costs may all need to be discussed. Additional information on possible reasons for nonadherence can be found in the medical record at times, but this information is usually incomplete and tends to be presented to demonstrate how the patient has behaved badly.

Once the specific reason(s) for the nonadherence is determined, the health psychology consultant can intervene to address or remove the barriers that are preventing adequate adherence. The goals of intervention when the patient has demonstrated problems with adherence are to increase motivation to perform the behavior and to generate plans to make performance of the behavior easier.

Plans to Improve Adherence

Specific interventions that are useful in addressing adherence problems (besides the education which is the most basic and critical component) include motivational interviewing (MI), developing behavioral plans, and improving communication with the medical providers. Often a combination of these interventions is warranted to address all of the relevant issues. Two large reviews of adherence interventions have reported improvements in adherence or outcomes after many types of adherence interventions (Conn, Ruppar, Enriquez, & Cooper, 2016; McDonald, Garg, & Haynes, 2002).

ENHANCE MOTIVATION

MI is "a skillful clinical style for eliciting from patients their own good motivations for making behavior changes in the interest of their health" (Rollnick, Miller, & Butler, 2008, p. 6). It involves a range of interviewing techniques that are designed to increase motivation to adhere to health recommendations. MI is related to the transtheoretical model (Prochaska et al., 1992) in which the goal is to move clients from ambivalence about change to a greater readiness to change. Developed initially to treat substance abuse, MI has now been used in many areas with many problems and health issues. Reviews have demonstrated positive effects of MI on behavioral changes in the context of diabetes, dental health, diet and exercise, asthma, hypertension, hyperlipidemia, heart disease, and others (B. L. Burke, Arkowitz, & Menchola, 2003; Knight, McGowan, Dickens, & Bundy, 2006; Martins & McNeil, 2009).

In the inpatient medical setting, specific interventions grounded in the principles of MI can be used to help patients move toward change. Patients can be asked about behaviors that can improve their health, why they would want to engage in these behaviors, and how they could begin to do so. Patients can be asked to rate their motivation and the likelihood they would institute the new behavior. One strategy is to delineate the inconsistency between a patient's health goals and current behavior and then to evaluate the risks and benefits of making changes. For example, many bariatric surgery patients express an eagerness to undergo surgery, a procedure that involves physical risk, in an effort to improve their health. Yet they are often less willing to quit smoking, an activity that involves significantly less risk but perhaps more effort. The discrepancy between undertaking one health behavior that involves significant risk while not undertaking another which involves no risk, although both have the potential for significant benefit, can be discussed. The patient can be asked to consider how quitting smoking could affect her health and how important it is, and to describe activities that could move her closer to making changes. The goal is to facilitate the patient moving toward the new behavior by eliciting her thoughts about why this is important and what she could do to make the changes. The clinician's role is to listen for and capitalize on statements that suggest change and to guide and encourage the patient to make the relevant changes. Specific techniques and examples of the use of MI can be found in Anstiss and Passmore (2012), Miller and Rollnick (2013), and Rollnick et al. (2008).

PROMOTE ADAPTIVE ILLNESS BELIEFS

Correcting any inaccurate beliefs is one way to improve adherence. As noted previously, education about the disease, the recommended medication or behavior, potential benefits, and also possible side effects should all be discussed with the patient. He should be made aware of potential consequences of nonadherence in terms of disease progression, quality of life, pain, and longevity. If the patient has any additional concerns, such as negative information he has heard from family or friends, these should all be addressed. Sometimes people have been told information that is blatantly wrong. Incorrect ideas need to be discussed and corrected so that the patient is not harboring potentially incorrect information that could influence adherence.

Patient beliefs about their ability to perform the required behavior should also be explored. Plans can be made to provide specific skills training to the patient (e.g., for self-administering insulin) or for strategies that can help the patient to integrate the new behavior into his daily routine. Patients should gain an understanding of the recommended behavior and its importance, as well as a sense of efficacy that they are capable of performing it as required for as long as it is necessary.

DEVELOP COGNITIVE–BEHAVIORAL TREATMENT PLANS

Once the patient has made a commitment to the regimen, the psychologist can help the patient to generate a compliance plan using cognitive and behavioral strategies to help him consistently engage in the behavior. The patient may be unwilling to discuss a detailed plan for adherence unless he understands that the goal is to organize the situation to make this as easy as possible. Often the plan can be simple and serves only to cue the patient to engage in the behavior. For example, if a patient forgets to take morning medications, perhaps placing the medication bottle next to her toothbrush or the coffee pot, putting a sticky note on the bathroom mirror, or setting an alarm on the patient's cell phone will serve as a sufficient reminder for the patient to take the medication. For a patient who needs to remember to walk each morning, placing tennis shoes on the floor next to the bed can remind her to put them on and go. Similarly, a plan to self-monitor the behavior with a simple chart may serve to cue the behavior. If the patient is agreeable with the regimen but forgets, simple reminders such as these may be enough to resolve the adherence problem.

However, some regimens need more complex planning, either due to the complexity of the regimen itself or because the barriers to adherence are more complicated. As with all behavior plans, it is critical to involve the patient in setting appropriate goals, developing the schedule, and selecting reinforcers. It is important to offer the patient as much control over the plan as possible, while keeping the plan realistic. For a patient who needs to begin an exercise regimen but has been nonadherent for the past 2 months, once understanding is established and the patient appears motivated to engage in exercise, plans can be made regarding how to get started. Attending to even small details will improve the likelihood that the plan will work; a common mistake on the part of the psychologist is to assume the patient has a better understanding of this process than he actually does. The patient and the psychologist will need to determine which days and what time of day the patient will begin to exercise, as well as what type and how much exercise she should do initially. It is common for patients to generate plans that are unrealistic (e.g., "Well, I'll just start exercising every day for 60 minutes"). Patients need to be encouraged to start slowly and gradually increase the exercise rather than starting with the ultimate goal. Plans to problem solve if something goes wrong can also be discussed. Monitoring of the behavior, usually with a simple calendar or chart, can help establish and also maintain the behavior.

The adherence plan will work best if reinforcement for the behavior is built into the plan. Patients will need help choosing rewards and developing the proper contingencies. They should be helped to develop small and frequent rewards initially (e.g., a relaxing hot bath after exercise, 30 minutes to play a computer game), followed by bigger rewards after larger accomplishments (e.g., see a movie or buy a new sweater after 2 weeks of following the regimen). Cognitive strategies can also be used to help the patient to maintain motivation (e.g., remind herself of the potential benefits and that she is doing a good job).

ENHANCE SOCIAL SUPPORT

Patients often do not take advantage of the social support available to them and need to be encouraged to do so. Family members may be unaware of a patient's medical regimen, but if the patient explains the requirements, family members can offer emotional support and reminders that may help the patient improve adherence. In some cases, a patient's wife (who does the cooking) is unaware that her husband needs to make dietary changes, but she can help with that if he explains to her what needs to be done. In other cases, grown children can help with shopping and cooking for elderly parents who live alone. Medication adherence generally improves if a significant other takes responsibility for the patient's medications. This could involve requesting and picking up refills in a timely manner, setting up a pill box, or actively dispensing the medications to the patient. The level of involvement of the family member will depend on the functioning of the patient, but family involvement generally works to increase adherence; family members can also alert providers to problems.

IMPROVE COMMUNICATION WITH THE PROVIDER

If communication is a problem, the health psychology consultant can work with the patient to communicate more effectively with the treatment team (see the section on communication in Chapter 6, this volume). In some cases, it is useful for the psychologist to talk with the treatment team on the patient's behalf to encourage mutual understanding and develop methods to facilitate contact between the provider and the patient.

DECREASE REGIMEN COMPLEXITY

There may be ways the physician can simplify the treatment regimen to improve patient adherence (e.g., by adjusting doses of medications, using extended-release versions, or substituting other medications that can be taken less frequently). If this is not possible, the health psychology consultant can work with the patient to simplify it in other ways. For example, if several medications are to be taken once daily, is it possible to take them all at the same time? Can the patient use his inhaler at the same time he takes his oral medications?

ONGOING MONITORING

Finally, patients need to be attentive to their own adherence, and strategies can be provided to increase their attention to this. For example, a diabetic patient should perhaps reevaluate diet and medication adherence on a monthly basis. On the first day of each month, she could review her adherence to the regimen. If she sees her adherence is lessening, she could then review her educational materials and develop a plan to resume the proper behaviors. If she is not successful, then she should call a member of her treatment team to request additional help. Patients are better able to solve adherence problems when they occur if they have plans in place to do so.

Pain 13

Inpatient health psychology consultations may not be specifically requested for pain management because physicians tend to think in terms of medication for the treatment of pain. However, referrals may be requested when medications are not sufficiently managing the pain or if there are issues of personality or psychopathology that interfere with the medical treatment. In addition, pain is often discovered as a problem when the health psychology consultant is evaluating a patient for some other reason.

Acute and Chronic Pain

Acute pain occurs frequently in the inpatient hospital setting (e.g., after a surgery, during a sickle cell pain crisis, in physical rehabilitation, or associated with mucositis after chemotherapy). There is generally a specific, known cause for the pain, which sends an adaptive signal to the individual that something is wrong in the body and should be addressed. Acute pain is expected to be time-limited, that is, the pain will decrease and stop completely as its cause is resolved. Treatments of acute pain include medication, ice or heat, and psychological interventions.

http://dx.doi.org/10.1037/0000108-014
Health Psychology Consultation in the Inpatient Medical Setting, by S. M. Labott

Chronic pain is pain that has continued for a longer time and/or at greater intensity than what is expected based on the physical examination and is most frequently treated in the outpatient setting. However, chronic pain patients may be seen in the hospital, often for an acute exacerbation of ongoing chronic pain, such as in the case of a sickle cell patient who experiences chronic pain but is admitted for an acute pain crisis.

Pain Assessment

Patients in pain may be irritable and unwilling to participate in an extended interview. However, if a patient believes the interview with the health psychologist can have a positive impact on their pain, they are more likely to cooperate. One way to facilitate the patient's engagement is to demonstrate appropriate attention to the pain. Therefore, if a patient complains about pain, the psychologist should stop the standard interview, assess the patient's pain, and provide some immediate intervention before returning to the interview. The psychologist should make the assessment of the pain a priority, limit nonpain interview questions to those required, and perhaps postpone the remainder of a comprehensive interview to a later time when the patient is feeling better. This approach can provide the patient with some immediate pain relief, may result in more or more accurate information being obtained from the patient, and will also facilitate rapport.

Pain is a subjective experience. Physicians have an idea of how much pain a patient is likely to experience based on the medical issues they are dealing with, but the patient's subjective report of his pain experience is the main factor in determining pain treatment. In the inpatient medical setting, the assessment of pain is often simple: Patients are asked how much pain they are experiencing on a scale from 0 to 10, with 0 being no pain at all and 10 being the worst pain they could imagine. The scale is straightforward and provides an easy method to get a rough estimate of pain from almost all patients, including those with poor literacy. This scale is used frequently by nurses and other medical personnel, so patients are familiar with it and can easily provide a pain rating; it can also be used to track changes in pain over time.

Interview items to be included in a brief pain assessment are listed in Exhibit 13.1. The health psychology consultant should know the answers to some of these items from the chart review, but some information will need to be confirmed by again asking the patient. (Reinterviewing patients about many items that have been discussed at length with other providers will be annoying to them; strategies for making it less annoying include saying, "I know you have explained this before, but it helps me to hear it directly from you.") Information about the location, intensity, type of pain, triggers, and factors that help to decrease the pain can provide a basic conceptualization for the psychologist to begin to intervene quickly. There are a variety of more thorough quantitative measures of pain that are most useful in the assessment of ongoing pain in the outpatient setting, such as the McGill Pain Questionnaire (Katz & Melzack, 2011) and the Multidimensional Pain Inventory (Kerns, Turk, & Rudy, 1985). These and other measures of pain and related variables are described in Hardin (2004) and Turk and Melzack (2011).

EXHIBIT 13.1

Basic Pain Assessment

Location of the pain
Intensity
Is there a known cause? An acute cause?
Continual or sporadic
Duration
What factors make it worse? Better?
What is being done to manage it
Is doctor/nurse aware?
Type of pain (e.g., stabbing, throbbing, aching)

Factors That Impact Pain

Turk, Wilson, and Swanson (2012) have provided an extensive description of psychological factors associated with chronic pain; many of these are also relevant for acute pain. These factors include negative emotions, cognitive factors, pain beliefs, coping, catastrophizing, perceived control, self-efficacy, and attention. Negative emotions, such as anxiety, anger, and depression, can exacerbate both acute and chronic pain. In the hospital, patients may be dealing with an unknown medical diagnosis and its potential impact on their lives, or they may already have been diagnosed with a frightening illness that could end their lives. Patients who experience pain are often fearful that the pain will increase and that it will not be managed effectively, increasing their current stress and discomfort. Feeling a lack of control over the pain or over the medical problem can also influence the patient's pain experience. These situations can be associated with negative emotions (such as fear, anxiety, or depression) that can decrease the patient's ability to cope effectively with the pain. Alternately, if a patient has just had a successful surgery, the pain associated with the healing process is less likely to elicit negative emotions because it is perceived differently.

The inpatient hospital milieu may also result in other discomforts (such as sleep deprivation) that can also impair coping and exacerbate pain. Other stressors associated with the hospital admission, such as insurance problems or fears of job loss and related financial problems, can also increase stress and affect pain. Families are often stressed by the patient's medical problem, and chronic family problems may intensify with a new medical crisis. Each of these can create additional stress for the patient that may be reflected in the experience of pain.

Lazarus and Folkman (1984) proposed a model of stress, appraisal, and coping that is relevant to a patient's experience of pain. In this model, people appraise the threat associated with an event (i.e., the pain), and their beliefs about their own ability to cope with or manage it. These appraisals and beliefs then determine what, if any, coping behaviors the patient will engage in to manage the threat.

Patients also make judgments about the meaning of their pain, and these appraisals can influence the experience of pain. Most people understand that pain signals that something is wrong in the body, and many believe that being healthy means there is never any pain experienced. Therefore, pain means that something bad is happening to them physically. Especially if the cause of the pain is undiagnosed, some people will catastrophize, believing their pain is a horrible threat that they are completely unable to manage. They may become overly distressed and upset, which can exacerbate the pain.

Patients' expectations also play a role in the experience of pain and may need to be addressed. In some cases, patients should not expect to be pain free. In these cases, they will do better if they understand that they may not be pain free but that medication and psychological interventions will enable them to manage their pain. If a patient's expectation is to be completely pain free, she will have more difficulty coping with the pain, especially if it is ongoing.

It can be extremely difficult for patients to focus their attention on other issues when they are in pain, especially if the pain is intense, but attention to the pain is likely to exacerbate it. Somatosensory amplification occurs when a patient is attentive to (sometimes minimal) bodily sensations and is upset by them. Studied most in the context of somatoform disorders, amplification has been associated with increased discomfort and also disability (Barsky, Goodson, Lane, & Cleary, 1988). Many of the psychological interventions for pain are based on distraction, and "attention management" (to include treatments such as mindfulness, imagery, and pain coping) has been shown to decrease the interference of pain, anxiety, and hypervigilance in chronic pain patients (Elomaa, de C. Williams, & Kalso, 2009).

Interventions to Address Pain

The health psychology consultant who undertakes the management of acute pain with medical inpatients needs to accept two realities: (a) people often do not understand that psychological interventions can help to decrease physical pain, and (b) psychological interventions are adjuncts to pain medication, rather than substitutes for them. The first issue can be addressed through education (as described subsequently), and the second is addressed through the psychologist's presentation of the interventions. That is, these should not be presented to the patient as the ultimate "fix" for the pain but as techniques that the patient can use to help herself manage the pain, in addition to the medication provided by physicians. (Background information on a physician's assessment of pain, medications available for its management, and dosing schedules are described in Nejad and Alpay, 2010.) Many patients will attest to the utility of the psychological interventions when medications are not sufficiently controlling their pain or when the medication wears off between doses. Psychological interventions also allow them some feeling of control over the pain. Patients should be encouraged to view these psychological interventions as skills they can learn and use as needed.

In the inpatient medical setting, the main interventions a health psychology consultant uses to treat acute pain are education, relaxation strategies, distraction, and stress and affect management. It is often also useful to advocate for the patient with the medical team. Each of these is discussed in more detail in the following sections.

EDUCATION

Patients typically do not understand how psychological and social variables can influence pain, nor do they understand that they personally can have an impact on it. Hunter, Goodie, Oordt, and Dobmeyer (2017) developed a handout to use with patients to teach them about the role of psychosocial factors in the experience of pain (see Figure 13.1). They described a gate control model of pain (based on Melzack & Wall, 1965) in which psychosocial factors, such as depression, anxiety, and social withdrawal, can "open the gate" or increase pain. Other factors, such as

FIGURE 13.1

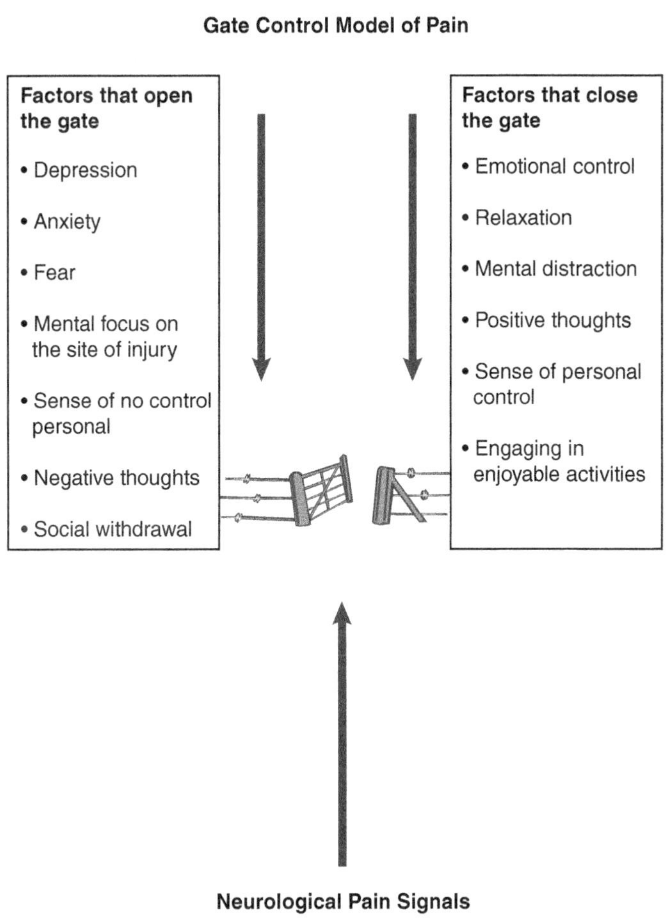

Gate control model of pain handout. From *Integrated Behavioral Health in Primary Care: Step-by-Step Guidance for Assessment and Intervention* (2nd ed., p. 166), by C. L. Hunter, J. L. Goodie, M. S. Oordt, and A. C. Dobmeyer, 2017, Washington, DC: American Psychological Association. Copyright 2017 by the American Psychological Association.

relaxation, feelings of control, and enjoyable activities can "close the gate" or help patients to decrease their experience of pain. These authors also provide a script for use in educating patients about the model and the relevant issues (Hunter et al., 2017, pp. 165–167).

Another useful conceptual model for use with patients is the pain–stress cycle described by Gatchel and Oordt (2003; see Figure 13.2). In this model, psychosocial factors are shown to affect pain and stress. The cyclical nature of pain and stress is clearly demonstrated here; for example, medical uncertainty can increase stress, which can then increase pain, which can then increase stress further. This model helps demonstrate to patients the importance of breaking the cycle.

Patients can often benefit from education about the proper use of pain medications. Many people avoid taking pain medications as prescribed because they fear addiction, but they are then more uncomfortable than they need to be, which can have a negative impact on their recovery and quality of life. They may avoid asking for prn (as needed) medications, refuse scheduled medications, or delay delivery of pain medications using a patient-controlled analgesia (PCA) pump. If there is any hint that the patient is not using pain medications properly, education can be provided about the importance of effective pain management to promote healing and how appropriate pain management in the short term will not result in addiction.

FIGURE 13.2

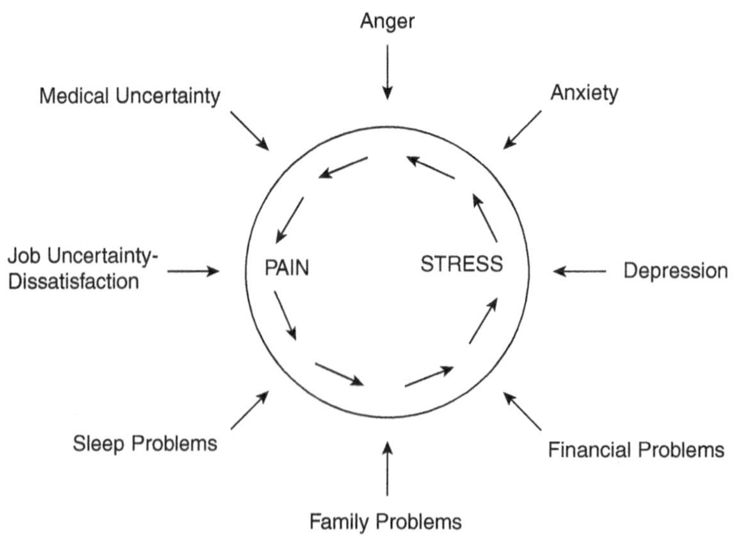

The pain–stress cycle, emphasizing the interaction of stress-related issues and the actual pain problem. From *Personality Characteristics of Patients With Pain* (p. 17), by R. J. Gatchel and J. N. Weisberg (Eds.), 2000, Washington, DC: American Psychological Association. Copyright 2000 by the American Psychological Association.

Patients may also need to be reminded of the need to ask for prn medications because nurses will generally not provide them unless the patient requests them. They may need additional instruction about how to deliver their own medications using the PCA as well as information about how the medical staff will evaluate their use of the pain medication and decrease the dose if the patient does not appear to need it. The psychologist should also be alert to patients who are delirious or forgetful and may need scheduled medications rather than prn or PCA dosing, and then relay that information to the medical team so that they can make appropriate adjustments.

There are times that a physician will not treat a patient's pain or will knowingly undertreat it. This is usually a temporary situation in which the doctor needs the reports of pain to help in the diagnosis of a new medical issue. Once the problem is correctly diagnosed, adequate pain control can be achieved and maintained. Although education does not improve the pain, this information may decrease the frustration a patient is experiencing if she feels her doctor is not managing the pain properly.

RELAXATION STRATEGIES

These strategies make up the main psychological interventions for acute pain management. When patients are experiencing pain, they often tense their muscles and "guard," which intensifies the pain, especially if they are tensing muscles in the area in which the pain originates. Various types of relaxation strategies can be useful (see the discussion of these in Chapter 7, this volume). Progressive muscle relaxation is often to be avoided because tensing muscles near an area in which a patient is experiencing pain is likely to exacerbate the pain. Even abdominal breathing may need to be modified, such as by decreasing the depth of the breathing, to accommodate the needs of specific patients. Other strategies can also be used; listening to calming and pleasant music is often a good way for patients to relax and can be easily done in the hospital setting without stressing the patient's body, for example.

Imagery and hypnosis are useful techniques to help promote relaxation (see Chapter 7 for more information on the use of imagery to decrease anxiety and promote relaxation), and a variety of techniques have been developed specifically for pain management. The basic procedures associated with imagery and hypnosis include focusing and deepening the patient's attention, visualization, and suggestion; specific suggestions to aid pain control include escaping from the pain, blocking it, or transforming it to something else (Syrjala & Abrams, 2002). For example, patients can learn to develop glove anesthesia (develop numbness at the pain site), "spread the pain" (expand the pain to outside of the body), and to use "radiant light" (to fill the body and then remove the pain; Pincus & Sheikh, 2009). Specific techniques and scripts for these and other imagery and hypnosis interventions for pain are provided by Pincus and Sheikh (2009) and Syrjala and Abrams (2002).

DISTRACTION

Distraction has also been previously discussed as an intervention for anxiety (Chapter 7); it can also be useful as an intervention for pain, largely because it is simple to use. As noted earlier, focusing on and attending to pain can exacerbate it, so anything a patient can do to distract himself from pain can decrease the experience of it. Therefore, helping patients to focus their attention on other issues can provide some relief. Patients can engage in a variety of activities while in the hospital to distract themselves, such as watching movies and TV, playing games, engaging in conversations with friends and family, and reading. These, and any other activities that take the patient's attention away from the pain, may also promote relaxation and can help patients to cope more effectively with the pain.

Sample 13.1 describes an inpatient evaluation of a patient with pain. For this patient, education was the most important factor in improving pain management. When this patient understood that his pain would be temporary and that the pain medication would help him to control it with no long-term adverse effects, he was better able to work with the medical team and achieved better pain control.

STRESS AND AFFECT MANAGEMENT

Turk et al. (2012) described the importance of emotional distress in the experience of pain in the following way: "Emotional distress may predispose people to experience pain, be a precipitant of symptoms, be a modulating factor amplifying or inhibiting the severity of pain, be a consequence of persistent pain, or be a perpetuating factor" (p. 154). It is completely understandable that people in the hospital would be stressed by their medical problems and also the hospital admission, and they may face anxiety and fear, sadness, anger, and other strong emotions as a result. The pain itself may also elicit negative emotions. Yet, as noted earlier, negative emotions and stress can exacerbate pain; therefore, helping patients to cope more effectively with emotions and stressors can help with pain management.

Assessing a patient's immediate stressors and then problem-solving to help address them can decrease the patient's stress level and help to moderate pain. Patients may also be overwhelmed with negative emotions due to the medical situation, and fearful about what it will mean for their future—or even if they will live to enjoy a future. Common stressors in the hospital setting are associated with the medical staff, the hospital milieu, and family concerns. Problems with the medical staff may involve misunderstandings that can be resolved by clearer communication. Stressors associated with the setting may relate to a lack of privacy, poor sleep, or decreased social contact. Patients may also have concerns about family members while they are in the hospital. Enlisting a trusted friend to help care for young children or to take some burden off a spouse can significantly decrease the patient's stress level while in the hospital. Concerns about possible job loss, financial problems, and insurance coverage are also sources of stress. Interventions that help the patient to generate possible solutions, to get more information, or to connect them with other resources (such as social work) can all serve to decrease stress and negative emotions and can also increase feelings of control and self-efficacy.

At times, nonpsychological interventions can help to decrease a patient's stress and pain. One elderly patient had been moved to a new room where the phone did not work. She was fearful that her daughter would call the old room and think she had died when she did not answer. There was an empty room next door, and the phone cords could be switched. This was done fairly quickly, and the patient was able to call her daughter to inform her of the room change. She was noticeably calmer and more comfortable when the issue was resolved (and was thus more open to the health psychology evaluation taking place).

ADVOCATE FOR THE PATIENT WITH THE MEDICAL TEAM

There are some cases in which patients and medical staff are not communicating well about the patient's pain. The psychologist can work with both parties to improve communication and can also act as an advocate for the patient. Because the medical staff members may not understand the patient's psychological concerns, the health psychology consultant can explain the patient's behavior and enlist the staff's support. For example, in the case of an anxious patient who is annoying the doctor with complaints of pain and worries, the psychologist might explain:

> Mrs. T is quite anxious and fearful about this pain and is worried it will increase and continue for the long term, and that is why she is so persistent in her requests for more meds. I am working with her to decrease her anxiety and also to develop additional strategies to help her manage her pain. In the meantime, if there is anything else you can do to help with the pain control . . .

Enlisting the provider's support through collaboration is always preferable to a situation in which a patient in pain accuses the provider of not providing adequate care.

There are rare cases in which the medical staff do not believe a patient's report of pain and therefore under treat it. This seems to happen in cases of patients who (a) have had repeat admissions for pain, (b) are demanding and difficult, or (c) do not have objective clinical findings that would account for their pain. These can be difficult cases because as the patient's complaints intensify, the medical staff tends to stop listening. If the issues are not resolved, these patients may leave the hospital against medical advice (AMA) because they feel they are not getting proper treatment for their medical problem. Sample 13.2 describes this situation in the case of a patient with sickle cell disease.

If a Pain Service is also seeing the patient, the psychologist would generally also want to discuss the patient with them. The patient's interactions with the pain team can often provide insight into the patient's psychological situation (e.g., a patient who appears to be in significant pain but who is irritable and always tells the pain service that he is "fine"). Similarly, the psychologist can provide suggestions that can help the pain team to work with the patient.

OTHER STRATEGIES TO MANAGE PAIN

There are also a variety of additional cognitive–behavioral interventions commonly used in the outpatient setting with chronic pain patients that can be adapted for use in the inpatient setting when appropriate. Turk (2002) presented an excellent description of the cognitive–behavioral approach to chronic pain, including interventions such as cognitive restructuring to address maladaptive thoughts; education about the associations between cognitions, emotions, and pain; challenges to maladaptive thinking; and problem-solving. He also discusses the importance of relaxation and activity pacing, which can be relevant to both acute and chronic pain management.

Biofeedback has also been used to help patients to develop some control over physiological responses that are associated with the pain. It is typically used to affect chronic pain in the outpatient setting and has been used most frequently for the treatment of headache, low back pain, and temporomandibular joint pain. Arena and Blanchard (2002) provided instruction on how to use biofeedback clinically with pain patients; at times, this can also be used in the inpatient setting.

In summary, the first-line treatment of pain in the hospital is medication, but medication alone does not provide sufficient pain management for all patients. The health psychology consultant can help patients work more effectively with the medical team on pain that is not adequately controlled while providing additional strategies to improve coping with and management of the pain.

Sample 13.1
Evaluation of an Inpatient With Pain

Patient referred by Dr. S for health psych evaluation for mood lability. He has been both irritable and tearful over the past 24 hours. Pt is a 69 y/o Caucasian man, s/p (*status post*) successful epigastric hernia repair.

Pt with hx HTN (*hypertension*), hypercholesterol, OSA (*obstructive sleep apnea*). No problems with medication, CPAP (*continuous positive airway pressure; treatment for OSA*), or medical appointment compliance. No hx drug or Etoh problems. Currently, pt smokes 1/2 ppd (*pack per day*) and drinks a few beers weekly. No leisure drug use.

Pt is widowed × 4 yrs, lives with his daughter and 2 teenage grandchildren. He is a retired construction worker who completed h.s. Pt manages his own ADLs (*activities of daily living*), is active socially, and keeps generally busy.

He denies any past inpatient or outpt psych tx, denies emotional problems throughout his life. Pt today denies depressed mood, sleep and appetite changes, decreased interest and motivation, suicidal ideation. He also denies anxiety, panic, paranoia, hallucinations. Pt reports significant worry and frustration re: post-op pain, that has made him both irritable and tearful at times since his surgery a few days ago. He reports experiencing significantly more pain that he had anticipated—this makes him concerned that something went wrong during the surgery and he is fearful he will need to live with this pain for the long-term.

Pt is on PCA (*patient-controlled analgesia*) for pain, with additional oral pain meds available for breakthrough pain as needed. Pain team has reviewed PCA use daily and has decreased dosage daily, as pt has been using very little; he has also requested no prn oral pain meds in the past 36 hrs.

On mental status exam pt was alert and oriented × 3. He appeared tense, and any movement appeared painful. Attention and concentration, judgment, long-term memory, and abstract thinking were all intact. Registration intact, short-term memory mildly impaired (2/3).

Impressions and Recommendations: Pt s/p GI surgery, with recent irritability and tearfulness. He has no psych hx and no significant psych issues currently. Cognition WNL. Pt is not using pain meds properly; he reports avoiding use of pain meds because he had a nephew who died of drug addiction and he is fearful of that. Discussed with pt the proper use of pain meds as a temporary measure to help his body to heal from the surgery. Discussed how this use is quite different from that of his nephew and unlikely to result in addiction. Reviewed with patient the use of the PCA pump as well as when to request additional meds from his nurse. Will also ask primary team to reevaluate his pain and medications in light of this, and also to review the outcome of the surgery with him. Pt understands and seems agreeable to using pain meds more frequently, as Rx'd. He administered from PCA during evaluation and soon appeared much more comfortable. Also discussed with pt additional pain management strategies, i.e., distraction and relaxation, and generated specific plans for him to use these also. We will follow to continue to monitor mood and pain management.

Sample 13.2 Report for a Patient Who Frequently Requests Pain Medication

Patient is a 22 y/o AA woman, referred by Dr. G due to pt's repeated hospital admissions for pain crises and repeated requests for pain meds. Pt has hx of sickle cell disease. No drug or alcohol hx or current use.

Pt lives with her mother and 8 y/o brother. She is unemployed, reports being unable to work due to sickle cell disease. She did not complete h.s., as she missed a lot of school due to illness (pain) and finally dropped out. She reports an "up and down" relationship with her boyfriend of 6 mts, and conflict with her mother over many issues.

Pt is known to health psych from many visits during past hospital admissions. Over the past year, she has not attended outpt sickle cell medical appointments but has been admitted to the hospital with pain crises every 3–5 weeks for the past 8 months.

Pt has no previous psych hospital admissions and no outpatient psych tx (although it has been recommended). She did have an episode of depression that lasted about 4 mts after her grandmother died when she was 16 y/o. She currently denies depression but reports significant frustration with her mother and boyfriend, and currently also with her nurses and doctors. Pt reports significant stress in her life and is aware that this exacerbates her sickle cell pain, but she does not know what to do for this (even though coping strategies have been discussed with her previously). She denies sleep and appetite problems and suicidal ideation, but reports poor energy and motivation. No anxiety, panic, worry, hallucinations, paranoia. No gross cognitive deficits noted during interview; formal mental status exam deferred for now.

Discussed with pt the importance of a comprehensive plan to address these issues. She agrees, and formal team meeting with pt and her mother, her doctor, social worker, and health psych consultant is scheduled for tomorrow.

Outcome: In the team meeting, the importance of a plan for good pain control on an outpt basis was discussed, and the patient's doctor presented a plan to begin methadone to help manage the daily pain she was experiencing. They also discussed the possibility of additional meds for when this was not sufficient. The pt was encouraged to attend outpt clinic apts regularly so that the tx plan could be adjusted as needed. The health psych consultant recommended outpt behavioral medicine treatment to help the pt to learn strategies to help manage her pain, as well as to cope with and perhaps resolve some of the ongoing interpersonal stressors. Over the next 3 mts, the pt complied with the methadone tx, and had only 1 hospital admission, although she did not attend outpt sickle cell clinic apts. She scheduled and rescheduled several outpt health psych apts, but had not yet attended one. The psychological tx plan was to continue to intervene with brief coping and pain management strategies at hospital admissions, and to continue to encourage attendance at outpt sickle cell and health psych apts.

End-of-Life Issues 14

Treating patients who are dying can be professionally stressful and emotionally painful. This chapter describes the management of end-of-life (EOL) referrals, with attention to the specific concerns of dying patients and efforts the health psychology consultant can make to help a patient have the best quality of death possible. Advance directives and physician orders for life-sustaining treatment are described, as well as Death With Dignity legislation. Managing the emotional aspects of this work is discussed in Chapter 16.

End-of-Life Referrals

EOL issues with dying patients is one aspect of inpatient health psychology work that consultants will be asked to manage. The emotional response to death has been conceptualized as occurring over time, in five predictable stages: denial, anger, bargaining, depression, and acceptance (Kübler-Ross, 1969). The stages may not occur in sequence, and the patient may vacillate among them rather than following an orderly progression.

Patients may stop progressing toward acceptance in any of the other phases. For example, a 35-year-old woman with three young children, divorced

http://dx.doi.org/10.1037/0000108-015
Health Psychology Consultation in the Inpatient Medical Setting, by S. M. Labott

and recently remarried, had been dealing with cancer for about 18 months, trying one treatment after another. When her physicians said they had no additional treatment options for her, she went to three other medical centers for additional opinions (which were all consistent with the first one) and then began seeking alternative treatments to cure the cancer. This patient denied her terminal illness throughout the process and did not progress through the other phases, even though she was clearly weaker and sicker as time progressed. Even when this reality was discussed directly with her, she acknowledged the illness but continued to be sure that she would "beat it." Her denial was so strong that she remained convinced she was not going to die until she became unresponsive prior to her death.

In the inpatient medical setting, the emotional stages remain relevant, but the consultant may participate in only a small part of the patient's emotional processing. The psychologist may be asked to see a patient to help her process the information immediately after the medical team has told her of a terminal illness, to be there with the medical team when they tell the patient she has a terminal illness, or to evaluate the patient's coping and resources to deal with EOL issues before discharge from the hospital.

For any consultation request dealing with EOL issues, it is critical to know what the patient has been told about the illness before interviewing the patient. The psychologist needs to know exactly what the patient knows, that is, do they understand this is a terminal illness, how much time they have left, and the expected course of the illness. When dealing with EOL issues, it is necessary to understand what the patient has been told by the medical team to properly address the patient's understanding, questions, and concerns.

Even after the consultant has discussed the patient's prognosis with the referral source and has a good understanding of what the patient has been told, information about the illness and associated issues should be obtained directly from the patient. That is, a consultant would not approach a patient saying that his physician has referred her to talk about EOL issues or even to talk about "bad news" about their medical situation. Although the medical team may have clearly discussed this with the patient, the patient may not have actually understood it. One psychology consultant was reassured by the medical team that the patient was aware that her cancer was inoperable and that she would die in a few months. The consultant began talking to the patient about how difficult the situation is and how she was there to support her, but the patient had no idea what she was talking about and became frightened. The psychologist had raised the issue and seemed to know more about the patient's medical situation than the patient did. She was then in the uncomfortable position of having to tell the patient she had a terminal illness, or stopping the interview and returning after the medical team had spoken to the patient again. Although it is common for the health psychology consultant to collaborate with the medical team to deliver information about a terminal illness to a patient and to help the patient ask questions so that she understands it, it is not the job of the psychologist to initially deliver the information. The physicians who have been treating the patient's illness are the best equipped to explain the medical situation to the patient and answer her questions about it.

The preferred way to address EOL issues if the patient does not raise the topic is to begin a typical interview, citing the stress of being in the hospital as an issue that warrants the visit. The consultant can then ask how the medical treatment is going, if it is progressing as the patient had hoped, and if he is communicating well with his doctors. When the patient explains more, the consultant can then ask what the patient's doctors have told him about the illness and its course. This is relevant information in most evaluations because it provides the psychologist with information about the patient's understanding of the situation, but when dealing with EOL issues, it avoids the problem of the psychologist assuming she is on the same page with the patient, then finding out she is not.

In many cases, the time afforded to the health psychology consultant to address the psychological impacts with the patient is short, although for different reasons. In one type of referral, the patient has developed a relatively recent problem that has required a hospital admission, with perhaps surgery or other procedures to diagnose the problem, and those results have now indicated that this is a terminal illness. The time people have remaining in their lives could range from a few days to a few years, but this is the first time they are aware that the illness will not be cured and that it will kill them. The psychologist needs to perform the inpatient evaluation and then provide brief intervention or referrals for outpatient treatment, if warranted. At this point, many patients are shocked by the news that they have a terminal illness, but the future implications are not yet clear to them. The patient may have some time to process and deal with the news of a terminal disease, although that will largely be done outside the hospital.

Consider a young mother who has recently been having stomach pain, difficulty tolerating food, and significant weight loss. A variety of outpatient tests were performed but were inconclusive, so she was admitted to the hospital for an exploratory abdominal surgery. During the surgery, her surgeons found what appeared to be a rare type of stomach cancer, too advanced to be operable. Biopsy results confirmed this diagnosis, and it was determined that the patient had 6 to 8 months to live. The referral was to evaluate the patient to assess her "coping," and then she was to be discharged home the same day. In this situation, the consultant could perform an abbreviated interview that is focused on how well the patient is dealing with the diagnosis and also what resources she has (or needs) to cope at home. See Sample 14.1 for the evaluation report.

Note that the evaluation referenced in Sample 14.1 did not cover all the major pieces of information that would be expected in a comprehensive interview. Here it was important to discuss the current situation with the patient, to assess how she was managing it, and to determine whether she required any resources after discharge. The discussion of her social situation was limited to that information necessary to contextualize her medical situation. Because there were no apparent substance use problems, this concern was not discussed, and past psychiatric history was abbreviated. Assessment of current psychological symptoms was limited to that information required to determine that she was safe and able to manage after discharge. Mental status was not formally assessed because there were no deficits noted during the interview or in other notes in the medical record. The patient's plans for coping were discussed in more detail, as was her concern about talking with her children about her illness. Because it appeared that she was managing adequately, no outpatient psychiatric or psychological follow-up was recommended, but the patient was given the consultant's contact information so that a referral for outpatient treatment could be obtained later (if warranted). If the patient had reported a history of significant depression and poor social support, the interview would have proceeded differently, and perhaps the outcome would have included a recommendation for outpatient follow-up to help her manage this difficult situation.

Another common scenario for an EOL referral in the inpatient medical setting involves a patient who has been ill with a known problem for a long time but is just now learning that there is nothing else medically to be done to treat the problem. The patient typically has had many procedures or treatments that have been difficult, with complications, side effects, and pain throughout a long process. At present, physicians have determined that further treatment is futile—that there are no other options for treatment that are likely to benefit this patient—and their focus then shifts to keeping the patient comfortable for the remainder of her time.

Consider a 50-year-old woman who developed acute leukemia a few years ago. She underwent several rounds of chemotherapy in the hospital and was quite sick each time. She then received an unrelated donor stem cell transplant (SCTP) and spent 3 months in the hospital for that. During the SCTP admission, she had several life-threatening infections as well as complications of graft versus host disease involving her skin and liver. While the stem cell transplant appeared to be successful initially, she then relapsed, and the leukemia returned. She is currently sick with fevers, fatigue, poor appetite, and significant weakness. She can undergo additional chemotherapy, but it is likely to make her sick again and will only add a few months to her life.

This patient was deteriorating quickly and was cognitively and physically unable to do much psychological processing. Her death could come quickly, so there was little time for the psychologist to work with her on EOL issues. Because the patient had been in and out of the hospital for a long time, she was known to the psychologist, and a complete evaluation had previously been completed and was in the medical record. The current consultation focused on the new challenges the patient was facing. See Sample 14.2 for this consult report.

For the remaining time that the leukemia patient (Sample 14.2) is in the hospital, the psychologist would follow up with her, with brief visits to monitor her mood and coping. This would take the form of the psychologist checking in to see how the patient is doing (emotionally and physically) as the disease progresses. Even though the patient is now aware that she will die, and perhaps soon, she will not want to discuss this issue all the time, so it is best for the psychologist to ask general questions and then follow the patient's lead to the areas she wants to discuss at each visit.

Concerns of Dying Patients

Many researchers have studied and reported on the most important concerns of dying patients as they approach the end of their lives (e.g., Barnato, Anthony, Skinner, Gallagher, & Fisher, 2009; Heyland et al., 2006; McPherson, Wilson, & Murray, 2007; Miccinesi, Bianchi, Brunelli, & Borreani, 2012; Singer, Martin, & Kelner, 1999).

EXHIBIT 14.1

Concerns of Dying Patients

Wishes to maintain control over decisions about medical treatment, including pain and symptom management
Avoid prolonging life
Avoid burdening family
Losses
Unfinished business
Choosing the place of death
Funeral and burial plans

Exhibit 14.1 summarizes these concerns. Individual patients weight these issues differently depending on the individual's specific medical and social situation.

In many cases, the role of the health psychology consultant is to listen and help the patient clarify his wishes about treatment at EOL and to aid the patient in explaining those preferences to the medical staff. One concern of dying patients involves symptom management; pain often is the main concern. Many patients are fearful about dying slowly and with significant pain. Even if they are not currently experiencing pain, the possibility of significant and poorly managed pain later can be a source of great worry. The role of the psychologist may be to help a patient deal with her fears of pain and to help her develop management plans. These plans may include discussions with medical providers and documentation of her wishes, so that the patient is comfortable that her concerns have been heard and will be respected if or when her pain increases. Certainly, if a patient's pain is not well managed at present, the psychologist can communicate that information to the medical team (especially if the patient is unable to do so) and can then also work with the patient on additional pain management strategies.

Patients consistently report that they do not want death to be prolonged and that they do not want to be kept alive on life support when recovery is not possible. Patients communicate these wishes to their medical team through living wills and by expressing their wishes directly to family members and medical staff. If the patient has not yet developed advance directives (which is common), it is often a difficult step for them to take immediately after being told they have a terminal illness. If the patient wishes to explicitly address their EOL wishes at this point, the health psychology consultant can help the patient to think through her wishes and make decisions about her care, then help the patient provide this information to her family and medical team so that these individuals can intervene in ways that improve her quality of life while she is dying.

Many patients have serious concerns about being a burden to family members, either because they need physical care, or for financial reasons, and these concerns can affect their decisions about EOL care. Although most patients prefer to die at home, some will choose to go to an inpatient hospice setting. An inpatient hospice or any other institution may be appropriate for the patient, but it may be difficult to determine whether this choice is what the patient prefers or if the choice is being made by the patient to avoid burdening family members with her care. Similarly, patients may refuse treatment so that their lives end more quickly to avoid burdening family with the emotional stress and financial burden of longer treatment. Some families may subtly pressure patients to make those choices because they do not want to take responsibility for the patient's care. In other cases, family members are clearly supportive, willing, and able to help; in cases like these the patient should be encouraged to discuss the issue of burden with them. Often families will deny feeling burdened and can remind the patient that she would do the same for them if the roles were reversed. This may help to assuage the patient's concerns about being a burden to them and may encourage her to make her EOL choices based on her own preferences.

As they approach the end of their lives, patients may grieve for activities they will miss, such as time spent with friends and family at holidays, tender moments with their spouse, or a great golf game. They may also feel cheated that they will miss special milestones of family and friends. It is common for patients to feel it is unfair that they will not see their children or grandchildren graduate from high school or college, get married, and have their own families. On occasion, patients will wish to write letters to a child, make a gift for a child to receive on a special day, or find some other activity to remain a part of the child's life even though she will no longer be physically present.

These discussions can be sad, as it *is* unfair that these people will not be able to share those special moments with their children. The psychologist can empathize with the feelings of loss, unfairness, and perhaps anger that the patient experiences. There may be actions the patient can take to feel less bad about missing these events (e.g., one woman made a list of "tips" for her daughter to read during adolescence to help her navigate growing up), but often the patient needs simply to express her sadness and to come to terms with the reality that she will not be there.

Dying patients may wish to address unfinished business, including old, interpersonal conflicts, often with an estranged family member. The patient may have been estranged from the family member for many years and now wishes to make amends before his death. Yet not all patients wish to address these unresolved issues and may handle the relationship with the estranged family member at the time of death exactly as they have handle it throughout their lives; one patient, for example, said: "I haven't wanted to see my son in 20 years, why would I want to talk to him now?"

For those patients who wish to attempt to repair the relationship, it can be emotional and complicated because the family member may be difficult to find or may not desire contact with the patient. The role of the health psychology consultant may be to help the patient make plans to contact and talk with the estranged family member, as well as to help the patient manage anxieties and disappointments that may occur during the process or when they do connect.

Dying patients often want to address new business raised by their impending death. Patients are often concerned about family members and their welfare after the patient's death, especially those patients who have been responsible for the family's financial support. Resolving the unfinished business in this situation may involve getting insurance paperwork in order, getting a will in place, or selling an old car. Although the psychologist will not be handling the details of these issues, he can help the patient organize the tasks and make plans for resolving them.

Some patients are eager to discuss their thoughts and concerns about their death, often including their wishes for their funeral and burial, and do so explicitly with family members. Patients who have strong feelings about what should (and should not) occur at their funeral and those wishing to make the process easiest on family members are those most likely to engage in planning of this sort. Others have no wish to think about funeral and burial plans at all, or may have families who will not discuss these issues. Mrs. J was an elderly patient who was told she had a terminal illness and would likely live only a few months. She had been an actress and had a flair for the dramatic. She began to plan her funeral in detail, even to include the music she wanted played when her body was taken away ("Ride of the Valkyries" by Wagner). She spent a great deal of time and thought on her funeral plans to make them consistent with her view of her life. Her family would not discuss these issues with her, and so she shared her wishes with the psychologist, making extensive notes that her family could use to implement her wishes for her funeral later. This patient had been organized and made plans over her entire life, and she was aware that others would not plan a funeral with the drama she craved, so she made her own plans that were consistent with her personality and the life she had lived.

For some patients, additional consultation will be helpful to determine the best EOL care. In some hospitals, a palliative care (PC) team can provide input. Often the focus is on pain management exclusively, but some PC teams address broader problems. Consultation with a hospital ethics committee may also be useful, especially in complicated cases involving decisional capacity or conflicts between family members, the patient, and the medical team. The health psychology consultant can recommend that the primary medical team obtain a consultation with either PC or Ethics, if that seems warranted for a particular patient. (Note that in almost all cases the psychologist would recommend that the primary team obtain any additional consultations. One exception to this may be Ethics: In some institutions anyone can request an ethics consultation. If requested by the psychologist, informing the medical team would still be appropriate.) If either PC or Ethics are involved with a patient's care, it will be important for the psychologist to collaborate with them to share information and develop a coordinated plan to address the medical, social, and psychological concerns.

Documentation of Patient Wishes for Medical Treatment

There are several methods to document patient wishes for EOL treatment, including advance directives and physician orders for life-sustaining treatment. These are often not used by patients, although a patient's preferences are more likely to be followed if formal documentation is in place.

ADVANCE DIRECTIVES

One of the main concerns of dying patients is that their wishes about EOL care are "heard," even if they are no longer able to express those wishes. Advance directives provide a method for individuals to document their wishes for treatment at the end of their lives. The Patient Self-Determination Act of 1990 (PSDA; https://www.congress.gov/bill/101st-congress/house-bill/4449/text) requires health care institutions such as hospitals, nursing homes, and hospice providers to provide patients with information on advance directives. This is done when patients are admitted to an institution but is not required for outpatient doctor visits. It explains the rights of patients to be involved in decisions about their health care, to accept or refuse health care treatment, and to make advance directives to direct their care at a later date if they are not able to make their own decisions at that time. It is not required that patients develop advance directives, but they are provided with the information and the forms to do so if they wish. If patients choose to outline advance directives, these are documented in the medical record. All states have some form of advance directive provisions and specific rules for implementation; the National Hospice and Palliative Care Organization provides information about advance care planning and relevant forms for each state (http://www.nhpco.org/advance-care-planning).

The PSDA was developed following the case of Nancy Cruzan, a young woman who had a car accident in 1983 and was in a persistent vegetative state for several years (Doukas & Brody, 1992). Her parents requested that nutrition and hydration be removed so that she could die, and the case went to a court in Missouri that agreed with the parents, then to the Missouri Supreme Court, which disagreed. The Missouri Supreme Court ruled that the State's goal is to preserve life and that "clear and convincing" evidence that Ms. Cruzan would have refused life-sustaining treatment if she had been able to had not been provided, so withdrawal of treatment could not be allowed. The U.S. Supreme Court agreed with the Missouri Supreme Court's decision. After a brief time, Ms. Cruzan's parents returned to the lower Missouri court, as the press from this long process had resulted in other friends of Ms. Cruzan coming forward who could provide evidence that she would have wished to terminate life-sustaining treatment in this situation. The Missouri court heard the new evidence and ruled that the "clear and convincing" evidence standard had now been met and allowed the termination of her treatment. Ms. Cruzan died in 1990—7 years after the car accident. The purpose of advance directives is to enable people to make clear what their wishes are so that they can be followed, even if the person is not able to express them at the time.

In theory, the advance directive seems to offer patients that which they want most: control over decisions about treatment at the end of their lives. Patients can write living wills in which they describe what measures they do or do not want if they are unable to make decisions at the time. They can also designate someone as their power of attorney (POA) for health care who will make decisions on their behalf.

One of the most common provisions in living wills is a DNR, or do not resuscitate order. In a DNR order, patients indicate that if they are terminally ill, they do not want CPR (cardiopulmonary resuscitation) if they stop breathing or have no pulse. The DNR order serves to protect people from painful and invasive procedures that will only temporarily prolong their lives. Variations of DNR orders can also be indicated, such as DNI (do not intubate). DNR, DNI, and other such designations are documented in the patient's medical record (and updated frequently) and followed by hospital staff if any of these events occurs in the hospital. Medical personnel are not allowed to move slowly if the person stops breathing if they don't have DNR orders in their medical record (known as a "slow code"), so it is important that the patient has these orders documented if he wants to avoid these procedures. Outside of the hospital, emergency personnel (such as emergency medical technicians) are not likely to have this information or to follow the advance directive if they are called to aid the patient in an emergency, so if a patient is sent home to die, families would not immediately call an ambulance to resuscitate him if he stops breathing.

Despite these opportunities for patients to achieve more control over their treatment, the PSDA has not achieved many of its overall goals to empower patients, ensure that their wishes are honored, and reduce the overtreatment of dying patients (Pope, 2013). One set of problems is due to implementation. Patients are often asked about advance directives for the first time when they are admitted to the hospital. If patients are admitted for an elective procedure, they may not see a need for advance directives because no life-threatening problems are expected. If they are admitted for an acute problem, they may be in too much pain or too distressed to consider EOL issues adequately. Further, the presentation of the advance directive materials is from someone they do not know and is done typically as part of the hospital admission process (along with a host of other paperwork), rather than being done by a trusted health care provider. Completion of thoughtful advance directives might be more likely if this topic is raised by the patient's outpatient physician in the course of routine treatment. The issues can then be discussed and the patient's preferences documented at an outpatient office visit, without the stress of an acute medical crisis. Although this happens in some physician practices, it is not required by PSDA.

Patient factors also influence the benefit a patient may obtain from an advance directive because the patient's understanding and trust in the medical system influence willingness to articulate an advance directive. White, educated, and older patients, and those with higher income are more likely to complete advance directives as a way to control their care (Rao, Anderson, Lin, & Laux, 2014), but poor, less educated, and non-White patients may avoid completing an advance directive because it may be perceived as an additional way for others to restrict their medical care (Mezey, Leitman, Mitty, Bottrell, & Ramsey, 2000). Often individuals do not complete advance directives due to a lack of awareness of what they are (Rao et al., 2014). Even if a patient understands the potential benefits of an advance directive, it may be difficult for the individual to anticipate what he will want in a particular situation in the future, making it impossible to formally communicate his wishes to others now.

An individual may also change his mind when the actual situation occurs. A patient may have decided and documented in an advance directive that he did not want to be kept alive on a ventilator ever. Several years later, when he is unable to breathe on his own due to a pneumonia that could potentially be cured, he may be willing to use a ventilator temporarily as the infection is being treated. Some researchers have argued that it is difficult for individuals to make predictions about their "preferences for an unspecifiable future confronted with unidentifiable maladies with unpredictable treatments" (Fagerlin & Schneider, 2004, p. 33).

Although patient discussions with family members about their wishes should be encouraged, documented advance directives are more likely to be followed than a family member's recollection of a conversation with the patient. A formal living will in the patient's medical record will carry more weight than a conversation a patient had with his brother a year ago. If there is no disagreement within the family, either could be followed exactly as the patient wished. If there is conflict in the patient's family about what should be done for the patient's EOL care, however, the patient's wishes may not be followed. Without a formal living will or POA for health care, the informal discussions could be overruled by family members who think they know better, and this typically results in additional life-sustaining treatment for the patient (Winter & Parks, 2008). Practically, the family can sue the physicians for withholding or withdrawing treatment, so their wishes may override those of the patient, especially in cases in which there is some doubt about what exactly the patient wanted. Many states now view the formal advanced directive as a binding legal document that is to be followed by medical staff, even if family members object. The critical point is that patients who prepare formal written advance directives are more likely to receive the type and quantity of care that they prefer at the end of their lives (Silveira, Kim, & Langa, 2010).

States differ in the rules they use to determine who makes decisions about a person's care if they are unable to do so themselves and if they do not have any formal advanced directive. Typically, a surrogate decision-maker, generally a spouse, parent, or adult child, is designated to make decisions on the patient's behalf. The job of a surrogate decision-maker (as well as that of a designated POA) can be difficult, especially if the patient has provided little information about her preferences to aid the surrogate in making decisions. Surrogates are expected to make decisions based on a "substituted judgment," that is, what the patient would have wanted, but surrogates are only accurate at predicting the patient's wishes 68% of the time (Shalowitz, Garrett-Mayer, & Wendler, 2006). Further, the time from hospital admission to a DNR order can be longer for patients with surrogate decision-makers, and patients are more likely to die in the hospital (Torke et al., 2011). Finally, surrogates often need to make decisions about withdrawing treatment, such as removing ventilator support or nutrition, if the situation changes and it is now clear that the patient would not want this treatment—and withdrawing an existing treatment is typically more emotionally difficult for family members than withholding the life-sustaining treatment in the first place.

PHYSICIAN ORDERS FOR LIFE-SUSTAINING TREATMENT

Physician orders for life-sustaining treatment (POLST) is a process in which patients who are ill or elderly can indicate their specific wishes for treatment (see Bomba, Kemp, & Black, 2012; Braun, 2016; Institute of Medicine, 2015; National POLST

Paradigm, n.d.; Pope & Hexum, 2012). It is a single-page document that summarizes a patient's (or surrogate's) discussions with a physician about medical treatments that are desired and those that are not (e.g., CPR), the extent of treatment (comfort only, limited intervention, full treatment), and nutrition. POLST travels with patients if they are transferred to a different health care facility, thus avoiding one of the problems with advance directives. POLST also provides more specific and actionable medical orders compared with the more general guidelines outlined in an advance directive. POLST should not replace advance directives but is intended for use by those who could die in the next year and provides more specific detail about a patient's wishes for treatment at present (Pope & Hexum, 2012). Many states have variations of POLST programs in place, and many others are under development (Braun, 2016; National POLST Paradigm, n.d.).

Bomba et al. (2012) reported that POLST has been effective at communicating patient preferences and is associated with the patient's wishes being followed. It has also resulted in the avoidance of unwanted treatments to prolong life. These authors also provided a good description of POLST, including a copy of a POLST document, and they presented a case that demonstrates how a patient's wishes for treatment are more likely to be followed if a POLST has been completed.

Death With Dignity Legislation

Death with dignity is the term applied to legislation on assisted suicide. By 2018, five states (Oregon, Washington, Vermont, Colorado, and California) and the District of Columbia had enacted death with dignity legislation. Each state has slightly different rules about how patients must proceed if they want help terminating their lives. The Oregon Death with Dignity Act (DWDA; Oregon Health Authority, 2017) was the first to be enacted in 1997 and has been used as a model for the others. It allows terminally ill patients to obtain a prescription from their doctor to end their life. Patients must meet certain criteria to participate in this program. Specifically, they need to be at least 18 years old, be an Oregon resident, be able to make their own decisions, and they must be diagnosed with an illness that is expected to cause their death within 6 months. They then must make two oral and one witnessed request to the physician, then two physicians must confirm the diagnosis and prognosis (i.e., that the patient has a terminal illness that will lead to death within 6 months) and also indicate that the patient is able to make his own medical decisions. If there is a question of impaired decision-making, the patient must have a psychological evaluation to confirm that his decision-making is not impaired. Physicians are required to discuss alternatives with the patient, and they need to provide all of this documentation to the state.

Because Oregon's DWDA has been in existence a relatively long time, a large amount of data has been collected on patients who have requested prescriptions to end their lives. Since 1997, 1,749 people have requested prescriptions, and 1,127 have died from taking them (Oregon Health Authority, 2017). Both the number of requests and the number of uses have increased over the years. Of the 133 deaths from DWDA prescriptions in 2016, most patients were over age 65, White, and well educated. Slightly more men than women died from DWDA prescriptions over all the years, and almost all patients chose to die at home. Only five patients in 2016 were referred for a psychological evaluation, with a total of 57 (5.1%) referred for a psychological evaluation over all the years (1998–2016). The most common concerns reported before their deaths by the patients who died from these prescription drugs were the loss of autonomy, an inability to engage in activities they enjoyed, and a loss of dignity (Oregon Health Authority, 2017). Data provided by other states with death with dignity legislation are similar (e.g., Washington State Department of Health, 2016).

Death with dignity legislation is likely to remain a topic of importance in the future, as many states are considering similar legislation, and there are ongoing legal challenges in some of the states that have already enacted it. Psychologists in states with this type of legislation will need to be familiar with the role they may be asked to play, including evaluations of "impaired judgment" or treatment to address a psychological disorder that may be causing impaired judgment. Information and educational materials for both patients and providers about EOL issues, advance directives, and death with dignity can be found at the website for Compassion & Choices (http://www.compassionandchoices.org), an organization that also provides consultation for patients and physicians about EOL decisions.

Promoting a "Good Death"

Individuals may die in hospitals, nursing homes, hospice settings, or at home. Each of these provides different experiences, both for family members and the individual who dies. There are pros and cons associated with each, and they are weighted differently depending on the individual's specific medical needs and social situation. If a patient is in the hospital and it has been decided that any further medical intervention is futile, the patient will likely be discharged. If it is expected that the patient will die within 6 months, they could be discharged to an inpatient hospice program or to hospice treatment at home. Hospice programs provide management of the patient's medical problems (although generally no active treatment) and also provide emotional support for the patient and the patient's family. Even with the support of hospice, caring for a patient at home can be both physically and emotionally taxing for the family.

Much attention has been focused on quality of life for medical patients—when patients are facing EOL issues the focus shifts to the quality of death. The process of dying involves many dimensions, such as physical changes and perhaps suffering, changes in or losses of relationships, fears of dying, and spiritual concerns, among others. "Good deaths" allow patients to die with dignity and respect and include plans to avoid the patient feeling alone, to provide adequate pain management, and to attend to the patient's wishes (Beckstrand, Callister, & Kirchhoff, 2006). The hospital setting generates a variety of barriers to achieving these goals (see Beckstrand et al., 2006), and the psychologist cannot control all of the variables that could provide a good death for a patient. Yet there are actions a psychologist can take to facilitate a good death for patients.

Exhibit 14.2 lists activities a psychologist can engage in to help improve the quality of the patient's death. If the patient remains able to engage with the health psychology consultant and has wishes to discuss EOL issues, there are typically many topics to discuss. Patients seem to approach this opportunity the way they have approached other options for psychological intervention previously. That is, some people have much to discuss and make good use of the psychologist's expertise, and others do not wish to discuss these issues at all or prefer to talk to a family member. Patients may wish to discuss their fears about death, decisions about additional treatment, concerns about their children, or worries about a spouse who will be left behind. They may be navigating relationship losses or conflicts and dealing with a multitude of changes in their lives as they progress toward death. The psychologist can help the patient to process and cope with these and many other concerns.

The patient should understand that anything can be discussed in the interactions with the psychologist. Frequently, family members are unable or unwilling to discuss EOL issues with patients, continuing to insist that patients remain "positive" and "hopeful" even when there is no longer any reason for optimism. The patient needs to be comfortable that any issue is open for discussion in meetings with the psychologist. When the patient wishes to engage with the psychologist, it is important that the conversation happens promptly because there may be no option to have the discussion tomorrow.

Even when the patient is no longer able to participate in conversation or engage with the psychologist, the psychologist should continue to see the patient. In this case, "seeing the patient" may involve a brief check-in visit to see whether the patient needs anything, or it may involve sitting with the patient for a few minutes of quiet support. The patient may not wish to talk or may be unable to communicate, yet the simple check-in by the health psychology consultant may be important to her. This

EXHIBIT 14.2

Facilitating a "Good Death"

- Interactions with the patient
  - Continue to check in to address any needs
  - Make it clear that anything the patient wants to discuss is acceptable
  - Support the patient
  - Share the burden: Address losses and worries
  - Work on coping
  - Help the patient make decisions about treatment
  - Connect the patient with chaplain or other clergy
- Advocate for the patient with the medical staff as needed
- Help family members cope with the patient's impending death

brief visit reinforces for the patient that she is not alone and that she has resources for support available if she wishes and is able to use them.

Once it is clear that medical intervention is futile, there is little for physicians to do instrumentally for the patient, and their previously frequent visits may stop completely. Although it is understandable that they have nothing else to offer the patient in terms of medical treatment, patients often feel an important connection to their physicians and take comfort from their presence. When those interactions stop, patients may feel abandoned by their providers and feel they have been left to die alone. The loss of this relationship is another sign of the many losses they are now facing, and some patients even feel they have failed the doctor because they have not been cured by the treatments that were attempted. The psychologist cannot fill the void but can help the patient to process this loss and also avoid amplifying it by continuing to follow the patient herself.

The work of the health psychology consultant may involve advocating for the patient. At times, this may involve working with medical staff on changes that can be made to improve the patient's death (e.g., increasing pain medication or avoiding interruptions of the patient's sleep). At other times, the psychologist may try to seek exceptions to the typical hospital rules to provide something of importance to the patient (e.g., to find a way for the patient's 8-year-old grandson to visit or allow a special meal to be brought to the patient). These are small acts that take additional effort and time on the part of the psychologist, but they go a long way toward improving a patient's quality of life as he approaches death.

The psychologist can also check with the patient on other needs that are perhaps not being met and can then intervene accordingly. For religious patients, the psychologist can notify the hospital chaplain if the patient wishes to be seen. Similarly, a patient may desire social work intervention or ask the health psychology consultant to contact a family member with a special request.

The patient may become unresponsive as death nears. Although the psychologist will then be unable to intervene directly with the patient, there may still be an advocacy role to fill. It will still be important to continue to follow the patient, checking on the patient's status to see whether there are additional needs to be met. In many cases, it is not clear how much of their surroundings patients are aware of when they are no longer alert and verbally responsive. Yet at some level, a patient may be aware of a touch on the shoulder and the familiar voice of a family member or the psychologist, and these actions may provide comfort. (If the patient is unaware, nothing is lost.)

If the psychologist has known the patient for some time, a relationship may have also developed with a spouse or other family member who has spent a significant amount of time with the patient. The psychologist may have been involved with the family member from previous discussions about the patient's history or symptoms and collaborative work on support for the patient if he has been delirious or upset; the psychologist may also have provided encouragement for the support person to continue to care for herself while providing support to the patient. At a time when the patient is no longer responsive, the psychologist's focus may shift almost exclusively to supporting the family member. While monitoring the patient, the psychologist may work with the family member on surrogate decision-making issues or on coping with the death of the loved one. (Some of the work with family members may need to occur outside the patient's room, especially if it is not known how much the patient is aware of what is going on around him.)

At some point, the dying patient will die, and the psychologist will either realize this when reviewing the patient's medical record before a visit or will stop by to check on the patient, and she will be gone. Nursing staff and medical records will be able to answer questions regarding what happened and when, and that will be all that is available to provide closure. Generally, the psychologist would not attend the patient's funeral because his presence may raise questions about the patient's psychological treatment. Even though the patient has died, it will still be important to maintain the patient's confidentiality (Dwyer, Deshields, & Nanna, 2012). Any support that the psychologist wishes to offer to the family can be done in a more private manner. If the support person was well known to the psychologist, a telephone call to that person might be warranted, typically a week or two later, after other family members have returned to their own lives. The goal of this call would be to offer sympathy and to provide resources if the support person appears to need them.

Sample 14.1 Evaluation of Patient With Terminal Cancer Diagnosis

Pt referred by Dr. J for health psych eval. She is a 34 y/o Caucasian woman, admitted for w/u of stomach pain. Pt diagnosed yesterday with terminal stomach CA (*cancer*), referred for assessment of coping.

Pt today was awake and alert with no gross cognitive deficits noted, tearful at times, and willing to discuss her terminal dx and its implications. She reports she has a supportive husband and 2 daughters (ages 2 and 4 y/o); pt's parents have been helping with their care. She had been working as a 3rd grade teacher until she became ill last fall.

Pt reported that she was not really surprised by the dx yesterday, as she had been thinking about this for a while and felt there was something "very wrong." She is both angry and sad as she feels she will be "cheated" of some experiences in life that are very important to her, e.g., seeing her daughters graduate from h.s., get married, and have their own families; growing old with her husband.

Today, pt is very eager for d/c (*discharge*) as she has not seen her kids in a week. She was concerned about what to tell her kids about her illness so we discussed that, as well as how to include family members as supports for her and for them. Pt denies anxiety, reports being comfortable with her MDs, and with their outpatient plans for her tx.

Pt denies any past psych hx. While she is profoundly sad about the diagnosis, she denied suicidal ideation, and she feels able to cope with the support of her family. She does not see a need for outpatient psych f/u, but she has my contact info if she has any questions or would like intervention later.

Conclusion: Pt with new dx terminal CA. She is sad, but coping well, and she has good social support. Pt to contact me as needed.

Thanks; please call with questions.

Susan Smith, PhD, pager xxxx

Sample 14.2 Report for Patient Whose Condition Is Rapidly Deteriorating

Pt referred by Dr. W for health psych eval to aid coping. She is a 50 y/o woman, dx'd with AML (*acute myeloid leukemia*) 3 yrs ago, s/p (*status post*) SCTP (*stem cell transplant*) last year. Pt has now relapsed, and medical team has d/w her the futility of additional tx. Pt is well-known to health psych due to frequent contacts to aid coping and adjustment during previous admissions. See initial consultation report from 5/12/xx.

Pt today was seen with her sister present (her primary support and caregiver). She was somnolent but arousable. She was able to briefly describe that she has been told there is nothing more to be done for her illness and that she doesn't have much time left. She denies significant symptoms of anxiety or depression, reporting that she is "so tired" and "unable to fight this anymore." She did not wish to talk at length, reporting that she is physically comfortable and that her sister is here to support her emotionally. Thinking was slow, but pt was oriented × 3.

Conclusion: Pt with no significant psych hx prior to leukemia dx several years ago. During the course of her illness, she has experienced some adjustment-related anxiety and depressed mood. Now, pt has been told her disease is terminal. She reports being tired, denying any significant emotional sx at present. We will follow to monitor mood and coping.

Thanks; please call with questions.
Sarah Stone, PhD, pager xxxx

ETHICS AND PROFESSIONAL ISSUES

V

The Ethics of Consultation With Medical Inpatients

15

The *Ethical Principles of Psychologists and Code of Conduct* (American Psychological Association [APA], 2017a), hereinafter referred to as the APA Ethics Code, applies to psychological work in the inpatient medical setting as well as elsewhere. Health psychology consultants need to adhere to the principles regarding beneficence and nonmaleficence, fidelity and responsibility, integrity, justice, and respect of patient rights and dignity just as they would in the outpatient setting. Yet the inpatient setting presents some additional challenges; some of these have been addressed in the *Guidelines for Psychological Practice in Health Care Delivery Systems* (APA, 2013). These Guidelines provide specific suggestions for the health care setting, specifically on (a) developing a distinct professional identity, (b) seeking appropriate privileges to practice in medical settings, (c) working toward collaborative care for patients, and (d) obtaining and maintaining competency in the work done in the medical setting. Several issues raised in the APA Ethics Code and in the Guidelines pose special challenges in the inpatient medical setting and are discussed more thoroughly in this chapter. Hanson, Kerkhoff, and Bush (2005) developed a casebook of ethical issues relevant to the health care setting, both inpatient and outpatient.

http://dx.doi.org/10.1037/0000108-016
Health Psychology Consultation in the Inpatient Medical Setting, by S. M. Labott

Privacy and Confidentiality

Federal regulations require that all health care providers protect a patient's personal health information; these regulations are provided in the Health Insurance Portability and Accountability Act of 1996 (HIPAA), formally described in the Code of Federal Regulations (45 C.F.R. Parts 160, 162, and 164). They can also be found in one combined document (see U.S. Department of Health and Human Services, 2013). These regulations provide standards for the use and transfer of electronic health information and require all entities that use protected health information (PHI) to develop guidelines for the use and transfer of this information. The APA Practice Organization provides a variety of resources about HIPAA compliance (see http://www.apapracticecentral.org/business/hipaa/index.aspx). For a health psychology consultant, the HIPAA rules dictate the proper use of medical record information. Specifically, medical center rules will regulate who can access medical records, which specific records can be accessed, what and where information can be printed, proper destruction of PHI, as well as many other issues (such as procedures and penalties if a breach occurs). The health psychology consultant needs to be aware of the privacy regulations, in general, as well as the specific rules of the setting in which he works.

The APA Ethics Code (APA, 2017a) stresses the importance of privacy and confidentiality (Ethical Standard 4.01). The inpatient medical setting presents challenges to the maintenance of a patient's privacy and confidentiality, especially because the health psychology consultant may have contacts with the patient's family and friends, roommates, and other members of the treatment team. Family members and friends are often present when the psychologist arrives to evaluate the patient or to provide follow-up treatment, and the psychologist will need to determine the patient's willingness to allow someone to stay for the health psychology visit. If the person present is a visitor who is not intimately involved with the patient's care, the health psychology consultant should either ask the person to step out briefly or should ascertain how long the visitor will be there and plan to return later to interview the patient. The purpose of the visit will also determine the best course of action (e.g., if the health psychology consultant needs only a few minutes with the patient, the visitor can be asked to step into the hallway briefly or to go get coffee for a few minutes to give the health psychology consultant some time alone with the patient). However, if a lot of time is needed with the patient (and if there is no emergency with the consult), it is preferable to return later. Although this is inconvenient for the consultant, many patients have visitors who have traveled long distances and have little time to spend. Although the health psychology evaluation is important, one should not underestimate the impact of social support on the patient's mental state and coping while in the hospital, so it is often appropriate to accommodate the patient's visitors.

Many times a spouse or adult child is present in the hospital with the patient most of the time and is involved in the patient's care. In these cases, the patient is generally comfortable with that person being allowed to witness and/or participate in an evaluation. These significant others know the patient well and can supply information the patient may have forgotten or provide a more objective perspective. Especially if the patient is cognitively impaired, history from the family can be invaluable for performing an evaluation and developing a treatment plan. Even if it is clear that the patient is comfortable with the significant other being present, the health psychology consultant should be sensitive to specific topics that would warrant asking this person to leave the room (e.g., when discussing a history of mental health treatment or abuse that the partner may be unaware of or conflicts in their relationship).

In some cases, a patient may be delirious or sedated and unable to complete an evaluation, and a family member who is present can provide a host of historical information. Although that person can probably not accurately report on the patient's current feelings and unobservable psychological symptoms, he can provide data on behavioral changes, and perhaps also on the patient's emotional state and cognitive functioning. The consultant will need to decide whether an interview with a family member can be done inside the patient's room or if it should occur where the patient cannot overhear.

In other cases, a family member may need to be called on the telephone and asked to provide information on the patient. Family members should only be contacted if the patient consents to the contact or if the patient is unable to provide information that is necessary for her treatment. When calling a family member, the health psychology consultant should immediately explain who she is and describe the purpose of the call because family members may fear that something bad has happened to the patient. The consultant can then ask for relevant background on the patient's social situation, substance use, past mental health treatment and current issues, and changes in emotional and cognitive functioning. When the patient is able to participate in an evaluation, the consultant will want to verify important information obtained from others. Some family members (even though designated as the closest contact) may be unaware of much of the patient's history or any recent changes in behavior or thinking, and if no one else is available, the consultant will need to work with incomplete information.

Roommates provide special challenges to patient privacy and confidentiality. Because most patients are unable to leave the room to find a private area, the evaluation needs to proceed with the roommate present. Generally there is a curtain that can be drawn to provide the illusion of privacy, and the health psychology consultant can move closer to the patient and speak quietly in an effort to keep the roommate from overhearing. If the roommate has her own visitors or has the television on, that also helps to decrease the likelihood of others hearing the discussion. There are some topics (e.g., sexuality, abuse) that should be avoided if it is clear the roommate is listening. If these are important to the patient's treatment, they will need to be discussed at another time. Yet none of this guarantees privacy or confidentiality; most health psychology consultants can describe situations in which they were performing a mental status examination with a patient, and the roommate yelled the correct answer to an item from the other side of the curtain!

The health psychology consultant needs to keep the primary medical team informed of her work because the consultant is treating their patient at their request. Typically, information is provided to the primary medical team after the initial evaluation, if something new happens with the patient (e.g., new cognitive changes or psychological symptoms, a change in medical status), and periodically at rounds or when the consultant runs into a member of the primary team in the hospital. Once the evaluation and treatment plan have been discussed with the primary team, much of the ongoing day-to-day treatment does not require a formal conversation and can simply be described in medical record notes.

Many of the discussions between providers about patients occur at the nurses' station or in the hallways and elevators of the hospital as teams move from one patient to another. In these settings, the psychologist should be aware of who is present and able to overhear the conversation. Once it is established which patient is being discussed, names and other identifiers can be avoided. Yet visitors and family members may be present or walking by. Although they may not know which patient is being discussed, they will make inferences about the care of patients in the hospital from the tone of a conversation they overhear. Many discussions about a specific patient occur outside the patient's room during rounds, and family members and the patient may be able to overhear the discussion among members of the treatment team. These conversations are not intended for them and can create additional stress and anxiety, so providers should close the door and talk quietly.

Developing, Practicing Within, and Maintaining Expertise

Expertise in clinical health psychology is developed through didactics and supervised experience, as in any other aspect of psychological practice. Boarding through the American Board of Professional Psychology (ABPP) is desirable in the hospital setting. As a part of their hospital credentialing process, physicians must be boarded in their specialty area. For psychologists who work in hospitals with physician colleagues, boarding in the psychologist's specialty area places them on a more equal footing with physicians. Earning diplomate status through ABPP also indicates competence in the provider's specialty area, beyond the minimal requirements for professional practice imposed by state licensing boards. Information on the process of becoming boarded in Clinical Health Psychology and other specialty areas can be found on the ABPP website (http://www.abpp.org).

Often, practicing within one's expertise as a health psychologist is easy in the hospital. There is no expectation that a health psychologist can do the work of a physical therapist or of a neurologist. Yet there is overlap, even with these professions: Both a neurologist and a health psychologist would give a mental status examination as part of their evaluation and could diagnose delirium and be involved in plans to address it. No one would expect a health psychologist to engage in the physical aspects of physical therapy with a patient, but the psychologist would need to understand what is going on in the physical therapy to be able to help with patient motivation and to develop plans (often in collaboration with the physical therapist) to address any problems the patient is having with PT.

Our medical colleagues, however, do not always see a clear distinction between a health psychology consultant and a psychiatrist, making it important for the psychologist to be aware of and enforce the boundaries of his competence (see Ethical Standard 2.01; APA, 2017a). For many years, psychiatrists have performed consultations in the hospital, and medical providers generally have a good understanding of the work they do. Health psychology is relatively new to inpatient consultation, and many physicians expect a health psychology consultant to have expertise similar to that of a psychiatrist. Over time and with experience, the expectations become more accurate, and physicians are more likely to consult a psychiatrist when they want help with psychotropic medication and a health psychologist when they want psychological intervention.

At times there may be pressure for the health psychology consultant to practice medicine. For example, in the case of a delirious patient with psychotic symptoms that are distressing to him and could result in safety concerns, the health psychology consultant could suggest that the primary team consider an antipsychotic to make the patient more comfortable and safe until the medical issue is resolved and the symptoms subside. This is no different from an outpatient psychologist suggesting that a patient consider starting medication for depression and then referring to a psychiatrist colleague for a medication evaluation. However, in the inpatient setting, a member of the primary medical team might ask the health psychologist specifically what medication to order for the patient. Even if the health psychology consultant knows that the first line of treatment for the symptoms of delirium is haloperidol, and even if she knows the particular dose at which to start (see Solai, 2009), providing that specific response could be construed as practicing medicine. The way in which the health psychology consultant responds to the question is important, and also serves to provide more information on the professional identity of the health psychology consultant. Consider this response: "As a health psychologist, medication is not my area of expertise, although often haloperidol is prescribed for symptoms like these, if that is medically appropriate. I could facilitate a referral to Psychiatry if you would like their recommendation." The primary physician may then request the referral to Psychiatry, may opt to order a psychotropic medication himself, or may decline the recommendation completely. In any case, the health psychology consultant has provided an appropriate recommendation without going outside the bounds of his expertise. The APA (2011) has also provided guidelines to help psychologists deal with pharmacological issues.

Competence for the hospital health psychology consultant needs to be broadly defined to include competence in both the practice of psychology and also in understanding relevant medical matters. Therefore, the psychologist should consider taking continuing education courses that broadly cover medical topics to include information on a wide range of medical issues typically addressed by health psychologists in the hospital. For example, health psychology consultants may need to attend conferences on psychooncology, new treatments in sickle cell disease, or various types of bariatric surgery. Although certainly the health psychologist does not need a level of medical knowledge that a physician working in one of these areas would need, the psychologist will need a fairly high level of medical knowledge to help patients deal with potential psychological reactions that can occur as a result of these treatments. Conferences that are more medical in nature may not be acceptable to state licensing boards as part of the required continuing education for a psychologist, and the consultant may need to take these courses in addition to those required for licensure as a psychologist. Relevant training is typically found through organizations dedicated to a particular disease, for example, the National Multiple Sclerosis Society, the American Lung Association, the American Cancer Society.

Respect for Other Hospital Staff Members

Interactions with patients and other staff members should communicate respect for other hospital employees. There are times that patients have complaints about staff members, for example, "the doctor doesn't listen and leaves too quickly," or "the cleaning lady doesn't do a good job of mopping the floor." Although the health psychology consultant can empathize with the patient's concerns, it is never appropriate to join in and reinforce the patient's complaints about another staff member, nor is it necessary to defend bad behavior on the part of staff members. At times the health psychology consultant can provide education if the patient misunderstands the behavior of a staff member (e.g., "the physical therapist is not trying to be mean, but she knows that pushing patients to do more helps them to improve more quickly and get back home sooner"). At other times, the health psychology consultant can help the patient problem-solve to develop strategies to help them get what they want (if appropriate). Chapter 4 of this volume discusses the management of patient complaints in more detail.

Working collaboratively (Ethical Standard 3.09; APA, 2017a) with other professionals is reflected in the development of joint treatment plans to address a patient issue and is also demonstrated as the health psychologist facilitates the work of other professionals (e.g., when allowing them to interrupt a psychological evaluation to get information they need; see Chapter 1). On rare occasions, the psychologist may be involved in a conflict with another staff member over a particular issue. Yet it is never appropriate to engage the patient in this, either explicitly or by making negative comments about the other staff member.

Relationships With Other Psychological Providers

In the outpatient setting, it would rarely be acceptable for a patient to see two psychologists at the same time, but this may occur when patients are admitted to the hospital. When a patient who is seeing an outpatient psychologist for ongoing treatment is admitted to the hospital, the medical team may request a consultation from the psychologist on staff in the hospital, who would then evaluate and treat the patient during the hospital stay. This scenario can be to the patient's benefit, especially if the inpatient health psychologist consults with the outpatient provider (with the patient's consent). The outpatient psychologist has usually had a longer relationship with the patient and knows him better, although the inpatient consultation will often yield new information that the outpatient provider was unaware of. Discussion with the outpatient provider can also ensure that the health psychology consultant does not interfere with the outpatient therapy. For example, if the outpatient psychologist has been seeing the patient for ongoing family concerns and dysthymia, the inpatient health psychology consultant could focus on the patient's coping with the hospital admission and adjustment to new medical issues. When the patient is discharged back to the outpatient provider, she and the patient may decide to integrate the inpatient issues into their ongoing outpatient treatment plan, but for the duration of the hospital stay, the health psychology consultant can work with the patient on the most pressing issues while in the hospital without interfering with the outpatient treatment.

Another concern involves the patient being seen by more than one psychologist during the hospital admission. In the outpatient setting, the relationship between the psychologist and the client is critical. In the inpatient setting, although still important, the relationship is diluted by the nature of the setting. Therefore, if the health psychology consultant has a bad cold, he might ask a colleague to follow his inpatients for a few days (to avoid spreading any infection to them). The covering health psychologist would pick up the treatment where the first psychologist left off and would act as a surrogate for the first consultant. This also occurs in emergencies; if the consultant working with a specific patient is unavailable, another will fill in. Because medical providers work in groups and even health psychologists often see patients with trainees, patients are generally accepting of this system because it provides continuity of care even when the primary psychologist is not available.

Culture and Diversity

The APA Ethics Code requires competence in "factors associated with age, gender, gender identity, race, ethnicity, culture, national origin, religion, sexual orientation, disability, language, or socioeconomic status" (APA, 2017a, Ethical Standard 2.01(b)). Multicultural Guidelines (APA, 2017b) focus specifically on cultural issues in treatment and research. These guidelines apply to interactions with patients in the hospital as well as other settings. Health psychology consultants in the medical setting may consult with a uniquely diverse group of individuals and are likely to gain expertise with many different populations. Yet there will be times when a health psychology consultant is faced with an individual from a culture or group in which he has no experience or training. In the inpatient setting, the correct response is to seek another provider who is competent to provide the psychological services. At times, however, there is no one else available, and the health psychologist will need to provide the services himself or the patient will get no psychological treatment. The APA Ethics Code considers this scenario and allows the health psychology consultant to provide services to ensure that services are not denied to the patient (Ethical Standard 2.02; APA, 2017a). Health psychology consultants undertaking this, however, should seek appropriate education and consultation to inform their work as soon as possible.

Some of the more common challenges seen when working with individuals of different backgrounds involve the patient's hesitation to discuss personal issues with individuals outside the culture or group, fears of stigma, poor understanding of psychological terminology, and language barriers. These will be discussed more fully here.

Some cultures and many individuals hold the belief that it is inappropriate to share personal information outside of the immediate group (or even outside the family). There may also be challenges specific to the health psychology consultant's age and culture (e.g., an elderly Mexican man may be unwilling to discuss personal issues with a psychologist who is young, White, and female). Some individuals may be taken aback by the psychologist's forthright request for personal information and may even be offended by it. Similarly, some patients may be concerned about stigma that could result from information they provide. In these cases, the health psychology consultant will need to take extra care and time to build rapport and trust and to explain her purposes to enlist the patient's cooperation in providing information needed for his treatment. In extreme cases, some information can be obtained from family members.

Psychological terminology is unfamiliar to many patients, often due to poor English fluency or education. Even individuals in the majority culture may not be familiar with terms such as *mania* and *delusions*, but people with less fluency may need explanations for more common words, such as *suicide*, *anxiety*, and *paranoia*. For all interviews, the health psychology consultant should explain any psychological terms used, but for patients with decreased psychological literacy, there may need to be a more extensive explanation of the terms, perhaps including examples.

Interviews with patients who do not speak English can be difficult, but larger medical centers have interpreters on staff or provide video or audio options to translate the interaction. Those interpreters who have experience with medical translation can be helpful and can often provide some additional cultural background or explanation that may help the consultant understand the patient.

In most cases, interpreters at medical centers are quite good and very professional, and relationships will be built with them over time. Because the health psychology interview is somewhat different from the medical interviews they are most experienced with, the health psychology consultant may need to provide some instruction regarding what is needed for the interview. It is also helpful if the consultant has a minimal understanding of the language being translated because this can facilitate the process. (Some medical centers offer classes in the languages most commonly spoken by their non–English-speaking patients that take little time and can be helpful.)

When interviewing patients through an interpreter, the health psychology consultant needs to (a) ask clear and brief questions and (b) address the patient when speaking (rather than the interpreter). Clear communication is always important, and long and convoluted questions and comments are difficult to translate. These introduce confusion and perhaps error. If a consultant would typically say, "Tell me where you are in life, like about your family and work," with a translator it is best to be more direct (e.g., "Who is in your family" and "What kind of work do you do?").

Further, for critical information, such as suicidal ideation, the consultant should always double-check to be sure the information obtained is correct.

The interpreter is usually seen by the patient as an ally, and the patient responds to him or her, often without regard to the consultant. Even so, it is important for the consultant to address the patient (and not the interpreter) to maintain the idea that the communication is between the patient and the consultant, with the interpreter as an aid to their communication.

The consultant should expect the interpreter to directly translate everything said by both the consultant and the patient, even if the interpreter does not feel the information is directly relevant. The interpreter should also understand that she is not to add her own input. In one case, the health psychology consultant asked a patient if she had ever had an episode of depression. The interpreter and patient talked back and forth for a few minutes, and the interpreter then translated the response as "no." Although perhaps the interpreter was only clarifying the question for the patient and the response provided was the correct answer, it is helpful to the consultant to understand all of the back-and-forth that went into the final answer. In another case, a young patient reported that she was considering suicide after an arm amputation. The interpreter stopped translating and began shaking his finger at the patient, telling her God would not approve of that. The consultant stopped the interpreter, reminding him simply to translate, and then regained control of the interview.

Right to Refuse Treatment

Patients have the right to refuse treatment, and those refusals often result in a consultation to health psychology. Patients may refuse chemotherapy because it will make them feel sick, hemodialysis because they feel it will negatively affect their quality of life, or any other treatment because they feel it will not work or because it will decrease their life quality. Patients may also decide to leave the hospital AMA (against medical advice). Although physicians prefer that their patients agree to the recommended treatment, they are respectful of a patient's decision—if the patient has capacity to make the decision. That is, if the patient has the capacity to make the decision, that patient's decision needs to be followed, even if it does not appear to be the "right" decision. Assessing decisional capacity is described in detail in Chapter 11.

If a patient maintains decisional capacity, she is also entitled to refuse a health psychology consultation and treatment. It is generally not a problem for a patient with capacity to refuse psychological treatment—the patient is able to explain the reason for the refusal, and the psychologist can make an effort to convince the patient to be seen. If the patient remains unwilling, the health psychology consultant can leave, providing a plan for recontact if the patient changes her mind. However, if the patient appears to be at risk of suicide, a danger to the hospital staff, or may not have decisional capacity, the situation is more difficult. In those cases, efforts must be made to obtain information to determine the patient's risk and capacity, even if a complete evaluation is not possible. Exhibit 15.1 describes a case in which a patient

EXHIBIT 15.1

Obtaining Useful Data When a Patient Refuses Psychology Consultation

Mr. G was a 53-year-old African American man with multiple medical problems, including diabetes mellitus (DM), end-stage renal disease (on hemodialysis [HD]), and hypertension. He was admitted to the hospital with AMS (*altered mental status*) and had missed HD for the past week. In the emergency department (ED), patient was mildly confused, did not know the date, and had poor memory. He was also crying but could not explain why. The health psychology consultation was requested with concerns about depression.

When entering the patient's room, he was again crying. The psychologist introduced herself and empathized that it can be difficult to be in the hospital, and then began to interview the patient. He immediately became irritable, yelled that he was not upset, and told the psychologist to leave. She tried to calm him, but he threw his lunch tray at her and began trying to climb out of bed to chase her away. The psychologist called the patient's nurse who was able to calm him (only with the psychologist outside the room).

The health psychology consultant was able to contact the patient's son, who lived with him. The son explained that the patient's behavioral changes began about 9 days ago when the patient had an argument with his nephew who was responsible for taking the patient to HD and to the pharmacy to pick up his medication. As a result, the patient would not go with the nephew to HD and was unable to get refills of two of his medications (son didn't know which ones). The son reported that the patient was initially angry at the nephew, but after a few days he began to cry and seemed confused. Son wasn't sure if patient was taking his remaining medications properly this past week. He brought the patient to the hospital when the patient threw an ashtray at him. Son reported the crying, confusion, and aggressiveness are atypical for the patient, who is usually "quiet and mellow." He also reported that patient has a history of alcohol abuse but that he has not had a drink in 7 years. Son is unaware of patient having any past emotional problems or psychiatric treatment.

On the basis of the patient's behavior, as described by his son and also the ED notes, a diagnosis of delirium was made. The patient's changes in cognition, emotion, and behavior seemed to result from him missing several HD sessions and also possible noncompliance with daily medications. While it was possible that the patient was experiencing anger and depressed mood following the conflict with his nephew, it was not possible to accurately assess that aspect (and also the possibility of depression) until the patient's cognition returned to baseline.

The patient was willing to comply with HD, medication, and other aspects of his current medical care in the hospital. The medical team was informed of this information, nursing staff made frequent checks on the patient to monitor his status, and the patient's son and daughter took turns staying with him. After 3 days, the patient appeared less confused and stopped crying. The psychologist returned, and the patient was willing to complete the evaluation. The conclusion was that the patient had been delirious at the time of the health psychology consultant's initial visit, but that 3 days later, the delirium had cleared. The patient acknowledged some stress associated with the argument with his nephew but denied symptoms of anxiety, depression, or psychosis. The son reported his father's behavior was back to baseline.

dramatically refused a consultation, as well as information on how the psychologist managed the evaluation and treatment. Note that the patient likely did not have decisional capacity when he initially refused the psychology evaluation, but the evaluation could not proceed without the patient's compliance anyway.

In this case, the psychologist was able to diagnose delirium from the patient's behavior and other data; even though the evaluation was incomplete, there was sufficient information to determine the appropriate treatment. Although the patient likely did not have decisional capacity, if the psychologist had forced the evaluation on him, it would have upset him further and provided minimal useful information. The psychologist respected the patient's refusal, monitored his status, and then returned when the patient was thinking more clearly to complete the evaluation.

Training, Billing, and Other Professional Issues

16

In the medical setting, psychologists need to attend to billing and productivity issues and may also need to implement plans for training students. The health psychology consultant will need to develop a professional identity that incorporates healthy boundaries, confidence in her own assessments, and a professional approach to patients and medical colleagues. The health psychologist will also need to attend to his own emotional reactions and self-care to maintain consistently good performance and to avoid burnout. These and other professional issues are discussed in this chapter.

Training Students

Inpatient psychology work with medical patients is interesting to many psychology students, and inpatient training experiences are offered by many externship, internship, and postdoctoral training programs. Yet trainees typically have little experience in the hospital setting, especially with respect to the interpretation of laboratory tests, medical diagnostic systems, pharmacology, delirium, and patient death (Ludwigsen & Albright, 1994; Schmaling, Giardino, Korslund, Roberts, & Sweeny, 2002). Dobmeyer and Rowan (2014) described core clinical competencies specific to psychologists who work in

http://dx.doi.org/10.1037/0000108-017
Health Psychology Consultation in the Inpatient Medical Setting, by S. M. Labott

medical settings (Table 16.1). A list of specific learning objectives for inpatient training has been developed by Schmaling et al. (2002) and is reprinted in Exhibit 16.1.

For many trainees, the hospital is a new world, and one that can be intimidating. Therefore, training in the health psychology methods described in this book should be viewed as specialized training that occurs after trainees have a good background and understanding of general clinical psychology and have basic skills in interviewing, therapy, and diagnostics. With such a background, trainees are prepared to integrate the additional skills required for successful hospital practice. Any trainee sent to evaluate an inpatient should have basic skills in place so that she can focus on the new medical aspects of the consultation and attend to the new requirements of the setting. The consultation is too overwhelming for a trainee who has not yet mastered the skills required to perform a basic psychological evaluation.

Successful training programs for inpatient consultation should include a seminar that is designed to (a) teach basic medical information, (b) demonstrate the overlap between psychological and medical issues, and (c) explicate psychological issues associated with medical diagnoses. The seminar can be geared to any trainee level but is often most successful when it includes externs, interns, postdocs, and faculty because all bring different perspectives. A good model is to have each member take a turn in presenting a topic (after initial modeling by a faculty member); outside speakers with expertise in specific areas of medicine can also contribute, with a psychologist filling in material on the relevant psychological issues. A new topic can be presented each week; the presentation could begin with a description of the medical problem and expected course of the disease, a discussion of associated psychological issues, and then

TABLE 16.1

Competencies for Psychologists in Medical Settings

Assessment	Psychologists in medical settings will have knowledge of psychological assessment measures specific to medical conditions. Psychologists in medical settings will understand the impact of medical symptoms and medications on standard psychological assessment measures developed and normed with nonmedical populations.
Advocacy	Psychologists in medical settings will effectively advocate for patients' needs and for appropriate psychological services to be available to medical patients.
Teaching	Psychologists in medical settings will effectively educate and train medical professionals from diverse disciplines in a biopsychosocial understanding of illness and in conceptualizing patients functionally rather than dualistically.
Professionalism	Psychologists in medical settings will pursue continuing education to increase knowledge and skill in topics related to health psychology. Psychologists in medical settings will demonstrate appropriate distress tolerance for working with patient populations in which physical disease, disability, or terminal illness are prevalent features.

Note. From *The Handbook of Clinical Psychology in Medical Settings: Evidence-Based Assessment and Intervention* (p. 82), by C. M. Hunter, C. L. Hunter, and R. Kessler (Eds.), 2014, New York, NY: Springer.

EXHIBIT 16.1

Learning Objectives for the Consultation–Liaison Rotation

Consult with staff to recommend behavioral plans and other strategies as needed for patient management.
Conduct brief, individual cognitive–behavior therapy with medical–surgical inpatients.
Engage in effective, assertive, and respectful team collaboration with physicians, social workers, medical assistants, and other professionals.
Communicate diagnostic and psychological information in a "consumer-friendly" manner to patients, referring physicians, and other professionals.
Demonstrate sensitivity to and competency in attending to issues of individual and cultural diversity.
Apply *Diagnostic and Statistical Manual of Mental Disorders* diagnoses reliably to adult problems with an emphasis on differential diagnosis.
Initiate discussions of ethical issues.
Practice efficient and thorough patient interviews including mental status exams as part of the team during rounds.
Enhance knowledge base as appropriate (review medical records; demonstrate a willingness to learn about unfamiliar illnesses and medications).
Formulate concise, clear, and organized oral case presentations to attendings.
Rapidly develop practical case conceptualization and treatment plans including treatment objectives and methods.
Develop self-confidence in the unique role of psychology in a medical setting and within an interdisciplinary team: Develop professional identity in this setting.
Demonstrate knowledge of the potential role (indications for, utility) of psychological assessment of patients in this setting.
Demonstrate familiarity with standard psychopharmacological treatments for adults, including methods of assessing drug effectiveness and side effects.
Seek exposure to the range of problems (both medical and psychiatric) seen in the medical center setting.
Participate in treatment planning as indicated (e.g., referral of the patient for psychotherapy, social work services, or other tests).
Write concise, organized, and complete initial evaluations and follow-up visit notes, reflecting the liaison role in a medical setting.

Note. Adapted from "The Utility of Interdisciplinary Training and Service: Psychology Training on a Psychiatry Consultation–Liaison Service," by K. B. Schmaling, N. D. Giardino, K. E. Korslund, L. J. Roberts, and S. Sweeny, 2002, *Professional Psychology: Research and Practice*, *33*, p. 417. Copyright 2002 by the American Psychological Association.

the presentation of a case that demonstrates these issues and leads to a discussion of the psychological evaluation and intervention. For example, for the topic of chronic obstructive pulmonary disease (COPD), the trainee could present a brief overview of emphysema and chronic bronchitis, explaining typical symptoms and disease course. Breathing symptoms and anxiety as they relate to the breathing disorder and psychological symptoms, as well as problems with differential diagnosis can then be explained. Last, a case of an inpatient with COPD could be described, including relevant medical information and presenting psychological symptoms, with a focus on determining the appropriate psychological intervention (e.g., anxiety management, depression treatment, adjustment and coping) while the patient remains in the hospital.

Although much education about health psychology inpatient consultation can be presented in a classroom setting, there is no substitute for the supervisor modeling the proper behaviors in the hospital with actual patients while the trainee observes. In most settings this will involve the supervisor initially doing all the work of the consultation and intervention, while the trainee follows along. The modeling by the supervisor should include every aspect of the consultation—receiving the referral, reviewing the medical record and any relevant literature, interviewing the patient, obtaining collateral information, report writing, providing feedback to the medical team, and planning follow-up intervention or monitoring. This allows the trainee to adjust to the hospital setting without pressure to perform so he can relax and gain some comfort with the supervisor and the setting. Further, there are many logistical details and professional interactions associated with this work that become second nature to the supervisor, who will not be able to address each specifically with the trainee. However, if the trainee is observing the supervisor, he will note many details and can ask questions to elicit more discussion from the supervisor. Through this method, the trainee will learn about the important clinical aspects of the work and will also learn practical details necessary for successful consultation (e.g., where to find the ward clerk, how to handle a doctor who wants immediate feedback before the trainee has had time to process the information, how to find the patient's nurse, where to write notes). A list of resources for trainees who are learning to do inpatient consultation is found in Exhibit 1.3 in Chapter 1 of this volume.

Over time, the trainee can become a more active participant and begin to review the patient's chart independently, manage part of the interview with the patient, and draft sections of the report. As the trainee gains knowledge and confidence, she can do more, and the supervisor can do more supervision and less direct evaluation and treatment. Ultimately, the trainee will do all aspects of the consultation alone, with supervision before and after each new consultation. The amount of time it will take a trainee to move through these steps will depend on her previous experience with these tasks.

Weekly individual supervision will also be important for the trainee to gain a healthy perspective on the work and to address ongoing intervention issues with hospitalized patients. Opportunities for group supervision are also useful because trainees can share experiences with patients and aspects of their training. The group meetings are also an important opportunity for trainees to provide support to each other because there is no shortage of stressful and emotional events they will need to cope with (e.g., the slow death of a favorite patient, mistreatment of a patient by a provider, family members who interfere with or sabotage a patient's psychological treatment). Trainees should also have access to a supervisor at all times to help them manage emergencies if they occur.

Billing and Productivity

Billing for inpatient health psychology services will depend on systems in place at the hospital as well as the psychologist's financial arrangements with the hospital. That is, the health psychology consultant may bill from a home department in the medical center, through the hospital billing department, privately, or as a service bundled with those of other providers. If services are billed to insurance companies, all psychologists will select from the same codes for use in billing; these are referred to as Current Procedural Terminology (CPT) codes.

Two main categories of codes can be used for inpatient billing (with additional codes available for specialized services, such as neuropsychological testing). Regardless of which codes are used for billing, the psychologist's documentation in the medical record needs to correctly reflect the services provided. Traditional psychotherapy codes can be used for both inpatient and outpatient billing and provide for a diagnostic evaluation as well as therapy sessions of varying lengths, as shown in Table 16.2. These codes are billed in conjunction with a diagnosis from the fifth edition of the *Diagnostic and Statistical Manual of Mental Disorders* (*DSM–5*; American Psychiatric Association, 2013). This can be problematic at times because many inpatients do not meet criteria for a psychiatric diagnosis. Services billed with these traditional psychotherapy codes are generally covered by the mental health portion of a patient's insurance.

Alternatively, health and behavior (H&B) codes can be used to bill for both inpatient and outpatient psychological services. H&B codes are billed in conjunction with the patient's medical diagnosis (e.g., multiple sclerosis, leukemia). The American Medical Association (2018) provides current medical diagnostic codes from the *International Statistical Classification of Diseases and Related Health Problems* (10th revision; known as ICD–10; Centers for Disease Control and Prevention, 2018). In choosing the medical diagnostic code for H&B billing, the psychologist should use a medical diagnosis that has been assigned by the medical team (because there are many subtle variations in the medical diagnostic codes, and the medical diagnosis for the health psychology treatment should correspond to that for the medical treatment). The H&B CPT codes are usually covered by the patient's medical rather than mental health insurance, and they cover both evaluation and intervention services. The focus of the treatment and evaluation is on the psychological issues as they relate to the medical diagnosis; that is, the health psychologist might be treating adjustment-related anxiety due to a new

TABLE 16.2

CPT Codes for Inpatient Health Psychology Billing

Traditional psychotherapy codes	
90791	Psychiatric diagnostic evaluation
90832	Psychotherapy, 30 minutes
90834	Psychotherapy, 45 minutes
90837	Psychotherapy, 60 minutes
Health & behavior (H&B) codes[a]	
96150	Initial H&B evaluation
96151	Reassessment of need for further treatment
96152	Intervention
96153	Intervention—group
96154	Intervention with patient and family
96155	Intervention with family without patient

Note. CPT = Current Procedural Terminology.
[a]All H&B codes are billed in 15-minute increments.

diagnosis of cancer rather than an ongoing anxiety disorder. The H&B codes can also capture brief visits, rarely require preauthorization from insurance companies, and avoid the potential of stigmatizing a patient with a psychiatric diagnosis. Yet even though these codes have been in existence since 2002, some institutions are not yet set up to use them effectively, and some insurance companies do not cover them.

There are some special circumstances in which the psychologist may not directly bill insurance companies for services provided to a patient. This is most likely to occur if the health psychology consultant is part of a specialty group, such as a transplant program, and provides a designated service, such as an evaluation, for all patients. For this work, special arrangements are made between the psychologist and the larger transplant program, so that several services are bundled into one bill and submitted to the insurance company by the larger program. For example, the transplant program could submit one bill that covers the evaluations provided by health psychology, social work, and nutrition. The insurance company pays the one bill, and the health psychologist (or his department) is then reimbursed a previously agreed-on amount for that service in that program.

Relative value units (RVUs) are used in the Medicare reimbursement system and define the amount of "value" that providers earn for a particular piece of work. RVUs can be thought of as "points" for performing a particular service; some services are worth more points than others. That is, a surgeon earns more RVUs for a 6-hour heart transplant procedure than a psychologist earns for a therapy session, but a longer therapy session is worth more RVUs than a shorter one. RVUs are often used by the institution to monitor the professional's productivity; a certain number of RVUs (usually based on the percentage of time spent in clinical work) are expected to be earned to demonstrate that the clinician has performed the required amount of clinical work. Although the actual RVU values are consistent across the country, the number of RVUs designated as "appropriate" productivity is not, and some hospitals and departments use other factors in addition to RVUs to describe productivity. That is, 30% clinical time in two institutions can translate into dramatically different RVUs that the psychologists at those institutions are expected to earn to remain in good standing. Some institutions use RVUs to monitor productivity exclusively, whereas others also consider nonbillable activities in evaluating a psychologist's productivity (e.g., supervision). Because of the discrepancies across institutions, health psychologists will need to clarify exactly what the expectations for productivity are within a specific institution. If a psychologist is not paid by the institution (as in the case of a private practitioner who consults to patients in the hospital part time), RVUs are generally not relevant.

Developing a Professional Identity

The health psychology consultant will do well to attend to the culture and politics of psychologists in the hospital, working within any established roles, then making changes as necessary. The role of the psychologist is partially dictated by his location; a psychologist who is from a freestanding Department of Psychology may have a different role from one who is a member of a Department of Psychiatry or from that of a psychologist who works in private practice outside of the hospital.

The role of the health psychology consultant is also dictated by expectations within the medical center. For example, a psychologist might see patients throughout the hospital, but not in the emergency department, especially if other mental health services are available there. If there is a separate psychiatry consultation service, there will likely be existing relationships and informal rules about how the services interact; work will go more smoothly if the health psychology consultant is aware of these arrangements.

Over time, the many and varied experiences that occur in the inpatient medical setting aid the health psychology consultant in defining his role; many seemingly trivial experiences help to develop the professional identity of a specific psychologist. Managing unwilling patients, uncooperative families, arrogant providers, and overworked nurses are only a few of the challenges the psychologist may face. How each of these is addressed will help to solidify both the role and the reputation of the psychologist. While all health psychology consultants perform similar work, individual psychologists have differing approaches to the work, their patients, and their colleagues, and these ultimately define the psychologist as an independent provider in the medical center.

The health psychologist will want to approach all issues in ways that reflect well on the profession of psychology and that also lend credibility to the psychologist's work in the medical center. Further, the psychologist needs to achieve an identity that is comfortable for her personally. A psychologist should consider her expectations of medical colleagues as well as her own responsibilities and obligations to patients and hospital staff. Much advice on how to manage this work has been provided throughout this book, but ultimately each psychologist needs to develop a role, identity, and relationships with colleagues and patients that are comfortable for her.

The health psychology consultant will need to manage the inpatient workflow differently than he would in an outpatient office practice. People are admitted to the hospital at all times of the day and night. As referral sources learn of the work of the health psychologist, they are often eager to make use of this service for their patients. That increases the number of referrals exponentially, and a lone health psychologist may need to set limits on the amount of time she is available or the types of referrals she can accommodate. If there is a consultation-liaison psychiatry service that is available 24 hours each day for emergencies, the psychologist can set specific hours and let referral sources know of his availability, requesting that they contact the emergency psychiatry service during night and weekend hours (and this should also be arranged with that service beforehand). If there are no emergency mental health services available in the hospital, the psychologist will need to make other arrangements for coverage when she is not available.

Psychologists will also need to develop a sense of what is possible in the setting in which they work and also deal with the limitations on what they can accomplish. For example, it is tempting to develop comprehensive treatment plans for inpatients and then plan to deliver this treatment personally while the patient is in the hospital or after discharge. Yet the best-laid inpatient treatment plans often do not come to fruition—for example, if the patient is discharged unexpectedly. Further, if the health psychology consultant plans to continue outpatient work with all appropriate inpatients, she will soon have no time available to see new inpatients. Appropriate referrals will need to be developed.

Self-Care

The work of the inpatient health psychology consultant can be emotionally draining because the work can be intense and stressful. Patients die, they may be discharged unexpectedly, and a variety of social and administrative factors can interfere with plans for a patient's treatment. Psychologists will need to develop ways to manage the emotional and stressful aspects of inpatient work; this will involve learning to grieve appropriately, manage frustration, and cope with ongoing stressors.

Psychologists will never be able to predict with 100% certainty when a patient will be discharged, but the anticipated length of stay needs to be considered when developing treatment plans to avoid the patient's discharge during an important phase of treatment. Experience in working with certain medical illnesses and also the discharge habits of specific physicians can provide important data to help a psychologist anticipate discharge, yet it is still not uncommon for the psychologist to be surprised by a patient's discharge. The health psychology consultant may be involved in treatment with a patient who is expected to be in the hospital for a while; then something changes medically, and the patient is discharged unexpectedly (often over a weekend), and the psychologist is unaware until returning to work on Monday. For some patients, the focus of the intervention was on dealing with the inpatient admission, which may become a nonissue after discharge. Other patients can be contacted and referred for continuation of treatment on an outpatient basis, but that is often not possible.

Even if appropriate plans are made with the patient for ongoing outpatient treatment, a variety of factors can interfere so that the treatment does not occur. Some of the more common barriers are transportation problems, family members who actively obstruct the patient's attendance, and patient illness and motivation. Attending to potential barriers throughout the inpatient admission can help to mitigate some of them, and at times, the psychologist can be creative in finding ways to continue to monitor the patient after discharge (e.g., seeing the patient when he comes to an outpatient visit with his pulmonologist), although those arrangements present additional challenges in terms of logistics and confidentiality. Many times there is nothing the psychologist can do to resolve these issues, and the patient is lost to outpatient follow-up.

A more emotionally difficult situation occurs when the patient dies; both anticipated and unexpected deaths can result in grief for the psychologist. As with other losses, the type and severity of the grief may relate to the length and intensity of the relationship with the patient, as well as other personal issues of the psychologist.

In graduate school, students receive training in the assessment and management of suicide, but rarely is any attention paid to the experience of having a patient die due to medical illness. Dwyer, Deshields, and Nanna (2012) provided recommendations for coping with a patient's death. These include considering the relationship with surviving family members (including decisions about providing treatment to them) and maintaining the confidentiality of the deceased. They also noted the importance of maintaining control over one's own grief, so that the focus remains on the family.

Time and experience will help the health psychology consultant learn to manage grief over the death of a patient. Successful negotiation of the grief is associated with proper management of the emotional relationship with the patient (before the death), developing a mixture of work activities, consultation with colleagues, and attention to coping.

Maintaining the proper emotional distance from a patient is necessary to preserve objectivity and promote client progress in treatment. Leitner (1995) used the term *optimal therapeutic distance* to describe the blend of connectedness and separateness with the client that is most associated with client growth. When applied to inpatient consultation, if the psychologist is too emotionally close to the patient, she is overinvolved and may be unable to maintain objectivity and to intervene successfully. If the relationship with the patient is too distant, the psychologist may be seen as cold and aloof and may have difficulty with rapport, resulting in less effective treatment. The proper emotional distance is associated with the most effective treatment and also helps to provide the psychologist with a healthy perspective from which to manage grief. The optimal emotional distance may not be consistent across patients and will almost certainly differ across psychologists, based on their personalities.

Particular challenges are presented by those patients who remind the psychologist of a significant person in his past or current life. It is not uncommon for trainees to recognize familiar aspects of their grandparents in elderly patients they treat. Similarly, psychologists often have difficulty managing a relationship with a patient who is similar to themselves in terms of gender, marriage, family, or lifestyle. A health psychology consultant needs to be aware of any issues and relationships in their own lives that may influence the relationship with and the treatment of a specific patient. Although these complications are to be expected, the health psychology consultant needs to develop an awareness of them as well as effective management strategies so that the psychologist's objectivity and the patient's treatment are not negatively affected.

For many psychologists, losses of multiple patients over a short period of time can accumulate and intensify the psychologist's emotional reaction. For this reason, many psychologists will develop a work life that includes a variety of activities. That is, the psychologist may divide her time among inpatient clinical work, research, and supervising students. While this means the psychologist may have professional demands of several types, this arrangement is often less emotionally taxing than spending all of her time working with very ill patients.

Consulting with colleagues is another way to mitigate the emotional feelings of loss when patients die. As with any other loss, discussing the events with supportive others can help the psychologist to gain some perspective and to move through the grief more rapidly. Dwyer et al. (2012) noted the importance of using professional support to help with grieving, as well as the development of a "grief ritual" (e.g., a time for reflection, a prayer) that the psychologist uses to help cope with patient deaths.

Health psychology consultants need to acknowledge that work with medical inpatients can be emotionally difficult and make plans to cope effectively at times of loss and stress. Although psychologists will ideally have stress management and coping activities built into their lives, the awareness of a new or impending loss should elicit additional coping to help the psychologist deal with it. The specific coping strategies should be designed to help the psychologist to relax, process the event, and manage painful affect.

Dealing With Pressure From Medical Colleagues

At times, physicians may have a specific psychiatric diagnosis in mind for a patient and may pressure the health psychology consultant to confirm it. In these cases, the psychologist should hear their opinions but will then complete his own evaluation and come to his own conclusion based on all the data. This situation may occur with a patient who demonstrates symptoms that warrant a hospital admission, but after thorough workup, the symptoms remain medically unexplained. If there is no clear physical reason for the symptom, some physicians will conclude the symptom must have a psychological etiology. Health psychology referrals may be received for cases in which a doctor is convinced the patient has a conversion disorder because there seems to be no medical cause for the symptom. There are several reasons to not be pressured into agreeing with this diagnosis. Conversion disorder is rare and difficult to diagnose from an inpatient interview alone. The *DSM–5* (American Psychiatric Association, 2013) provides additional detail on the diagnosis of conversion disorder (known currently also as functional neurological symptom disorder).

Further, many medically unexplained symptoms are subclinical at the time patients initially seek treatment and are undetectable on current laboratory tests, but with time the symptoms progress and a medical disorder is diagnosed (e.g., multiple sclerosis often takes many years for a clear diagnosis to emerge). Finally, if the patient is given a conversion disorder diagnosis, physicians may stop seeking a medical cause and may also stop treating the physical symptoms, referring for psychiatric treatment instead. The diagnosis will continue to be missed, and the patient will not get proper medical treatment.

If the health psychology consultant is unable to conclusively diagnose a conversion disorder (which is likely to happen much of the time), that should be clearly, but tactfully, stated, together with additional recommendations for the patient's treatment. The following is an example of recommendations for a case like this:

> Summary: Pt with medically unexplained neurological sx, but no conclusive evidence of conversion disorder obtained. D/w pt how the stress of unexplained sx can exacerbate sx and discussed strategies to aid her coping. Both medical and psychological providers should continue to follow, to monitor pt's sx and clinical findings over time.

A similar situation occurs when the patient has been diagnosed with a medical problem and has also developed acute mental status changes (delirium). At times, the medical symptoms are treated successfully, but the delirium is slower to resolve. Physicians are under pressure to discharge patients as soon as they can, so may be eager to send the patient home, often without consulting the psychologist who has been following the patient. In the case of mild cognitive changes and a supportive family that is present to help and monitor the patient, discharge may be safe. If the patient will be alone, however, and if the cognitive changes are more severe, the health psychology consultant may need to insist that the patient remain in the hospital longer until the cognitive symptoms improve and he is safe to be home alone.

Dealing With Incomplete Information

Many times, patients are unable to provide adequate information to aid in their evaluation, family members are unavailable, and no historical information is available in the medical record. In some cases, the health psychology consultant can draw reasonable conclusions without much history by observing the patient's current behavior. In other cases, few conclusions can be drawn until more information is obtained, and the psychologist will need to withhold judgment until more information becomes available. Patients may also report events that cannot be corroborated and treatment will need to proceed with incomplete information (Exhibit 16.2).

The health psychology consultant will always want to believe what the patient reports, or believe *they* believe it and are upset by it, even if it is not objectively true. In this case, we could never be 100% certain that the patient was not abused or certain that this represented a delusion that was a symptom of delirium. All relevant parties continued to monitor the patient frequently, and her daughter spent 3 more nights with her. Over the next few days, the patient's confusion disappeared, and her memory improved. It was striking that she was later unconcerned about the reported abuse incident, and she was no longer fearful of being in the hospital. The ultimate goals were to ensure that the patient felt safe and that she was treated fairly, and those goals were accomplished.

Marketing Health Psychology Inpatient Services

In a large medical center, due to the rotation schedules of attendings, fellows, and residents, word may spread quickly that the health psychology consultant is available to see patients. Physicians are often eager to enlist psychological support for their patients because they may feel poorly equipped to address the psychological concerns of their patients adequately.

Tovian (2014) described useful strategies for marketing psychological services, most of which are relevant to the hospital setting. These include strategies for

EXHIBIT 16.2

Managing a Consultation With Incomplete Information

Ms. N was a 62 y/o Hispanic woman, admitted to the neurology unit a week ago after a stroke. A psychology consultation was requested for poststroke adjustment. The patient had some weakness and few physical limitations, but she demonstrated mild confusion and disorientation on evaluation. She appeared nervous during the evaluation but denied any psychological symptoms or mental health history. She appeared to be holding something back but denied it when asked by the psychologist. Several hours later, nursing staff paged the psychologist, reporting that the patient's daughter was angry because the patient told her she was fondled by a male nurse last night. Daughter reported the incident to hospital administration who began to investigate. Nursing staff requested that the psychologist return and speak with the patient as they felt this event did not truly happen and could not understand why the patient would make up something like this.

The psychologist returned to see the patient who explained in a whisper that a male nurse, mid-30s, African American, had come into her room the night before and told her to be quiet. He raised her hospital gown, listened to her heart, then fondled her breasts and told her not to tell anyone or he would kill her. She denied being physically harmed but was distressed and afraid he would return and hurt her. The patient's mental status was WNL *(within normal limits)*, except for mild impairment in short-term recall (two of three items after 3 minutes).

The psychologist discussed the case with the patient, her daughter, the patient's nurse, and the unit charge nurse and developed the following plan: The patient's daughter will spend the night with the patient for a few nights to provide support and to increase her comfort level. The nurses will check on the patient more frequently, and she will only be cared for by female nurses. The charge nurse will work with the hospital administration to review staffing on the unit last night for anyone fitting the patient's description of her abuser. All these plans were discussed with the patient, and she was comfortable with the plan. She was assured of her safety and staff plans to keep her safe throughout her hospital admission.

At this point, it was unclear whether the patient had actually been fondled by a nurse or if it was a delusion that the patient had experienced. At times, delirious patients report that they have been taken to a mall, a bank, or a party and then returned to the hospital in the morning. It is fairly easy to determine the reality of these events because staff can attest to the patient being present in the hospital all night. Further, patients often cannot explain details of the events they believe they have attended (e.g., how they traveled to the party, where they got street clothes). In this case, however, because the patient had not reported leaving the hospital, it was possible that the event had occurred as she described it.

In the next 24 hours, nursing administration was able to confirm that there were no male nurses on duty on the patient's floor during the night in question. (However, it was still possible that an extraneous person came to the floor and perpetrated the abuse.) The patient's daughter noted that she became slightly agitated the next night and called nursing staff. They, in turn, called the resident on call, who gave the patient low dose Haldol. This calmed her; she relaxed and slept well, denying any incidents the next morning. The patient's doctors also noted some fluctuation in her mental status throughout the day and attributed it to poststroke delirium.

educating referral sources, establishing competence, and also demonstrating an ability to collaborate effectively. Anytime the psychologist evaluates a patient, education can be provided about what she has to offer to the primary medical team. That is, the health psychology consultant can define referral questions that specific providers may have that she can address. Health psychology consultants can also volunteer to give lectures and presentations to medical staff on issues that are relevant to them (e.g., depression in patients with diabetes).

Good communication about patient issues is critical. Communication needs to be clear, accurate, brief, prompt, and useful to the referral source. Some doctors have preferences for certain types of communication or for contacts at certain times; the health psychology consultant should accommodate their preferences as much as possible. (See Tovian, 2006, for additional suggestions on communication with physicians.) The psychologist will also need to demonstrate an awareness of medical issues and evidence-based practices, as well as professionalism and flexibility when working with patients. Once relationships are established with referral sources, they need to be nurtured over time. Tovian (2014) provided more detail on these topics, as well as other suggestions regarding the marketing of psychological services.

Summary

There is much that psychologists can offer to hospitalized patients who are dealing with difficult medical issues. Health psychology consultants perform evaluation and intervention, provide education and strategies to minimize the stress of hospitalization, promote adjustment to the medical issue, and enhance coping with medical or end of life issues. Psychologists can normalize the patient's hospital experience, circumvent trauma, and also provide support to patients and their families. They can help to provide safe passage as patients navigate through their medical issues and the hospital system, providing a combination of services that are not offered by any other professionals in the hospital. With attention to the norms and rules of the hospital milieu and professional and ethical issues, the health psychology consultant can successfully adapt traditional clinical psychology interventions to enhance the quality of life of hospitalized medical patients.

Appendix A

Common Medical Abbreviations

AA	African American
AAF	African American female
AAM	African American male
ABG	arterial blood gases
Abx	antibiotics
ADL	activities of daily living
Ad lib	as desired
Adm	admitting
AFib	atrial fibrillation
AICD	automatic implantable cardioverter-defibrillator
AKA	above-the-knee amputation
ALL	acute lymphocytic leukemia
AMA	against medical advice
AML	acute myelocytic leukemia
AMS	altered mental status
ANC	absolute neutrophil count
Ant	anterior
A&O	alert and oriented
A&O × 3	alert and oriented in three spheres (time, place, person)
A/P	assessment/plan
ARF	acute renal failure
ASA	acetylsalicylic acid (aspirin)
ASHD	arteriosclerotic heart disease
BCLS	basic cardiac life support
BG	blood glucose

BID	twice a day
Bil	bilateral
BKA	below-knee amputation
BMI	body mass index
Bx	biopsy
CA	carcinoma; cancer
Ca	calcium
CABG	coronary artery bypass graft
CAD	coronary artery disease
CAPD	continuous ambulatory peritoneal dialysis
CAT	computerized axial tomography
CBC	complete blood count
CC	chief complaint
CF	cystic fibrosis
CHF	congestive heart failure
CKD	chronic kidney disease
c/o	complains of
COPD	chronic obstructive pulmonary disease
CP	cerebral palsy; chest pain
CPAP	continuous positive airway pressure
CPR	cardiopulmonary resuscitation
CR	complete remission
CRF	chronic renal failure
CT scan	computer-assisted tomography
CVA	cerebrovascular accident
CVD	cardiovascular disease
c/w	consistent with
CXR	chest x-ray
d/c	discharge; discontinue
DJD	degenerative joint disease
DKA	diabetic ketoacidosis
DM	diabetes mellitus
DME	durable medical equipment
DNR	do not resuscitate
DOE	dyspnea on exertion
DVT	deep vein thrombosis
Dx	diagnosis
DZ	disease
ECG	electrocardiogram
Echo	echocardiogram
ED	emergency department
EEG	electroencephalogram
EENT	eye, ear, nose, and throat
EF	ejection fraction

EKG	electrocardiogram
ENT	ear, nose, and throat
ESRD	end-stage renal disease
ETOH	alcohol
Fe	iron
Fhx	family history
FT	feeding tube
FTT	failure to thrive
FU, f/u	follow-up
FUO	fever of unknown origin
Fx	fracture
GERD	gastroesophageal reflux disease
GI	gastrointestinal
GSW	gunshot wound
G tube	gastrostomy tube
HA	headache
HBV	hepatitis B virus
HCV	hepatitis C virus
HD	hemodialysis
HF	Hispanic female
HM	Hispanic male
h/o	history of
HOH	hard of hearing
H&P	history and physical
HPI	history of present illness
HR	heart rate
Hs	at bedtime
HTN	hypertension
Hx	history
I&O	intake and output
IBW	ideal body weight
ICU	intensive care unit
IM	intramuscular
Inpt	inpatient
IPD	inpatient department
IV	intravenous
IVDA	intravenous drug abuse
J tube	jejunostomy tube
K	potassium
L	left
L&D	labor and delivery
LBP	low back pain
LE	lower extremity
LFTs	liver function tests
LLE	left lower extremity

LLL	left lower lobe
LLQ	left lower quadrant
LOC	loss of consciousness
LP	lumbar puncture
LUE	left upper extremity
LUL	left upper lobe
LUQ	left upper quadrant
LVAD	left ventricular assist device
Meds	medications
Met	metastatic
Mg	milligram, magnesium
MI	myocardial infarction
MICU	medical intensive care unit
MJ	marijuana
MMP	multiple medical problems
MRI	magnetic resonance imaging
MRSA	methicillin resistant *Staphylococcus aureus*
MS	multiple sclerosis
MSE	mental status examination
MV	mitral valve
MVA	motor vehicle accident
MVI	multivitamin
NAD	no acute distress
NGT	nasogastric tube
NH	nursing home
NIDDM	non–insulin dependent diabetes mellitus
NKA	no known allergies
NKDA	no known drug allergies
NOS	not otherwise specified
NPO	nothing by mouth
NSAID	nonsteroidal anti-inflammatory drug
NSR	normal sinus rhythm
N&V	nausea and vomiting
O2	oxygen
O2 sat	oxygen saturation
OA	osteoarthritis
OC	oral contraceptives
OPD	outpatient department
OSH	outside hospital
Outpt	outpatient
PA	physician's assistant
PC	after meals
PCA	patient-controlled analgesia
PCP	primary care physician
PD	peritoneal dialysis

PE	pulmonary embolism; physical examination
Peds	pediatrics
PERRLA	pupils equal, round, reactive to light and accommodation
PET	positron emission tomography
PFT	pulmonary function test
PICU	pediatric intensive care unit
PID	pelvic inflammatory disease
PMH	past medical history
PO	by mouth
POD	postoperative day
PPD	packs per day
PR	partial remission
Prn	as necessary
PSH	past social history
pt	patient
PT	physical therapy
PTA	prior to admission
PUD	peptic ulcer disease
PVD	peripheral vascular disease
Q	every
Qam	every morning
Qd	every day
Qhs	every evening at bedtime
QID	four times daily
R	right
RA	rheumatoid arthritis
RBC	red blood count
RD	registered dietician
RLE	right lower extremity
RLL	right lower lobe
RLQ	right lower quadrant
r/o	rule out
ROM	range of motion
ROS	review of systems
RSR	regular sinus rhythm
RT	respiratory therapy; radiation therapy
RTC	return to clinic
RTW	return to work
RUE	right upper extremity
RUL	right upper lobe
RUQ	right upper quadrant
Rx	treatment or prescription
SAH	subarachnoid hemorrhage
SBO	small bowel obstruction

SBP systolic blood pressure
SCD sickle cell disease
SH social history
SICU surgical intensive care unit
SLE systemic lupus erythematosus
SNF skilled nursing facility
SOAP subjective objective assessment plan
SOB shortness of breath
S/P status post
STAT immediately
SW social work
Sx symptoms
Sz seizure
TB tuberculosis
THA total hip arthroplasty
TIA transient ischemic attack
TID three times a day
TKA total knee arthroplasty
TMAX maximum temperature
TPN total parenteral nutrition
Trach tracheostomy
Tx treatment
TX transplant
UA urinalysis
UE upper extremity
URI upper respiratory infection
US ultrasound
UTI urinary tract infection
VDRL venereal disease research lab
V/S vital signs
WBC white blood cell; white blood cell count
WC wheelchair
WF White female
WM White male
WNL within normal limits
w/o without
w/u workup

Symbols

c with
s without
– negative
+ positive

Appendix B

Common Laboratory Tests and Their Interpretation

The following list and the interpretations provided are not comprehensive and intended only to provide a general sense of some common tests and their meanings. More detail on these and other tests can be found at WebMD (https://www.webmd.com) and Medline Plus (https://medlineplus.gov/labtests.html).

Blood Panel

Complete blood count (CBC): provides levels of a variety of different cells in the blood

White blood cell count (WBC): white cells help fight infection; WBC is elevated with infections and some kinds of leukemia

Neutrophils: a type of WBC, high with infection, inflammation; low in response to chemo drugs or radiation

Red blood cell count (RBC): red blood cells carry oxygen from lungs to cells.

Hemoglobin (Hgb) and *Hematocrit (Hct):* components of RBC; high with dehydration, low in anemia

Platelets (PLT): responsible for blood clotting; high in certain cancers and anemias; low in bone marrow diseases

Metabolic Panel

Glucose (blood sugar): high in diabetes, with certain drugs (steroids, tricyclic antidepressants, diuretics), chronic renal failure; low with endocrine disorders, hypothyroid, hypopituitarism

Blood urea nitrogen (BUN): high values with impaired kidney function; low values due to diet, liver disease, malnutrition, pregnancy
Creatinine: high with high protein intake, kidney infection; low in conditions that are associated with decreased muscle mass
Sodium (Na): high values in dehydration, kidney disease; low values with excess water retention (heart failure, cirrhosis) and certain drugs
Potassium (K): high with certain drugs, renal failure, injuries; low due to diuretics, diarrhea, vomiting, dehydration
Albumin: used to screen for liver and kidney disorders and to evaluate nutritional status; high in dehydration; low in kidney and liver disease, malnutrition
Bilirubin: elevated in liver disease and alcohol abuse
Thyroid-stimulating hormone (TSH): hypothyroid (underactive thyroid gland) is associated with weight gain, tiredness, dry skin, feeling cold; hyperthyroid (overactive thyroid gland) is associated with weight loss, rapid heart rate, nervousness

Lipid Panel

Cholesterol: high values associated with increased risk for heart disease; low values associated with decreased risk for heart disease, malnutrition, liver disease
High-density lipoprotein (HDL): high values associated with decreased risk for heart disease (the "good" cholesterol)
Low-density lipoprotein (LDL): high values associated with increased risk of heart disease, pregnancy (the "bad" cholesterol)

Toxicology Screens

These screens provide information about the presence and quantity of specific drugs of abuse (e.g., cocaine, opiates, barbiturates, methadone) or prescription drugs (e.g., acetaminophen, barbiturates, benzodiazepines, phenytoin)

Urinalysis

This test provides levels for a variety of components of the urine. In many cases, of most importance is WBC level, which is elevated with infection.

References

Affleck, G., & Tennen, H. (1996). Construing benefits from adversity: Adaptational significance and dispositional underpinnings. *Journal of Personality, 64,* 899–922. http://dx.doi.org/10.1111/j.1467-6494.1996.tb00948.x

Aggarwal, B., Liao, M., Allegrante, J. P., & Mosca, L. (2010). Low social support level is associated with non-adherence to diet at 1 year in the Family Intervention Trial for Heart Health (FIT Heart). *Journal of Nutrition Education and Behavior, 42,* 380–388. http://dx.doi.org/10.1016/j.jneb.2009.08.006

Ajzen, I., & Manstead, A. S. R. (2007). Changing health-related behaviours: An approach based on the theory of planned behaviour. In M. Hewstone, H. A. W. Schut, J. B. F. De Wit, K. Van Den Bos, & M. S. Stroebe (Eds.), *The scope of social psychology: Theory and applications* (pp. 43–63). New York, NY: Psychology Press.

Alaja, R., & Seppä, K. (2003). Six-month outcomes of hospital-based psychiatric substance use consultations. *General Hospital Psychiatry, 25,* 103–107. http://dx.doi.org/10.1016/S0163-8343(03)00002-1

Amato, L., Minozzi, S., Vecchi, S., & Davoli, M. (2010). Benzodiazepines for alcohol withdrawal. *The Cochrane Database of Systematic Reviews, 3,* CD005063.

American Bar Association Commission on Law and Aging & American Psychological Association. (2008). *Assessment of older adults with diminished capacity: A handbook for psychologists.* Washington, DC: Author.

American Medical Association. (2018). *ICD–10–CM 2018: The complete official codebook.* Chicago, IL: Author.

American Psychiatric Association. (2013). *Diagnostic and statistical manual of mental disorders* (5th ed.). Arlington, VA: Author.

American Psychological Association. (2011). Practice guidelines regarding psychologists' involvement in pharmacological issues. *American Psychologist, 66,* 835–849. http://dx.doi.org/10.1037/a0025890

American Psychological Association. (2013). Guidelines for psychological practice in health care delivery systems. *American Psychologist, 68,* 1–6. http://dx.doi.org/10.1037/a0029890

American Psychological Association. (2017a). *Ethical principles of psychologists and code of conduct* (2002, Amended June 1, 2010 and January 1, 2017). Retrieved from http://www.apa.org/ethics/code/ethics-code-2017.pdf

American Psychological Association. (2017b). *Multicultural guidelines: An ecological approach to context, identity, and intersectionality.* Retrieved from http://www.apa.org/about/policy/multicultural-guidelines.pdf

American Psychological Association, Committee on Professional Practice of the Board of Professional Affairs. (1985). *A hospital practice primer for psychologists.* Washington, DC: Author.

Anstiss, T., & Passmore, J. (2012). Motivational interviewing. In M. Neenan & S. Palmer (Eds.), *Cognitive behavioural coaching in practice: An evidence based approach* (pp. 33–52). New York, NY: Routledge/Taylor & Francis.

Aoki, T., Sato, T., & Hosaka, T. (2004). Role of consultation-liaison psychiatry toward shortening of length of stay for medically ill patients with depression. *International Journal of Psychiatry in Clinical Practice, 8,* 71–76. http://dx.doi.org/10.1080/13651500310004957

Appelbaum, P. S., & Grisso, T. (1988). Assessing patients' capacities to consent to treatment. *The New England Journal of Medicine, 319,* 1635–1638. http://dx.doi.org/10.1056/NEJM198812223192504

Arena, J. G., & Blanchard, E. B. (2002). Biofeedback training for chronic pain disorders: A primer. In D. C. Turk & R. J. Gatchel (Eds.), *Psychological approaches to pain management: A practitioner's handbook* (2nd ed., pp. 159–186). New York, NY: Guilford Press.

Arinzon, Z., Peisakh, A., Schrire, S., & Berner, Y. N. (2011). Delirium in long-term care setting: Indicator to severe morbidity. *Archives of Gerontology and Geriatrics, 52,* 270–275. http://dx.doi.org/10.1016/j.archger.2010.04.012

Arnett, P. A., & Randolph, J. J. (2006). Longitudinal course of depression symptoms in multiple sclerosis. *Journal of Neurology, Neurosurgery & Psychiatry, 77,* 606–610. http://dx.doi.org/10.1136/jnnp.2004.047712

Arozullah, A. M., Yarnold, P. R., Bennett, C. L., Soltysik, R. C., Wolf, M. S., Ferreira, R. M., . . . Davis, T. (2007). Development and validation of a short-form, rapid estimate of adult literacy in medicine. *Medical Care, 45,* 1026–1033. http://dx.doi.org/10.1097/MLR.0b013e3180616c1b

Asnis, G. M., & De La Garza, R., 2nd. (2005). Interferon-induced depression: Strategies in treatment. *Progress in Neuro-Psychopharmacology & Biological Psychiatry, 29,* 808–818.

Auerbach, S. M., & Gramling, S. E. (1998). *Stress management.* Upper Saddle River, NJ: Prentice Hall.

Aujla, N., Walker, M., Sprigg, N., Abrams, K., Massey, A., & Vedhara, K. (2016). Can illness beliefs, from the common-sense model, prospectively predict adherence to self-management behaviours? A systematic review and meta-analysis. *Psychology & Health, 31,* 931–958. http://dx.doi.org/10.1080/08870446.2016.1153640

Balboni, T. A., Vanderwerker, L. C., Block, S. D., Paulk, M. E., Lathan, C. S., Peteet, J. R., & Prigerson, H. G. (2007). Religiousness and spiritual support among advanced cancer patients and associations with end-of-life treatment preferences and quality of life. *Journal of Clinical Oncology: Official Journal of the American Society of Clinical Oncology, 25,* 555–560.

Barat, I., Andreasen, F., & Damsgaard, E. M. (2001). Drug therapy in the elderly: What doctors believe and patients actually do. *British Journal of Clinical Pharmacology, 51,* 615–622.

Barnato, A. E., Anthony, D. L., Skinner, J., Gallagher, P. M., & Fisher, E. S. (2009). Racial and ethnic differences in preferences for end-of-life treatment. *Journal of General Internal Medicine, 24,* 695–701. http://dx.doi.org/10.1007/s11606-009-0952-6

Barreira, P. J. (1994). Depression. In S. E. Hyman & G. E. Tesar (Eds.), *Manual of psychiatric emergencies* (3rd ed., pp. 117–128). Boston, MA: Little, Brown.

Barsky, A. J., Goodson, J. D., Lane, R. S., & Cleary, P. D. (1988). The amplification of somatic symptoms. *Psychosomatic Medicine, 50,* 510–519. http://dx.doi.org/10.1097/00006842-198809000-00007

Beal, C. C., Stuifbergen, A. K., & Brown, A. (2007). Depression in multiple sclerosis: A longitudinal analysis. *Archives of Psychiatric Nursing, 21,* 181–191. http://dx.doi.org/10.1016/j.apnu.2007.02.008

Beck, A. T., Steer, R. A., & Brown, G. (1996). *Beck depression inventory—II.* Retrieved from PsycTests. http://dx.doi.org/10.1037/t00742-000

Beckstrand, R. L., Callister, L. C., & Kirchhoff, K. T. (2006). Providing a "good death": Critical care nurses' suggestions for improving end-of-life care. *American Journal of Critical Care, 15,* 38–45.

Bélanger, L., & Ducharme, F. (2011). Patients' and nurses' experiences of delirium: A review of qualitative studies. *Nursing in Critical Care, 16,* 303–315. http://dx.doi.org/10.1111/j.1478-5153.2011.00454.x

Belar, C. D., & Deardorff, W. W. (2009). *Clinical health psychology in medical settings: A practitioner's guidebook* (2nd ed.). Washington, DC: American Psychological Association. http://dx.doi.org/10.1037/11852-000

Bhatti, A. B., Usman, M., & Kandi, V. (2016). Current scenario of HIV/AIDS, treatment options, and major challenges with compliance to antiretroviral therapy. *Cureus, 8,* e515.

Billings, A. G., & Moos, R. H. (1981). The role of coping responses and social resources in attenuating the stress of life events. *Journal of Behavioral Medicine, 4,* 139–157. http://dx.doi.org/10.1007/BF00844267

Bomba, P. A., Kemp, M., & Black, J. S. (2012). POLST: An improvement over traditional advance directives. *Cleveland Clinic Journal of Medicine, 79,* 457–464. http://dx.doi.org/10.3949/ccjm.79a.11098

Bourne, E. J. (2015). *The anxiety & phobia workbook* (6th ed.). Oakland, CA: New Harbinger.

Boustani, M., Peterson, B., Harris, R., Lux, L. J., Krasnov, C., Sutton, S. F., . . . Lohr, K. N. (2003, June). *Screening for dementia* (Systematic Evidence Reviews No. 20). Rockville, MD: Agency for Healthcare Research and Quality.

Braun, U. K. (2016). Experiences with POLST: Opportunities for improving advance care planning: Editorial & comment on: "Use of Physician Orders for Life-Sustaining Treatment Among California Nursing Home Residents." *Journal of General Internal Medicine, 31,* 1111–1112. http://dx.doi.org/10.1007/s11606-016-3795-y

Bravo, G., & Hébert, R. (1997). Age- and education-specific reference values for the Mini-Mental and modified Mini-Mental State Examinations derived from a non-demented elderly population. *International Journal of Geriatric Psychiatry, 12,* 1008–1018. http://dx.doi.org/10.1002/(SICI)1099-1166(199710)12:10<1008::AID-GPS676>3.0.CO;2-A

Breitbart, W., & Cohen, K. R. (1998). Delirium. In J. C. Holland (Ed.), *Psycho-Oncology* (pp. 564–575). New York, NY: Oxford University Press.

Breitbart, W., Rosenfeld, B., Roth, A., Smith, M. J., Cohen, K., & Passik, S. (1997). The memorial delirium assessment scale. *Journal of Pain and Symptom Management, 13,* 128–137.

Broadbent, E., Donkin, L., & Stroh, J. C. (2011). Illness and treatment perceptions are associated with adherence to medications, diet, and exercise in diabetic patients. *Diabetes Care, 34,* 338–340. http://dx.doi.org/10.2337/dc10-1779

Burke, B. L., Arkowitz, H., & Menchola, M. (2003). The efficacy of motivational interviewing: A meta-analysis of controlled clinical trials. *Journal of Consulting and Clinical Psychology, 71,* 843–861. http://dx.doi.org/10.1037/0022-006X.71.5.843

Burke, L. E., Dunbar-Jacob, J. M., & Hill, M. N. (1997). Compliance with cardiovascular disease prevention strategies: A review of the research. *Annals of Behavioral Medicine: A Publication of the Society of Behavioral Medicine, 19,* 239–263.

Burns, J. M., Sneddon, I., Lovell, M., McLean, A., & Martin, B. J. (1992). Elderly patients and their medication: A post-discharge follow-up study. *Age and Ageing, 21,* 178–181. http://dx.doi.org/10.1093/ageing/21.3.178

Byatt, N., Rothschild, A. J., Riskind, P., Ionete, C., & Hunt, A. T. (2011). Relationships between multiple sclerosis and depression. *The Journal of Neuropsychiatry and Clinical Neurosciences, 23,* 198–200. http://dx.doi.org/10.1176/jnp.23.2.jnp198

Caeiro, L., Ferro, J. M., Santos, C. O., & Figueira, M. L. (2006). Depression in acute stroke. *Journal of Psychiatry & Neuroscience, 31,* 377–383. http://search.proquest.com/docview/621655887?accountid=14552

Calhoun, L. G., & Tedeschi, R. G. (2001). Posttraumatic growth: The positive lessons of loss. In R. A. Neimeyer (Ed.), *Meaning reconstruction & the experience of loss* (pp. 157–172). Washington, DC: American Psychological Association. http://dx.doi.org/10.1037/10397-008

Camacho, A., & Ng, B. (2006). Methylphenidate for alpha-interferon induced depression. *Journal of Psychopharmacology, 20,* 687–689.

Cao, D., Srisuma, S., Bronstein, A. C., & Hoyte, C. O. (2016). Characterization of edible marijuana product exposures reported to United States poison centers. *Clinical Toxicology, 54,* 840–846. http://dx.doi.org/10.1080/15563650.2016.1209761

Carroll, K. M., Rounsaville, B. J., & Bryant, K. J. (1993). Alcoholism in treatment-seeking cocaine abusers: Clinical and prognostic significance. *Journal of Studies on Alcohol, 54,* 199–208. http://dx.doi.org/10.15288/jsa.1993.54.199

Carver, C. S., Scheier, M. F., & Segerstrom, S. C. (2010). Optimism. *Clinical Psychology Reviews, 30,* 879–889.

Carver, C. S., Scheier, M. F., & Weintraub, J. K. (1989). Assessing coping strategies: A theoretically based approach. *Journal of Personality and Social Psychology, 56,* 267–283. http://dx.doi.org/10.1037/0022-3514.56.2.267

Center for Behavioral Health Statistics and Quality. (2015). *Behavioral health trends in the United States: Results from the 2014 National Survey on Drug Use and Health* (HHS Publication No. SMA 15-4927, NSDUH Series H-50). Retrieved from http://www.samhsa.gov/data

Centers for Disease Control and Prevention. (2017). *Annual surveillance report of drug-related risks and outcomes.* Retrieved from https://www.cdc.gov/drugoverdose/pdf/pubs/2017-cdc-drug-surveillance-report.pdf

Centers for Disease Control and Prevention. (2018). *International classification of diseases, tenth revision, clinical modification* (ICD–10–CM). Retrieved from https://www.cdc.gov/nchs/icd/icd10cm.htm

Chang, C. H., Chen, S. J., & Liu, C. Y. (2015). Adjuvant treatments of breast cancer increase the risk of depressive disorders: A population-based study. *Journal of Affective Disorders, 182,* 44–49. http://dx.doi.org/10.1016/j.jad.2015.04.027

Chen, A. M. H., Yehle, K. S., Albert, N. M., Ferraro, K. F., Mason, H. L., Murawski, M. M., & Plake, K. S. (2014). Relationships between health literacy and heart failure knowledge, self-efficacy, and self-care adherence. *Research in Social & Administrative Pharmacy, 10,* 378–386. http://dx.doi.org/10.1016/j.sapharm.2013.07.001

Ciraulo, D. A., & Sarid-Segal, O. (2009). Sedative-, hypnotic-, or anxiolytic-related disorders. In B. J. Sadock, V. A. Sadock, & P. Ruiz (Eds.), *Kaplan & Sadock's comprehensive textbook of psychiatry* (9th ed., pp. 1397–1418). Philadelphia, PA: Wolters Kluwer.

Claxton, A. J., Cramer, J., & Pierce, C. (2001). A systematic review of the associations between dose regimens and medication compliance. *Clinical Therapeutics, 23,* 1296–1310.

Colbert, A. M., Sereika, S. M., & Erlen, J. A. (2013). Functional health literacy, medication-taking self-efficacy and adherence to antiretroviral therapy. *Journal of Advanced Nursing, 69,* 295–304. http://dx.doi.org/10.1111/j.1365-2648.2012.06007.x

Colón, E. A., & Popkin, M. K. (2002). Anxiety and panic. In M. G. Wise & J. R. Rundell (Eds.), *The American Psychiatric Publishing textbook of consultation-liaison psychiatry: Psychiatry in the medically ill* (2nd ed., pp. 393–415). Washington, DC: American Psychiatric Association.

Conn, V. S., Ruppar, T. M., Enriquez, M., & Cooper, P. S. (2016). Patient-centered outcomes of medication adherence interventions: Systematic review and meta-analysis. *Value in Health, 19,* 277–285. http://dx.doi.org/10.1016/j.jval.2015.12.001

Cooney, N. L., Kadden, R. M., & Steinberg, H. R. (2008). Assessment of alcohol problems. In D. M. Donovan & G. A. Marlatt (Eds.), *Assessment of addictive behaviors* (pp. 71–112). New York, NY: Guilford Press.

Cordina, M., Fenech, A. G., Vassallo, J., & Cacciottolo, J. M. (2009). Anxiety and the management of asthma in an adult outpatient population. *Therapeutic Advances in Respiratory Disease, 3,* 227–233. http://dx.doi.org/10.1177/1753465809347038

Costa, V., Pereira, M. G., & Pedras, S. (2012). Partner support, social-cognitive variables and their role in adherence to self-monitoring of blood glucose in type 2 diabetes. *European Diabetes Nursing, 9,* 81–86. http://dx.doi.org/10.1002/edn.212

Culpepper, L. (2009). Generalized anxiety disorder and medical illness. *The Journal of Clinical Psychiatry, 70*(Suppl. 2), 20–24.

Curtis, R., Groarke, A., Coughlan, R., & Gsel, A. (2004). The influence of disease severity, perceived stress, social support and coping in patients with chronic illness: A 1 year follow up. *Psychology Health & Medicine, 9,* 456–475. http://dx.doi.org/10.1080/13548500420000267058

Dalton, E. J., & Heinrichs, R. W. (2005). Depression in multiple sclerosis: A quantitative review of the evidence. *Neuropsychology, 19,* 152–158. http://dx.doi.org/10.1037/0894-4105.19.2.152

De Mello, M. T., Lemos, V. A., Antunes, H. K. M., Bittencourt, L., Santos-Silva, R., & Tufik, S. (2013). Relationship between physical activity and depression and anxiety symptoms: A population study. *Journal of Affective Disorders, 149,* 241–246. http://dx.doi.org/10.1016/j.jad.2013.01.035

Dempster, M., Howell, D., & McCorry, N. K. (2015). Illness perceptions and coping in physical health conditions: A meta-analysis. *Journal of Psychosomatic Research, 79,* 506–513. http://dx.doi.org/10.1016/j.jpsychores.2015.10.006

de Ridder, D., Geenen, R., Kuijer, R., & van Middendorp, H. (2008). Psychological adjustment to chronic disease. *The Lancet, 372,* 246–255. http://dx.doi.org/10.1016/S0140-6736(08)61078-8

Dewalt, D. A., Berkman, N. D., Sheridan, S., Lohr, K. N., & Pignone, M. P. (2004). Literacy and health outcomes: A systematic review of the literature. *Journal of General Internal Medicine, 19,* 1228–1239.

Di Marco, F., Verga, M., Santus, P., Giovannelli, F., Busatto, P., Neri, M., . . . Centanni, S. (2010). Close correlation between anxiety, depression, and asthma control. *Respiratory Medicine, 104,* 22–28. http://dx.doi.org/10.1016/j.rmed.2009.08.005

DiMatteo, M. R. (2004). Social support and patient adherence to medical treatment: A meta-analysis. *Health Psychology, 23,* 207–218. http://dx.doi.org/10.1037/0278-6133.23.2.207

DiMatteo, M. R., Haskard-Zolnierek, K. B., & Martin, L. R. (2012). Improving patient adherence: A three-factor model to guide practice. *Health Psychology Review, 6,* 74–91. http://dx.doi.org/10.1080/17437199.2010.537592

Dobmeyer, A. C., & Rowan, A. B. (2014). Core competencies for psychologists: How to succeed in medical settings. In C. M. Hunter, C. L. Hunter, & R. Kessler (Eds.), *The handbook of clinical psychology in medical settings: Evidence-based assessment and intervention* (pp. 77–98). New York, NY: Springer.

Donovan, D. M. (2008). Assessment of addictive behaviors for relapse prevention. In D. M. Donovan & G. A. Marlatt (Eds.), *Assessment of addictive behaviors* (pp. 1–48). New York, NY: Guilford Press.

Douaihy, A., Daley, D. C., Stowell, K. R., & Park, T. W. (2007). Relapse prevention: Clinical strategies for substance use disorders. In K. Witkiewitz & G. A. Marlatt (Eds.), *Therapist's guide to evidence-based relapse prevention* (pp. 37–71). Burlington, MA: Academic Press. http://dx.doi.org/10.1016/B978-012369429-4/50033-1

Doukas, D. J., & Brody, H. (1992). After the Cruzan case: The primary care physician and the use of advance directives. *The Journal of the American Board of Family Practice, 5,* 201–205.

Druss, R. G., & Douglas, C. J. (1988). Adaptive responses to illness and disability. Healthy denial. *General Hospital Psychiatry, 10,* 163–168. http://dx.doi.org/10.1016/0163-8343(88)90015-1

Duangdao, K. M., & Roesch, S. C. (2008). Coping with diabetes in adulthood: A meta-analysis. *Journal of Behavioral Medicine, 31,* 291–300. http://dx.doi.org/10.1007/s10865-008-9155-6

Dunbar-Jacob, J., Gemmell, L. A., & Schlenk, E. A. (2009). Predictors of patient adherence: Patient characteristics. *The handbook of health behavior change* (3rd ed., pp. 398–410). New York, NY: Springer.

Dunbar-Jacob, J., & Schlenk, E. A. (1996). Treatment adherence and clinical outcome: Can we make a difference? In R. J. Resnick & R. H. Rozensky (Eds.), *Health psychology through the life span: Practice and research opportunities* (pp. 323–343). Washington, DC: American Psychological Association.

Dunbar-Jacob, J., & Schlenk, E. (2001). Patient adherence to treatment regimen. In A. Baum, T. A. Revenson, & J. E. Singer (Eds.), *Handbook of health psychology* (pp. 571–580). Mahwah, NJ: Erlbaum.

Dunbar-Jacob, J., Schlenk, E., & McCall, M. (2012). *Patient adherence to treatment regimen.* New York, NY: Psychology Press.

Dunn, L. B., Nowrangi, M. A., Palmer, B. W., Jeste, D. V., & Saks, E. R. (2006). Assessing decisional capacity for clinical research or treatment: A review of instruments. *The American Journal of Psychiatry, 163,* 1323–1334.

Dwyer, M. L., Deshields, T. L., & Nanna, S. K. (2012). Death is a part of life: Considerations for the natural death of a therapy patient. *Professional Psychology: Research and Practice, 43,* 123–129. http://dx.doi.org/10.1037/a0026614

Edelstein, B. (2000). Challenges in the assessment of decision-making capacity. *Journal of Aging Studies, 14,* 423–437. http://dx.doi.org/10.1016/S0890-4065(00)80006-7

Elomaa, M. M., de C. Williams, A. C., & Kalso, E. A. (2009). Attention management as a treatment for chronic pain. *European Journal of Pain, 13,* 1062–1067. http://dx.doi.org/10.1016/j.ejpain.2008.12.002

Ely, E. W., Margolin, R., Francis, J., May, L., Truman, B., Dittus, R., . . . Inouye, S. K. (2001). Evaluation of delirium in critically ill patients: Validation of the Confusion Assessment Method for the Intensive Care Unit (CAM–ICU). *Critical Care Medicine, 29,* 1370–1379. http://dx.doi.org/10.1097/00003246-200107000-00012

Engel, G. L. (1977). The need for a new medical model: A challenge for biomedicine. *Science, 196,* 129–136. http://dx.doi.org/10.1126/science.847460

Engel, G. L. (1980). The clinical application of the biopsychosocial model. *The American Journal of Psychiatry, 137,* 535–544. http://dx.doi.org/10.1176/ajp.137.5.535

Eriksson, I., Gustafson, Y., Fagerström, L., & Olofsson, B. (2011). Urinary tract infection in very old women is associated with delirium. *International Psychogeriatrics, 23,* 496–502. http://dx.doi.org/10.1017/S1041610210001456

Erlangsen, A., Vach, W., & Jeune, B. (2005). The effect of hospitalization with medical illnesses on the suicide risk in the oldest old: A population-based register study. *Journal of the American Geriatrics Society, 53,* 771–776. http://dx.doi.org/10.1111/j.1532-5415.2005.53256.x

Etchells, E., Darzins, P., Silberfeld, M., Singer, P. A., McKenny, J., Naglie, G., . . . Strang, D. (1999). Assessment of patient capacity to consent to treatment. *Journal of General Internal Medicine, 14,* 27–34. http://dx.doi.org/10.1046/j.1525-1497.1999.00277.x

Ewing, J. A. (1984). Detecting alcoholism: The CAGE questionnaire. *JAMA, 252,* 1905–1907. http://dx.doi.org/10.1001/jama.1984.03350140051025

Faaij, R. A., Ziere, G., Zietse, R., & Van der Cammen, T. J. (2009). Delirium due to a drug–drug interaction of lithium and an NSAID. *The Journal of Nutrition, Health & Aging, 13,* 275–276. http://dx.doi.org/10.1007/s12603-009-0072-3

Fagerberg, I., & Jonhagen, M. E. (2002). Temporary confusion: A fearful experience. *Journal of Psychiatric and Mental Health Nursing, 9,* 339–346. http://dx.doi.org/10.1046/j.1365-2850.2002.00498.x

Fagerlin, A., & Schneider, C. E. (2004). Enough: The failure of the living will. *The Hastings Center Report, 34,* 30–42. http://dx.doi.org/10.2307/3527683

Fernandes, L., Fonseca, J., Martins, S., Delgado, L., Pereira, A. C., Vaz, M., & Branco, G. (2010). Association of anxiety with asthma: Subjective and objective outcome measures. *Psychosomatics, 51,* 39–46. http://dx.doi.org/10.1016/S0033-3182(10)70657-5

Fick, D. M., Agostini, J. V., & Inouye, S. K. (2002). Delirium superimposed on dementia: A systematic review. *Journal of the American Geriatrics Society, 50,* 1723–1732.

Fischbach, F., & Dunning, M. B., III. (2015). *A manual of laboratory and diagnostic tests.* Philadelphia, PA: Wolters Kluwer.

Flaherty, J. H. (2011). The evaluation and management of delirium among older persons. *The Medical Clinics of North America, 95,* 555–577, xi. http://dx.doi.org/10.1016/j.mcna.2011.02.005

Fletcher, C., Flight, I., Chapman, J., Fennell, K., & Wilson, C. (2017). The information needs of adult cancer survivors across the cancer continuum: A scoping review. *Patient Education and Counseling, 100,* 383–410. http://dx.doi.org/10.1016/j.pec.2016.10.008

Folkman, S., & Lazarus, R. S. (1985). If it changes it must be a process: Study of emotion and coping during three stages of a college examination. *Journal of Personality and Social Psychology, 48,* 150–170. http://dx.doi.org/10.1037/0022-3514.48.1.150

Folkman, S., Lazarus, R. S., Dunkel-Schetter, C., DeLongis, A., & Gruen, R. J. (1986). Dynamics of a stressful encounter: Cognitive appraisal, coping, and encounter outcomes. *Journal of Personality and Social Psychology, 50,* 992–1003. http://dx.doi.org/10.1037/0022-3514.50.5.992

Folstein, M. F., Folstein, S. E., & McHugh, P. R. (1975). "Mini-Mental State." A practical method for grading the cognitive state of patients for the clinician. *Journal of Psychiatric Research, 12,* 189–198. http://dx.doi.org/10.1016/0022-3956(75)90026-6

Fond, G., Loundou, A., Hamdani, N., Boukouaci, W., Dargel, A., Oliveira, J., . . . Boyer, L. (2014). Anxiety and depression comorbidities in irritable bowel syndrome (IBS): A systematic review and meta-analysis. *European Archives of Psychiatry and Clinical Neuroscience, 264,* 651–660. http://dx.doi.org/10.1007/s00406-014-0502-z

Fong, T. G., Tulebaev, S. R., & Inouye, S. K. (2009). Delirium in elderly adults: Diagnosis, prevention and treatment. *Nature Reviews: Neurology, 5,* 210–220. http://dx.doi.org/10.1038/nrneurol.2009.24

Forissier, T. (2011). *Patient adherence: The next frontier in patient care.* New York, NY: Capgemini Consulting.

Fournier, M., de Ridder, D., & Bensing, J. (2002). How optimism contributes to the adaptation of chronic illness: A prospective study into the enduring effects of optimism on adaptation moderated by the controllability of chronic illness. *Personality and Individual Differences, 33,* 1163–1183. http://dx.doi.org/10.1016/S0191-8869(02)00006-5

Fox, S. A., Heritage, J., Stockdale, S. E., Asch, S. M., Duan, N., & Reise, S. P. (2009). Cancer screening adherence: Does physician–patient communication matter? *Patient Education and Counseling, 75,* 178–184. http://dx.doi.org/10.1016/j.pec.2008.09.010

Fragoso, Y. D., Frota, E. R. C., Lopes, J. S., Noal, J. S., Giacomo, M. C., Gomes, S., . . . Finkelsztejn, A. (2010). Severe depression, suicide attempts, and ideation during the use of interferon beta by patients with multiple sclerosis. *Clinical Neuropharmacology, 33,* 312–316. http://dx.doi.org/10.1097/WNF.0b013e3181f8d513

Franklin, J. E., Jr., Leamon, M. H., & Frances, R. J. (2002). Substance-related disorders. In M. G. Wise & J. R. Rundell (Eds.), *The American Psychiatric Publishing textbook of consultation-liaison psychiatry: Psychiatry in the medically ill* (2nd ed., pp. 417–453). Washington, DC: American Psychiatric Association.

Friedlander, M. M., Brayman, Y., & Breitbart, W. S. (2004). Delirium in palliative care. *Oncology, 18,* 1541–1550; discussion 1551–1553.

Frontera, J. A. (2012). Metabolic encephalopathies in the critical care unit. *Continuum, 18,* 611–639.

Furnham, A. (2003). Belief in a just world: Research progress over the past decade. *Personality and Individual Differences, 34,* 795–817. http://dx.doi.org/10.1016/S0191-8869(02)00072-7

Gadkari, A. S., & McHorney, C. A. (2012). Unintentional non-adherence to chronic prescription medications: How unintentional is it really? *BMC Health Services Research, 12,* 98. Retrieved from https://bmchealthservres.biomedcentral.com/articles/10.1186/1472-6963-12-98

Gall, T. L., & Guirguis-Younger, M. (2013). Religious and spiritual coping: Current theory and research. In K. I. Pargament (Ed.), *APA handbook of psychology, religion, and spirituality: Vol. 1. Context, theory, and research* (pp. 349–364). Washington, DC: American Psychological Association. http://dx.doi.org/10.1037/14045-019

Gallant, M. P. (2003). The influence of social support on chronic illness self-management: A review and directions for research. *Health Education & Behavior, 30,* 170–195. http://dx.doi.org/10.1177/1090198102251030

Gatchel, R. J., & Oordt, M. S. (2003). *Clinical health psychology and primary care.* Washington, DC: American Psychological Association.

Gelberg, L., Andersen, R. M., Afifi, A. A., Leake, B. D., Arangua, L., Vahidi, M., . . . Baumeister, S. E. (2015). Project QUIT (Quit Using Drugs Intervention Trial): A randomized controlled trial of a primary care-based multi-component brief intervention to reduce risky drug use. *Addiction, 110,* 1777–1790. http://dx.doi.org/10.1111/add.12993

Gill, J. R. (2014). The syndrome of excited delirium. *Forensic Science, Medicine, and Pathology, 10,* 223–228. http://dx.doi.org/10.1007/s12024-014-9530-2

Giordano, A., Granella, F., Lugaresi, A., Martinelli, V., Trojano, M., Confalonieri, P., . . . Solari, A., & the SIMS-Trial group. (2011). Anxiety and depression in multiple sclerosis patients around diagnosis. *Journal of the Neurological Sciences, 307,* 86–91. http://dx.doi.org/10.1016/j.jns.2011.05.008

Glass, J. E., Hamilton, A. M., Powell, B. J., Perron, B. E., Brown, R. T., & Ilgen, M. A. (2015). Specialty substance use disorder services following brief alcohol intervention: A meta-analysis of randomized controlled trials. *Addiction, 110,* 1404–1415. http://dx.doi.org/10.1111/add.12950

Glidden-Tracey, C. E. (2005). *Counseling and therapy with clients who abuse alcohol or other drugs: An integrative approach.* Mahwah, NJ: Erlbaum.

Goldston, K., & Baillie, A. J. (2008). Depression and coronary heart disease: A review of the epidemiological evidence, explanatory mechanisms and management approaches. *Clinical Psychology Review, 28,* 288–306. http://dx.doi.org/10.1016/j.cpr.2007.05.005

Goodwin, R. D., & Stein, M. B. (2002). Generalized anxiety disorder and peptic ulcer disease among adults in the United States. *Psychosomatic Medicine, 64,* 862–866.

Goodwin, R. D., Talley, N. J., Hotopf, M., Cowles, R. A., Galea, S., & Jacobi, F. (2013). A link between physician-diagnosed ulcer and anxiety disorders among adults. *Annals of Epidemiology, 23,* 189–192. http://dx.doi.org/10.1016/j.annepidem.2013.01.003

Greenberg, L. S. (2004). Emotion-focused therapy. *Clinical Psychology & Psychotherapy, 11,* 3–16. http://dx.doi.org/10.1002/cpp.388

Grisso, T., Appelbaum, P. S., & Hill-Fotouhi, C. (1997). The MacCAT–T: A clinical tool to assess patients' capacities to make treatment decisions. *Psychiatric Services, 48,* 1415–1419. http://dx.doi.org/10.1176/ps.48.11.1415

Grover, S., & Kate, N. (2012). Assessment scales for delirium: A review. *World Journal of Psychiatry, 2,* 58–70. http://dx.doi.org/10.5498/wjp.v2.i4.58

Gulseren, S., Gulseren, L., Hekimsoy, Z., Cetinay, P., Ozen, C., & Tokatlioglu, B. (2006). Depression, anxiety, health-related quality of life, and disability in patients with overt and subclinical thyroid dysfunction. *Archives of Medical Research, 37,* 133–139.

Hagger, M. S., & Orbell, S. (2003). A meta-analytic review of the common-sense model of illness representations. *Psychology & Health, 18,* 141–184. http://dx.doi.org/10.1080/0887044031000081321

Hall, H. (2003). Imagery and cancer. In A. A. Sheikh (Ed.), *Healing images* (pp. 408–426). Amityville, NY: Baywood.

Hall, W. D., & Degenhardt, L. (2009). Cannabis-related disorders. In B. J. Sadock, V. A. Sadock, & P. Ruiz (Eds.), *Kaplan & Sadock's comprehensive textbook of psychiatry* (9th ed., pp. 1309–1318). Philadelphia, PA: Wolters Kluwer.

Haller, D. L., Acosta, M. C., Newville, H., & Herron, A. (2015). Drug use and abuse. In F. Andrasik, J. L. Goodie, & A. L. Peterson (Eds.), *Biopsychosocial assessment in clinical health psychology* (pp. 87–116). New York, NY: Guilford Press.

Haney, M. (2005). The marijuana withdrawal syndrome: Diagnosis and treatment. *Current Psychiatry Reports, 7,* 360–366. http://dx.doi.org/10.1007/s11920-005-0036-1

Hanson, S. L., Kerkhoff, T. R., & Bush, S. S. (2005). *Health care ethics for psychologists: A casebook.* Washington, DC: American Psychological Association. http://dx.doi.org/10.1037/10845-000

Hardin, K. N. (2004). Chronic pain management. In P. M. Camic & S. J. Knight (Eds.), *Clinical handbook of health psychology: A practical guide to effective interventions* (2nd rev. and exp. ed., pp. 75–99). Ashland, OH: Hogrefe & Huber.

Härter, M. C., Conway, K. P., & Merikangas, K. R. (2003). Associations between anxiety disorders and physical illness. *European Archives of Psychiatry and Clinical Neuroscience, 253*, 313–320. http://dx.doi.org/10.1007/s00406-003-0449-y

Haskard Zolnierek, K. B., & DiMatteo, M. R. (2009). Physician communication and patient adherence to treatment: A meta-analysis. *Medical Care, 47*, 826–834. http://dx.doi.org/10.1097/MLR.0b013e31819a5acc

Helgeson, V. S., Snyder, P., & Seltman, H. (2004). Psychological and physical adjustment to breast cancer over 4 years: Identifying distinct trajectories of change. *Health Psychology, 23*, 3–15. http://dx.doi.org/10.1037/0278-6133.23.1.3

Heyland, D. K., Dodek, P., Rocker, G., Groll, D., Gafni, A., Pichora, D., . . . Lam, M. (2006). What matters most in end-of-life care: Perceptions of seriously ill patients and their family members. *Canadian Medical Association Journal, 174*, 627–633. http://dx.doi.org/10.1503/cmaj.050626

Hildebrandt, H., & Eling, P. (2014). A longitudinal study on fatigue, depression, and their relation to neurocognition in multiple sclerosis. *Journal of Clinical and Experimental Neuropsychology, 36*, 410–417. http://dx.doi.org/10.1080/13803395.2014.903900

Hill, K. P. (2014). Medical marijuana: More questions than answers. *Journal of Psychiatric Practice, 20*, 389–391. http://dx.doi.org/10.1097/01.pra.0000454786.97976.96

Hipp, D. M., & Ely, E. W. (2012). Pharmacological and nonpharmacological management of delirium in critically ill patients. *Neurotherapeutics, 9*, 158–175. http://dx.doi.org/10.1007/s13311-011-0102-9

Hoyt, M. A., & Stanton, A. L. (2012). Adjustment to chronic illness. In A. Baum, T. A. Revenson, & J. Singer (Eds.), *Handbook of health psychology* (2nd ed., pp. 219–246). New York, NY: Psychology Press.

Hsieh, S. J., Ely, E. W., & Gong, M. N. (2013). Can intensive care unit delirium be prevented and reduced? Lessons learned and future directions. *Annals of the American Thoracic Society, 10*, 648–656. http://dx.doi.org/10.1513/AnnalsATS.201307-232FR

Hunter, C. L., Goodie, J. L., Oordt, M. S., & Dobmeyer, A. C. (2017). *Integrated behavioral health in primary care: Step-by-step guidance for assessment and intervention* (2nd ed.). Washington, DC: American Psychological Association.

Hyman, S. E. (1994). Alcohol-related emergencies. In S. E. Hyman & G. E. Tesar (Eds.), *Manual of psychiatric emergencies* (3rd ed., pp. 294–303). Boston, MA: Little, Brown.

Ibrahim, S. A., Kwoh, C. K., & Krishnan, E. (2007). Factors associated with patients who leave acute-care hospitals against medical advice. *American Journal of Public Health, 97*, 2204–2208.

Ingersoll, K. S., & Cohen, J. (2008). The impact of medication regimen factors on adherence to chronic treatment: A review of literature. *Journal of Behavioral Medicine, 31*, 213–224. http://dx.doi.org/10.1007/s10865-007-9147-y

Inouye, S. K., van Dyck, C. H., Alessi, C. A., Balkin, S., Siegal, A. P., & Horwitz, R. I. (1990). Clarifying confusion: The confusion assessment method. A new method for detection of delirium. *Annals of Internal Medicine, 113*, 941–948. http://dx.doi.org/10.7326/0003-4819-113-12-941

Inouye, S. K., Westendorp, R. G. J., & Saczynski, J. S. (2014). Delirium in elderly people. *The Lancet, 383*, 911–922. http://dx.doi.org/10.1016/S0140-6736(13)60688-1

Institute of Medicine. (2015). *Dying in America: Improving quality and honoring individual preferences near the end of life*. Washington, DC: National Academies Press.

Institute of Medicine Committee on Health Literacy. (2004). *Health literacy: A prescription to end confusion*. Washington, DC: National Academies Press.

Irwin, S. A., Pirrello, R. D., Hirst, J. M., Buckholz, G. T., & Ferris, F. D. (2013). Clarifying delirium management: Practical, evidenced-based, expert recommendations for clinical practice. *Journal of Palliative Medicine, 16*, 423–435. http://dx.doi.org/10.1089/jpm.2012.0319

Jacobsen, J., Kvale, E., Rabow, M., Rinaldi, S., Cohen, S., Weissman, D., & Jackson, V. (2014). Helping patients with serious illness live well through the promotion of adaptive coping: A report from the Improving Outpatient Palliative Care (IPAL–OP) Initiative. *Journal of Palliative Medicine, 17*, 463–468.

Jensen, M. P., Molton, I. R., Gertz, K. J., Bombardier, C. H., & Rosenberg, D. E. (2012). Physical activity and depression in middle and older-aged adults with multiple sclerosis. *Disability and Health Journal, 5*, 269–276. http://dx.doi.org/10.1016/j.dhjo.2012.05.006

Johansen, A., Holmen, J., Stewart, R., & Bjerkeset, O. (2012). Anxiety and depression symptoms in arterial hypertension: The influence of antihypertensive treatment. The HUNT study, Norway. *European Journal of Epidemiology, 27*, 63–72. http://dx.doi.org/10.1007/s10654-011-9641-y

Jones, R. T. (2009). Hallucinogen-related disorders. In B. J. Sadock, V. A. Sadock, & P. Ruiz (Eds.), *Kaplan & Sadock's comprehensive textbook of psychiatry* (9th ed., pp. 1331–1340). Philadelphia, PA: Wolters Kluwer.

Kahn, D. R., Bourgeois, J. A., Klein, S. C., & Iosif, A. M. (2009). A prospective observational study of decisional capacity determinations in an academic medical center. *International Journal of Psychiatry in Medicine, 39*, 405–415. http://dx.doi.org/10.2190/PM.39.4.e

Kalish, V. B., Gillham, J. E., & Unwin, B. K. (2014). Delirium in older persons: Evaluation and management. *American Family Physician, 90*, 150–158.

Kaner, E. F., Dickinson, H. O., Beyer, F., Pienaar, E., Schlesinger, C., Campbell, F., . . . Heather, N. (2009). The effectiveness of brief alcohol interventions in primary care settings: A systematic review. *Drug and Alcohol Review, 28*, 301–323. http://dx.doi.org/10.1111/j.1465-3362.2009.00071.x

Katz, J., & Melzack, R. (2011). The McGill Pain Questionnaire. In D. C. Turk & R. Melzack (Eds.), *Handbook of pain assessment* (3rd ed., pp. 45–66). New York, NY: Guilford Press.

Kenna, H. A., Poon, A. W., de los Angeles, C. P., & Koran, L. M. (2011). Psychiatric complications of treatment with corticosteroids: Review with case report. *Psychiatry and Clinical Neurosciences, 65*, 549–560. http://dx.doi.org/10.1111/j.1440-1819.2011.02260.x

Kerns, R. D., Turk, D. C., & Rudy, T. E. (1985). The West Haven–Yale Multidimensional Pain Inventory (WHYMPI). *Pain, 23*, 345–356. http://dx.doi.org/10.1016/0304-3959(85)90004-1

Kerr, C. W., Drake, J., Milch, R. A., Brazeau, D. A., Skretny, J. A., Brazeau, G. A., & Donnelly, J. P. (2012). Effects of methylphenidate on fatigue and depression: A randomized, double-blind, placebo-controlled trial. *Journal of Pain and Symptom Management, 43,* 68–77. http://dx.doi.org/10.1016/j.jpainsymman.2011.03.026

Kim, S. Y. H., Karlawish, J. H. T., & Caine, E. D. (2002). Current state of research on decision-making competence of cognitively impaired elderly persons. *The American Journal of Geriatric Psychiatry, 10,* 151–165. http://dx.doi.org/10.1097/00019442-200203000-00006

King, A., & Hoppe, R. B. (2013). "Best practice" for patient-centered communication: A narrative review. *Journal of Graduate Medical Education, 5,* 385–393. http://dx.doi.org/10.4300/JGME-D-13-00072.1

Knight, K. M., McGowan, L., Dickens, C., & Bundy, C. (2006). A systematic review of motivational interviewing in physical health care settings. *British Journal of Health Psychology, 11*(Pt 2), 319–332. http://dx.doi.org/10.1348/135910705X52516

Koenig, H. G., Larson, D. B., & Larson, S. S. (2001). Religion and coping with serious medical illness. *The Annals of Pharmacotherapy, 35,* 352–359. http://dx.doi.org/10.1345/aph.10215

Kouimtsidis, C., Reynolds, M., Hunt, M., Lind, J., Beckett, J., Drummond, C., & Ghodse, H. (2003). Substance use in the general hospital. *Addictive Behaviors, 28,* 483–499. http://dx.doi.org/10.1016/S0306-4603(01)00263-5

Kraut, A., Fransoo, R., Olafson, K., Ramsey, C. D., Yogendran, M., & Garland, A. (2013). A population-based analysis of leaving the hospital against medical advice: Incidence and associated variables. *BMC Health Services Research, 13,* 415-6963-13-415.

Kripalani, S., Gatti, M. E., & Jacobson, T. A. (2010). Association of age, health literacy, and medication management strategies with cardiovascular medication adherence. *Patient Education and Counseling, 81,* 177–181. http://dx.doi.org/10.1016/j.pec.2010.04.030

Krishnan, V., Leung, L. Y., & Caplan, L. R. (2014). A neurologist's approach to delirium: Diagnosis and management of toxic metabolic encephalopathies. *European Journal of Internal Medicine, 25,* 112–116. http://dx.doi.org/10.1016/j.ejim.2013.11.010

Krueger, K. P., Berger, B. A., & Felkey, B. (2005). Medication adherence and persistence: A comprehensive review. *Advances in Therapy, 22,* 313–356.

Kübler-Ross, E. (1969). *On death and dying.* New York, NY: Macmillan.

Labott, S. (2006). Understanding a patient's wishes to die. *Clinical Case Studies, 5,* 220–230. http://dx.doi.org/10.1177/1534650104264923

Laederach-Hofmann, K., & Bunzel, B. (2000). Noncompliance in organ transplant recipients: A literature review. *General Hospital Psychiatry, 22,* 412–424.

Larson, C. O., Nelson, E. C., Gustafson, D., & Batalden, P. B. (1996). The relationship between meeting patients' information needs and their satisfaction with hospital care and general health status outcomes. *International Journal for Quality in Health Care: Journal of the International Society for Quality in Health Care, 8,* 447–456.

Larson, E. (1988). A causal link between handwashing and risk of infection? Examination of the evidence. *Infection Control and Hospital Epidemiology, 9,* 28–36. http://dx.doi.org/10.2307/30144131

Lau, D. T., & Nau, D. P. (2004). Oral antihyperglycemic medication nonadherence and subsequent hospitalization among individuals with type 2 diabetes. *Diabetes Care, 27,* 2149–2153.

Lazarus, R. S., & Folkman, S. (1984). *Stress, appraisal, and coping.* New York, NY: Springer.

Lee, S. Y., Bender, D. E., Ruiz, R. E., & Cho, Y. I. (2006). Development of an easy-to-use Spanish health literacy test. *Health Services Research, 41,* 1392–1412.

Lee, Y.-Y., & Lin, J. L. (2009). The effects of trust in physician on self-efficacy, adherence and diabetes outcomes. *Social Science & Medicine, 68,* 1060–1068. http://dx.doi.org/10.1016/j.socscimed.2008.12.033

Leitner, L. M. (1995). Optimal therapeutic distance: A therapist's experience of personal construct psychotherapy. In R. A. Neimeyer & M. J. Mahoney (Eds.), *Constructivism in psychotherapy* (pp. 357–370). Washington, DC: American Psychological Association. http://dx.doi.org/10.1037/10170-015

Leo, R. J. (1999). Competency and the capacity to make treatment decisions: A primer for primary care physicians. *Primary Care Companion to the Journal of Clinical Psychiatry, 1,* 131–141. http://dx.doi.org/10.4088/PCC.v01n0501

Leonard, M. M., Agar, M., Spiller, J. A., Davis, B., Mohamad, M. M., Meagher, D. J., & Lawlor, P. G. (2014). Delirium diagnostic and classification challenges in palliative care: Subsyndromal delirium, comorbid delirium-dementia, and psychomotor subtypes. *Journal of Pain and Symptom Management, 48,* 199–214. http://dx.doi.org/10.1016/j.jpainsymman.2014.03.012

Leventhal, H., Brissette, I., & Leventhal, E. A. (2003). The common-sense model of self-regulation of health and illness. *The self-regulation of health and illness behaviour* (pp. 42–65). New York, NY: Routledge.

Leventhal, H., McCarthy, D. E., Leventhal, E. A., & Bold, K. W. (2015). Medication adherence. In F. Andrasik, J. L. Goodie, & A. L. Peterson (Eds.), *Biopsychosocial assessment in clinical health psychology* (pp. 21–46). New York, NY: Guilford Press.

Leventhal, H., Phillips, L. A., & Burns, E. (2016). The Common-Sense Model of Self-Regulation (CSM): A dynamic framework for understanding illness self-management. *Journal of Behavioral Medicine, 39,* 935–946. Advance online publication. http://dx.doi.org/10.1007/s10865-016-9782-2

Lewinsohn, P. M., & Graf, M. (1973). Pleasant activities and depression. *Journal of Consulting and Clinical Psychology, 41,* 261–268. http://dx.doi.org/10.1037/h0035142

Lewis, L. M., Miller, D. K., Morley, J. E., Nork, M. J., & Lasater, L. C. (1995). Unrecognized delirium in ED geriatric patients. *The American Journal of Emergency Medicine, 13,* 142–145. http://dx.doi.org/10.1016/0735-6757(95)90080-2

Lin, C. E., & Mao, W. C. (2010). Mania complicated with delirium following cessation of long-term lithium therapy. *General Hospital Psychiatry, 32,* 102–104. http://dx.doi.org/10.1016/j.genhosppsych.2009.09.003

Linn, A. J., van Weert, J. C. M., van Dijk, L., Horne, R., & Smit, E. G. (2016). The value of nurses' tailored communication when discussing medicines: Exploring the relationship between satisfaction, beliefs and adherence. *Journal of Health Psychology, 21,* 798–807. http://dx.doi.org/10.1177/1359105314539529

Liptzin, B., & Levkoff, S. E. (1992). An empirical study of delirium subtypes. *The British Journal of Psychiatry, 161,* 843–845. http://dx.doi.org/10.1192/bjp.161.6.843

Litman, J. A. (2006). The COPE inventory: Dimensionality and relationships with approach- and avoidance-motives and positive and negative traits. *Personality and Individual Differences, 41,* 273–284. http://dx.doi.org/10.1016/j.paid.2005.11.032

Litman, J. A., & Lunsford, G. D. (2009). Frequency of use and impact of coping strategies assessed by the COPE inventory and their relationships to post-event health and well-being. *Journal of Health Psychology, 14,* 982–991. http://dx.doi.org/10.1177/1359105309341207

Ludwigsen, K. R., & Albright, D. (1994). Training psychologists for hospital practice: A proposal. *Professional Psychology: Research and Practice, 25,* 241–246. http://dx.doi.org/10.1037/0735-7028.25.3.241

Mackenzie, T. B., & Popkin, M. K. (1987). Suicide in the medical patient. *International Journal of Psychiatry in Medicine, 17,* 3–22. http://dx.doi.org/10.2190/EF4F-9KV7-1MLM-MYXQ

Madras, B. K., Compton, W. M., Avula, D., Stegbauer, T., Stein, J. B., & Clark, H. W. (2009). Screening, brief interventions, referral to treatment (SBIRT) for illicit drug and alcohol use at multiple healthcare sites: Comparison at intake and 6 months later. *Drug and Alcohol Dependence, 99,* 280–295. http://dx.doi.org/10.1016/j.drugalcdep.2008.08.003

Maes, S., Leventhal, H., & de Ridder, D. T. D. (1996). Coping with chronic diseases. In M. Zeidner & N. S. Endler (Eds.), *Handbook of coping: Theory, research, applications* (pp. 221–251). New York, NY: Wiley.

Magrin, M. E., D'Addario, M., Greco, A., Miglioretti, M., Sarini, M., Scrignaro, M., . . . Crocetti, E. (2015). Social support and adherence to treatment in hypertensive patients: A meta-analysis. *Annals of Behavioral Medicine, 49,* 307–318. http://dx.doi.org/10.1007/s12160-014-9663-2

Maldonado, J. R. (2008). Delirium in the acute care setting: Characteristics, diagnosis and treatment. *Critical Care Clinics, 24,* 657–722, vii. http://dx.doi.org/10.1016/j.ccc.2008.05.008

Maldonado, J. R. (2010). An approach to the patient with substance use and abuse. *The Medical Clinics of North America, 94,* 1169–1205.

Mammen, G., & Faulkner, G. (2013). Physical activity and the prevention of depression: A systematic review of prospective studies. *American Journal of Preventive Medicine, 45,* 649–657. http://dx.doi.org/10.1016/j.amepre.2013.08.001

Marlatt, G. A., & Witkiewitz, K. (2005). Relapse prevention for alcohol and drug problems. In G. A. Marlatt & D. M. Donovan (Eds.), *Relapse prevention: Maintenance strategies in the treatment of addictive behaviors* (2nd ed., pp. 1–44). New York, NY: Guilford Press.

Marson, D. C., Ingram, K. K., Cody, H. A., & Harrell, L. E. (1995). Assessing the competency of patients with Alzheimer's disease under different legal standards: A prototype instrument. *Archives of Neurology, 52,* 949–954. http://dx.doi.org/10.1001/archneur.1995.00540340029010

Martin, L. R., Haskard-Zolnierek, K. B., & DiMatteo, M. R. (2010). *Health behavior change and treatment adherence: Evidence-based guidelines for improving healthcare.* New York, NY: Oxford University Press.

Martins, R. K., & McNeil, D. W. (2009). Review of motivational interviewing in promoting health behaviors. *Clinical Psychology Review, 29,* 283–293. http://dx.doi.org/10.1016/j.cpr.2009.02.001

Mausbach, B. T., Chattillion, E. A., Moore, R. C., Roepke, S. K., Depp, C. A., & Roesch, S. (2011). Activity restriction and depression in medical patients and their caregivers: A meta-analysis. *Clinical Psychology Review, 31,* 900–908. http://dx.doi.org/10.1016/j.cpr.2011.04.004

McAuley, E., Mullen, S. P., Szabo, A. N., White, S. M., Wójcicki, T. R., Mailey, E. L., . . . Kramer, A. F. (2011). Self-regulatory processes and exercise adherence in older adults: Executive function and self-efficacy effects. *American Journal of Preventive Medicine, 41,* 284–290. http://dx.doi.org/10.1016/j.amepre.2011.04.014

McCann, U. D., & Ricaurte, G. A. (2009). Amphetamine (or amphetamine-like)-related disorders. In B. J. Sadock, V. A. Sadock, & P. Ruiz (Eds.), *Kaplan & Sadock's comprehensive textbook of psychiatry* (9th ed., pp. 1288–1296). Philadelphia, PA: Wolters Kluwer.

McDonald, H. P., Garg, A. X., & Haynes, R. B. (2002). Interventions to enhance patient adherence to medication prescriptions: Scientific review. *JAMA, 288,* 2868–2879. http://dx.doi.org/10.1001/jama.288.22.2868

McNicoll, L., Pisani, M. A., Zhang, Y., Ely, E. W., Siegel, M. D., & Inouye, S. K. (2003). Delirium in the intensive care unit: Occurrence and clinical course in older patients. *Journal of the American Geriatrics Society, 51,* 591–598. http://dx.doi.org/10.1034/j.1600-0579.2003.00201.x

McPherson, C. J., Wilson, K. G., & Murray, M. A. (2007). Feeling like a burden to others: A systematic review focusing on the end of life. *Palliative Medicine, 21,* 115–128. http://dx.doi.org/10.1177/0269216307076345

McWilliams, L. A., Goodwin, R. D., & Cox, B. J. (2004). Depression and anxiety associated with three pain conditions: Results from a nationally representative sample. *Pain, 111,* 77–83. http://dx.doi.org/10.1016/j.pain.2004.06.002

Meagher, D. J., Leonard, M., Donnelly, S., Conroy, M., Adamis, D., & Trzepacz, P. T. (2011). A longitudinal study of motor subtypes in delirium: Relationship with other phenomenology, etiology, medication exposure and prognosis. *Journal of Psychosomatic Research, 71,* 395–403. http://dx.doi.org/10.1016/j.jpsychores.2011.06.001

Meagher, D. J., O'Hanlon, D., O'Mahony, E., Casey, P. R., & Trzepacz, P. T. (2000). Relationship between symptoms and motoric subtype of delirium. *The Journal of Neuropsychiatry and Clinical Neurosciences, 12,* 51–56.

Medline Plus. (n.d.). *Vital signs.* Retrieved from https://medlineplus.gov/ency/article/002341.htm

Meichenbaum, D., & Turk, D. C. (1987). *Facilitating treatment adherence: A practitioner's guidebook.* New York, NY: Plenum Press.

Melchert, T. P. (2015). *Biopsychosocial practice: A science-based framework for behavioral health care.* Washington, DC: American Psychological Association. http://dx.doi.org/10.1037/14441-000

Melzack, R., & Wall, P. D. (1965). Pain mechanisms: A new theory. *Science, 150,* 971–979. http://dx.doi.org/10.1126/science.150.3699.971

Mezey, M. D., Leitman, R., Mitty, E. L., Bottrell, M. M., & Ramsey, G. C. (2000). Why hospital patients do and do not execute an advance directive. *Nursing Outlook, 48,* 165–171.

Miccinesi, G., Bianchi, E., Brunelli, C., & Borreani, C. (2012). End-of-life preferences in advanced cancer patients willing to discuss issues surrounding their terminal condition. *European Journal of Cancer Care, 21,* 623–633. http://dx.doi.org/10.1111/j.1365-2354.2012.01347.x

Miller, T. A. (2016). Health literacy and adherence to medical treatment in chronic and acute illness: A meta-analysis. *Patient Education and Counseling, 99,* 1079–1086. http://dx.doi.org/10.1016/j.pec.2016.01.020

Miller, W. R., & Rollnick, S. (2013). *Motivational interviewing: Helping people change.* New York, NY: Guilford Press.

Mills, P. D., Watts, B. V., & Hemphill, R. R. (2014). Suicide attempts and completions on medical-surgical and intensive care units. *Journal of Hospital Medicine, 9,* 182–185. http://dx.doi.org/10.1002/jhm.2141

Miodownik, C., Alkatnany, A., Frolova, K., & Lerner, V. (2008). Delirium associated with lithium-quetiapine combination. *Clinical Neuropharmacology, 31,* 176–179. http://dx.doi.org/10.1097/WNF.0b013e31814a619d

Misak, C. J. (2004). The critical care experience: A patient's view. *American Journal of Respiratory and Critical Care Medicine, 170,* 357–359. http://dx.doi.org/10.1164/rccm.200403-309OE

Misono, S., Weiss, N. S., Fann, J. R., Redman, M., & Yueh, B. (2008). Incidence of suicide in persons with cancer. *Journal of Clinical Oncology, 26,* 4731–4738. http://dx.doi.org/10.1200/JCO.2007.13.8941

Mitchell, A. J., Shukla, D., Ajumal, H. A., Stubbs, B., & Tahir, T. A. (2014). The Mini-Mental State Examination as a diagnostic and screening test for delirium: Systematic review and meta-analysis. *General Hospital Psychiatry, 36,* 627–633. http://dx.doi.org/10.1016/j.genhosppsych.2014.09.003

Mittal, V., Muralee, S., Williamson, D., McEnerney, N., Thomas, J., Cash, M., & Tampi, R. R. (2011). Review: *Delirium in the elderly: A comprehensive review. American Journal of Alzheimer's Disease and Other Dementias, 26,* 97–109. http://dx.doi.org/10.1177/1533317510397331

Moore, P., Hirst, C., Harding, K. E., Clarkson, H., Pickersgill, T. P., & Robertson, N. P. (2012). Multiple sclerosis relapses and depression. *Journal of Psychosomatic Research, 73,* 272–276. http://dx.doi.org/10.1016/j.jpsychores.2012.08.004

Morris, N. S., MacLean, C. D., Chew, L. D., & Littenberg, B. (2006, March). The Single Item Literacy Screener: Evaluation of a brief instrument to identify limited reading ability. *BMC Family Practice, 7,* 21. http://dx.doi.org/10.1186/1471-2296-7-21

Moskowitz, J. T., Hult, J. R., Bussolari, C., & Acree, M. (2009). What works in coping with HIV? A meta-analysis with implications for coping with serious illness. *Psychological Bulletin, 135,* 121–141. http://dx.doi.org/10.1037/a0014210

Moye, J., Karel, M. J., Azar, A. R., & Gurrera, R. J. (2004). Capacity to consent to treatment: Empirical comparison of three instruments in older adults with and without dementia. *The Gerontologist, 44,* 166–175. http://dx.doi.org/10.1093/geront/44.2.166

Moyers, T. B., & Houck, J. (2011). Combining motivational interviewing with cognitive-behavioral treatments for substance abuse: Lessons from the COMBINE research project. *Cognitive and Behavioral Practice, 18,* 38–45. http://dx.doi.org/10.1016/j.cbpra.2009.09.005

Muller, J. E., Koen, L., & Stein, D. J. (2005). Anxiety and medical disorders. *Current Psychiatry Reports, 7,* 245–251. http://dx.doi.org/10.1007/s11920-005-0077-5

National Institute on Drug Abuse. (2015, November). *Prescription and over-the-counter medications.* Retrieved from https://www.drugabuse.gov/drugs-abuse/prescription-drugs-over-counter-medicines

National Institute on Drug Abuse. (n.d.). *NIDA drug screening tool.* Retrieved from http://drugabuse.gov/nmassist

National POLST Paradigm. (n.d.). Retrieved from http://polst.org

Nejad, S. H., & Alpay, M. (2010). Pain patients. In T. A. Stern, G. L. Fricchione, N. H. Cassem, M. S. Jellinek, & J. F. Rosenbaum (Eds.), *Massachusetts General Hospital handbook of general hospital psychiatry* (6th ed., pp. 211–236). Philadelphia, PA: Saunders.

Nes, L. S., & Segerstrom, S. C. (2006). Dispositional optimism and coping: A meta-analytic review. *Personality and Social Psychology Review, 10,* 235–251. http://dx.doi.org/10.1207/s15327957pspr1003_3

Office of State Guardian [Illinois]. *Health Care Surrogate Act (effective 1998).* Retrieved from http://www2.illinois.gov/sites/gac/OSG/Pages/HCSA.aspx

Oliveira, V. C., Refshauge, K. M., Ferreira, M. L., Pinto, R. Z., Beckenkamp, P. R., Negrao Filho, R. F., & Ferreira, P. H. (2012). Communication that values patient autonomy is associated with satisfaction with care: A systematic review. *Journal of Physiotherapy, 58,* 215–229. http://dx.doi.org/10.1016/S1836-9553(12)70123-6

O'Mahony, R., Murthy, L., Akunne, A., & Young, J. (2011). Synopsis of the national institute for health and clinical excellence guideline for prevention of delirium. *Annals of Internal Medicine, 154,* 746–751. http://dx.doi.org/10.7326/0003-4819-154-11-201106070-00006

Oregon Health Authority, Public Health Division, Center for Health Statistics. (2017). *Oregon Death With Dignity Act: Data summary 2016.* Retrieved from https://public.health.oregon.gov/ProviderPartnerResources/EvaluationResearch/DeathwithDignityAct/Documents/year19.pdf

Oslin, D. W., Pettinati, H., & Volpicelli, J. R. (2002). Alcoholism treatment adherence: Older age predicts better adherence and drinking outcomes. *The American Journal of Geriatric Psychiatry, 10,* 740–747. http://dx.doi.org/10.1097/00019442-200211000-00013

Ossig, C., & Storch, A. (2015). Depression in Huntington's disease. In H. Reichmann (Ed.), *Neuropsychiatric symptoms of movement disorders* (pp. 201–209). Cham, Switzerland: Springer International.

Osterberg, L., & Blaschke, T. (2005). Adherence to medication. *The New England Journal of Medicine, 353,* 487–497. http://dx.doi.org/10.1056/NEJMra050100

Paasche-Orlow, M. K., Parker, R. M., Gazmararian, J. A., Nielsen-Bohlman, L. T., & Rudd, R. R. (2005). The prevalence of limited health literacy. *Journal of General Internal Medicine, 20,* 175–184.

Pagana, K. D., & Pagana, T. J. (2014). *Mosby's manual of diagnostic and laboratory tests* (5th ed.). St. Louis, MO: Elsevier.

Pakenham, K. I., & Rinaldis, M. (2001). The role of illness, resources, appraisal, and coping strategies in adjustment to HIV/AIDS: The direct and buffering effects. *Journal of Behavioral Medicine, 24,* 259–279. http://dx.doi.org/10.1023/A:1010718823753

Pargament, K. I., Koenig, H. G., & Perez, L. M. (2000). The many methods of religious coping: Development and initial validation of the RCOPE. *Journal of Clinical Psychology, 56,* 519–543. http://dx.doi.org/10.1002/(SICI)1097-4679(200004)56:4<519::AID-JCLP6>3.0.CO;2-1

Pargament, K. I., Smith, B. W., Koenig, H. G., & Perez, L. (1998). Patterns of positive and negative religious coping with major life stressors. *Journal for the Scientific Study of Religion, 37,* 710–724. http://dx.doi.org/10.2307/1388152

Patten, S. B., Beck, C. A., Williams, J. V. A., Barbui, C., & Metz, L. M. (2003). Major depression in multiple sclerosis: A population-based perspective. *Neurology, 61,* 1524–1527. http://dx.doi.org/10.1212/01.WNL.0000095964.34294.B4

Pauli, P., Wiedemann, G., Dengler, W., Blaumann-Benninghoff, G., & Kühlkamp, V. (1999). Anxiety in patients with an automatic implantable cardioverter defibrillator: What differentiates them from panic patients? *Psychosomatic Medicine, 61,* 69–76. http://dx.doi.org/10.1097/00006842-199901000-00012

Penn, C., Watermeyer, J., & Evans, M. (2011). Why don't patients take their drugs? The role of communication, context and culture in patient adherence and the work of the pharmacist in HIV/AIDS. *Patient Education and Counseling, 83,* 310–318. http://dx.doi.org/10.1016/j.pec.2011.02.018

Peterson, L. G., & Popkin, M. K. (1980). Neuropsychiatric effects of chemotherapeutic agents for cancer. *Psychosomatics, 21,* 141–153.

Phelps, A. C., Maciejewski, P. K., Nilsson, M., Balboni, T. A., Wright, A. A., Paulk, M. E., . . . Prigerson, H. G. (2009). Religious coping and use of intensive life-prolonging care near death in patients with advanced cancer. *JAMA, 301,* 1140–1147. http://dx.doi.org/10.1001/jama.2009.341

Pincus, D., & Sheikh, A. A. (2009). *Imagery for pain relief: A scientifically grounded guidebook for clinicians.* New York, NY: Routledge.

Pinto, B. M., Rabin, C., & Dunsiger, S. (2009). Home-based exercise among cancer survivors: Adherence and its predictors. *Psycho-Oncology, 18,* 369–376. http://dx.doi.org/10.1002/pon.1465

Popa, S. L., & Dumitrascu, D. L. (2015). Anxiety and IBS revisited: Ten years later. *Clujul Medical (1957), 88,* 253–257.

Pope, T. M. (2013). Legal briefing: The new patient self-determination act. *The Journal of Clinical Ethics, 24,* 156–167.

Pope, T. M., & Hexum, M. (2012). Legal briefing: POLST: Physician orders for life-sustaining treatment. *The Journal of Clinical Ethics, 23,* 353–376.

Portenoy, R. K. (1994). Opioid therapy for chronic nonmalignant pain: Current status. In H. L. Fields & J. C. Liebeskind (Eds.), *Progress in pain research and management* (pp. 247–287). Seattle, WA: IASP Press.

President's Commission for the Study of Ethical Problems in Medicine and Biomedical and Behavioral Research. (1982). *Making health care decisions: A report on the ethical and legal implications of informed consent in the patient–practitioner relationship.* Washington, DC: U.S. Government Printing Office.

Prochaska, J. O., DiClemente, C. C., & Norcross, J. C. (1992). In search of how people change: Applications to addictive behaviors. *American Psychologist, 47,* 1102–1114. http://dx.doi.org/10.1037/0003-066X.47.9.1102

Rao, J. K., Anderson, L. A., Lin, F. C., & Laux, J. P. (2014). Completion of advance directives among U.S. consumers. *American Journal of Preventive Medicine, 46,* 65–70. http://dx.doi.org/10.1016/j.amepre.2013.09.008

Rasmussen, H. N., Wrosch, C., Scheier, M. F., & Carver, C. S. (2006). Self-regulation processes and health: The importance of optimism and goal adjustment. *Journal of Personality, 74,* 1721–1747. http://dx.doi.org/10.1111/j.1467-6494.2006.00426.x

Rentsch, D., Dumont, P., Borgacci, S., Carballeira, Y., deTonnac, N., Archinard, M., & Andreoli, A. (2007). Prevalence and treatment of depression in a hospital department of internal medicine. *General Hospital Psychiatry, 29,* 25–31. http://dx.doi.org/10.1016/j.genhosppsych.2006.08.008

Reuben, D. B., Inouye, S. K., Bogardus, S. T., Jr., Baker, D. I., Leo-Summers, L., & Cooney, L. M., Jr. (2000). The Hospital Elder Life Program: A model of care to prevent cognitive and functional decline in older hospitalized patients. *Journal of the American Geriatrics Society, 48,* 1697–1706. http://dx.doi.org/10.1111/j.1532-5415.2000.tb03885.x

Reynolds, N. R., Martin, F., Nanyonga, R. C., & Alonzo, A. A. (2012). *Self-regulation: The common-sense model of illness representation.* Thousand Oaks, CA: Sage.

Rimm, D. C., & Masters, J. C. (1974). *Behavior therapy: Techniques and empirical findings.* New York, NY: Academic Press.

Robiner, W. N., Dixon, K. E., Miner, J. L., & Hong, B. A. (2010). Hospital privileges for psychologists in the era of competencies and increased accountability. *Journal of Clinical Psychology in Medical Settings, 17,* 301–314. http://dx.doi.org/10.1007/s10880-010-9203-6

Robinson, J. D., & Baker, J. (2006). Psychological consultation and services in a general medical hospital. *Professional Psychology: Research and Practice, 37,* 264–267. http://dx.doi.org/10.1037/0735-7028.37.3.264

Roesch, S. C., Adams, L., Hines, A., Palmores, A., Vyas, P., Tran, C., . . . Vaughn, A. A. (2005). Coping with prostate cancer: A meta-analytic review. *Journal of Behavioral Medicine, 28,* 281–293. http://dx.doi.org/10.1007/s10865-005-4664-z

Roesch, S. C., & Weiner, B. (2001). A meta-analytic review of coping with illness: Do causal attributions matter? *Journal of Psychosomatic Research, 50,* 205–219. http://dx.doi.org/10.1016/S0022-3999(01)00188-X

Rollnick, S., Miller, W. R., & Butler, C. C. (2008). *Motivational interviewing in health care: Helping patients change behavior*. New York, NY: Guilford Press.

Rosenstock, I. M., Strecher, V. J., & Becker, M. H. (1994). The health belief model and HIV risk behavior change. In R. J. DiClemente & J. L. Peterson (Eds.), *Preventing AIDS: Theories and methods of behavioral interventions* (pp. 5–24). New York, NY: Plenum Press. http://dx.doi.org/10.1007/978-1-4899-1193-3_2

Roy, A. (2009). Characteristics of cocaine dependent patients who attempt suicide. *Archives of Suicide Research, 13,* 46–51. http://dx.doi.org/10.1080/13811110802572130

Roy-Byrne, P. P., Davidson, K. W., Kessler, R. C., Asmundson, G. J., Goodwin, R. D., Kubzansky, L., . . . Stein, M. B. (2008). Anxiety disorders and comorbid medical illness. *General Hospital Psychiatry, 30,* 208–225. http://dx.doi.org/10.1016/j.genhosppsych.2007.12.006

Rush, A. J., & Nierenberg, A. A. (2009). Mood disorders: Treatment of depression. In B. J. Sadock, V. A. Sadock, & P. Ruiz (Eds.), *Kaplan & Sadock's comprehensive textbook of psychiatry* (9th ed., pp. 1734–1743). Philadelphia, PA: Wolters Kluwer.

Sabatino, C. P. (1994). The New Uniform Health Care Decisions Act: Paving a health care decisions superhighway? *Maryland Law Review, 53,* 1238–1254.

Safran, D. G., Taira, D. A., Rogers, W. H., Kosinski, M., Ware, J. E., & Tarlov, A. R. (1998). Linking primary care performance to outcomes of care. *The Journal of Family Practice, 47,* 213–220. Retrieved from http://search.proquest.com/docview/619374161?accountid=14552

Saitz, R. (2014). Screening and brief intervention for unhealthy drug use: Little or no efficacy. *Frontiers in Psychiatry, 5,* 121.

Saitz, R., Ciraulo, D. A., Shader, R. I., & Ciraulo, A. M. (2003). Treatment of alcohol withdrawal. In R. I. Shader (Ed.), *Manual of psychiatric therapeutics* (3rd ed., pp. 143–168). Philadelphia, PA: Lippincott Williams & Wilkins.

Saitz, R., Palfai, T. P. A., Cheng, D. M., Alford, D. P., Bernstein, J. A., Lloyd-Travaglini, C. A., . . . Samet, J. H. (2014). Screening and brief intervention for drug use in primary care: The ASPIRE randomized clinical trial. *JAMA, 312,* 502–513. http://dx.doi.org/10.1001/jama.2014.7862

Saunders, J. B., Aasland, O. G., Babor, T. F., de la Fuente, J. R., & Grant, M. (1993). Development of the alcohol use disorders identification test (AUDIT): WHO collaborative project on early detection of persons with harmful alcohol consumption: II. *Addiction, 88,* 791–804. http://dx.doi.org/10.1111/j.1360-0443.1993.tb02093.x

Sawyer, A. M., Gooneratne, N. S., Marcus, C. L., Ofer, D., Richards, K. C., & Weaver, T. E. (2011). A systematic review of CPAP adherence across age groups: Clinical and empiric insights for developing CPAP adherence interventions. *Sleep Medicine Reviews, 15,* 343–356. http://dx.doi.org/10.1016/j.smrv.2011.01.003

Schaefer, G. R., Matus, H., Schumann, J. H., Sauter, K., Vekhter, B., Meltzer, D. O., & Arora, V. M. (2012). Financial responsibility of hospitalized patients who left against medical advice: Medical urban legend? *Journal of General Internal Medicine, 27,* 825–830. http://dx.doi.org/10.1007/s11606-012-1984-x

Schaefer, M., Schwaiger, M., Garkisch, A. S., Pich, M., Hinzpeter, A., Uebelhack, R., . . . Berg, T. (2005). Prevention of interferon-alpha associated depression in psychiatric risk patients with chronic hepatitis C. *Journal of Hepatology, 42,* 793–798.

Schmaling, K. B., Giardino, N. D., Korslund, K. E., Roberts, L. J., & Sweeny, S. (2002). The utility of interdisciplinary training and service: Psychology training on a psychiatry consultation–liaison service. *Professional Psychology: Research and Practice, 33,* 413–417. http://dx.doi.org/10.1037/0735-7028.33.4.413

Schnoll, S. H., & Weaver, M. F. (2003). Addiction and pain. *The American Journal on Addictions, 12*(Suppl. 2), S27–35.

Schoenthaler, A., Chaplin, W. F., Allegrante, J. P., Fernandez, S., Diaz-Gloster, M., Tobin, J. N., & Ogedegbe, G. (2009). Provider communication effects medication adherence in hypertensive African Americans. *Patient Education and Counseling, 75,* 185–191. http://dx.doi.org/10.1016/j.pec.2008.09.018

Schuckit, M. A. (2009). Alcohol-related disorders. In B. J. Sadock, V. A. Sadock, & P. Ruiz (Eds.), *Kaplan & Sadock's comprehensive textbook of psychiatry* (9th ed., pp. 1268–1288). Philadelphia, PA: Wolters Kluwer.

Schüz, B., Marx, C., Wurm, S., Warner, L. M., Ziegelmann, J. P., Schwarzer, R., & Tesch-Römer, C. (2011). Medication beliefs predict medication adherence in older adults with multiple illnesses. *Journal of Psychosomatic Research, 70,* 179–187. http://dx.doi.org/10.1016/j.jpsychores.2010.07.014

Searight, H. R. (1992). Assessing patient competence for medical decision making. *American Family Physician, 45,* 751–759.

Selzer, M. L. (1971). The Michigan alcoholism screening test: The quest for a new diagnostic instrument. *The American Journal of Psychiatry, 127,* 1653–1658. http://dx.doi.org/10.1176/ajp.127.12.1653

Sessums, L. L., Zembrzuska, H., & Jackson, J. L. (2011). Does this patient have medical decision-making capacity? *JAMA, 306,* 420–427. http://dx.doi.org/10.1001/jama.2011.1023

Shalowitz, D. I., Garrett-Mayer, E., & Wendler, D. (2006). The accuracy of surrogate decision makers: A systematic review. *Archives of Internal Medicine, 166,* 493–497.

Siegel, J. D., Rhinehart, E., Jackson, M., Chiarello, L., & Health Care Infection Control Practices Advisory Committee. (2007). 2007 guideline for isolation precautions: Preventing transmission of infectious agents in health care settings. *American Journal of Infection Control, 35*(Suppl. 2), S65–164. http://dx.doi.org/10.1016/j.ajic.2007.10.007

Siegel, S. D., Turner, A. P., & Haselkorn, J. K. (2008). Adherence to disease-modifying therapies in multiple sclerosis: Does caregiver social support matter? *Rehabilitation Psychology, 53,* 73–79. http://dx.doi.org/10.1037/0090-5550.53.1.73

Silveira, M. J., Kim, S. Y. H., & Langa, K. M. (2010). Advance directives and outcomes of surrogate decision making before death. *The New England Journal of Medicine, 362,* 1211–1218. http://dx.doi.org/10.1056/NEJMsa0907901

Simioni, N., Cottencin, O., & Rolland, B. (2015). Interventions for increasing subsequent alcohol treatment utilisation among patients with alcohol use disorders from somatic inpatient settings: A systematic review. *Alcohol and Alcoholism, 50,* 420–429. http://dx.doi.org/10.1093/alcalc/agv017

Simon, N. M., Blacker, D., Korbly, N. B., Sharma, S. G., Worthington, J. J., Otto, M. W., & Pollack, M. H. (2002). Hypothyroidism and hyperthyroidism in anxiety disorders revisited: New data and literature review. *Journal of Affective Disorders, 69,* 209–217.

Simoni, J. M., Frick, P. A., & Huang, B. (2006). A longitudinal evaluation of a social support model of medication adherence among HIV-positive men and women on antiretroviral therapy. *Health Psychology, 25,* 74–81. http://dx.doi.org/10.1037/0278-6133.25.1.74

Singer, P. A., Martin, D. K., & Kelner, M. (1999). Quality end-of-life care: Patients' perspectives. *JAMA, 281,* 163–168. http://dx.doi.org/10.1001/jama.281.2.163

Slooter, A. J., Van De Leur, R. R., & Zaal, I. J. (2017). Delirium in critically ill patients. *Handbook of Clinical Neurology, 141,* 449–466.

Solai, L. K. K. (2009). Delirium. In B. J., Sadock, V. A. Sadock, & P. Ruiz, P. (Eds.), *Kaplan & Sadock's comprehensive textbook of psychiatry* (9th ed., pp. 1153–1167). Philadelphia, PA: Wolters Kluwer.

Spaulding, A., & Silverblatt, F. J. (1993). Using grids to document laboratory results. *Annals of Internal Medicine, 119,* 863. http://dx.doi.org/10.7326/0003-4819-119-8-199310150-00028

Specker, S., Meller, W. H., & Thurber, S. (2009). Psychiatric consultation and substance use disorders. *Substance Abuse: Research and Treatment, 3,* 93–98. http://dx.doi.org/10.4137/SART.S3457

Stapleton, J. A., Russell, M. A., Feyerabend, C., Wiseman, S. M., Gustavsson, G., Sawe, U., & Wiseman, D. (1995). Dose effects and predictors of outcome in a randomized trial of transdermal nicotine patches in general practice. *Addiction, 90,* 31–42. http://dx.doi.org/10.1046/j.1360-0443.1995.901316.x

Stein, L. A. R., & Lebeau-Craven, R. (2002). Motivational interviewing and relapse prevention for DWI: A pilot study. *Journal of Drug Issues, 32,* 1051–1070. http://dx.doi.org/10.1177/002204260203200403

Stocky, A. (1991). Ranitidine and depression. *Australian and New Zealand Journal of Psychiatry, 25,* 415–418. http://dx.doi.org/10.3109/00048679109062644

Strain, E. C., Lofwall, M. R., & Jaffe, J. H. (2009). Opioid-related disorders. In B. J. Sadock, V. A. Sadock, & P. Ruiz (Eds.), *Kaplan & Sadock's comprehensive textbook of psychiatry* (9th ed., pp. 1360–1387). Philadelphia, PA: Wolters Kluwer.

Strub, R. L., & Black, F. W. (2000). *The mental status examination in neurology* (4th ed.). Philadelphia, PA: F. A. Davis.

Substance Abuse and Mental Health Services Administration. (2011). *Screening, brief intervention and referral to treatment (SBIRT) in behavioral healthcare.* Retrieved from samhsa.gov/sites/default/files/sbirtwhitepaper_0.pdf

Substance Abuse and Mental Health Services Administration. (2015). *About screening, brief intervention, and referral to treatment (SBIRT).* Retrieved from www.samhsa.gov/sbirt/about

Substance Abuse and Mental Health Services Administration. (2016, September 8). *Prescription drug use and misuse in the United States: Results from the 2015 National Survey on Drug Use and Health.* http://www.samhsa.gov/data/sites/default/files/NSDUH-FFR2-2015/NSDUH-FFR2-2015.htm

Swain, S., Hariharan, M., Rana, S., Chivukula, U., & Thomas, M. (2015). Doctor–patient communication: Impact on adherence and prognosis among patients with primary hypertension. *Psychological Studies, 60,* 25–32. http://dx.doi.org/10.1007/s12646-014-0291-5

Syrjala, K. L., & Abrams, J. R. (2002). Hypnosis and imagery in the treatment of pain. In D. C. Turk & R. J. Gatchel (Eds.), *Psychological approaches to pain management: A practitioner's handbook* (2nd ed., pp. 187–209). New York, NY: Guilford Press.

Taha, F., Lipsitz, J. D., Galea, S., Demmer, R. T., Talley, N. J., & Goodwin, R. D. (2014). Anxiety disorders and risk of self-reported ulcer: A 10-year longitudinal study among US adults. *General Hospital Psychiatry, 36,* 674–679. http://dx.doi.org/10.1016/j.genhosppsych.2014.07.005

Tavoli, A., Mohagheghi, M. A., Montazeri, A., Roshan, R., Tavoli, Z., & Omidvari, S. (2007). Anxiety and depression in patients with gastrointestinal cancer: Does knowledge of cancer diagnosis matter? *BMC Gastroenterology, 7,* 28.

Tawadrous, D., Dixon, S., Shariff, S. Z., Fleet, J., Gandhi, S., Jain, A. K., . . . Garg, A. X. (2014). Altered mental status in older adults with histamine2-receptor antagonists: A population-based study. *European Journal of Internal Medicine, 25,* 701–709. http://dx.doi.org/10.1016/j.ejim.2014.06.021

Tawk, R., Freels, S., & Mullner, R. (2013). Associations of mental, and medical illnesses with against medical advice discharges: The National Hospital Discharge Survey, 1988–2006. *Administration and Policy in Mental Health, 40,* 124–132.

Tedeschi, R. G., & Calhoun, L. G. (2004). Target article: Posttraumatic growth: Conceptual foundations and empirical evidence. *Psychological Inquiry, 15,* 1–18. http://dx.doi.org/10.1207/s15327965pli1501_01

Teng, E. L., & Chui, H. C. (1987). The Modified Mini-Mental State (3MS) examination. *The Journal of Clinical Psychiatry, 48,* 314–318.

Torke, A. M., Sachs, G. A., Helft, P. R., Petronio, S., Purnell, C., Hui, S., & Callahan, C. M. (2011). Timing of do-not-resuscitate orders for hospitalized older adults who require a surrogate decision-maker. *Journal of the American Geriatrics Society, 59,* 1326–1331. http://dx.doi.org/10.1111/j.1532-5415.2011.03480.x

Tovar, E., Rayens, M. K., Gokun, Y., & Clark, M. (2015). Mediators of adherence among adults with comorbid diabetes and depression: The role of self-efficacy and social support. *Journal of Health Psychology, 20,* 1405–1415. http://dx.doi.org/10.1177/1359105313512514

Tovian, S. M. (2006). Interdisciplinary collaboration in outpatient practice. *Professional Psychology: Research and Practice, 37,* 268–272. http://dx.doi.org/10.1037/0735-7028.37.3.268

Tovian, S. M. (2014). Marketing health psychology. In C. M. Hunter, C. L. Hunter, & R. Kessler (Eds.), *Handbook of clinical psychology in medical settings: Evidence-based assessment and intervention* (pp. 151–168). New York, NY: Springer.

Trachsel, M., Hermann, H., & Biller-Andorno, N. (2015). Cognitive fluctuations as a challenge for the assessment of decision-making capacity in patients with dementia. *American Journal of Alzheimer's Disease and Other Dementias, 30,* 360–363. http://dx.doi.org/10.1177/1533317514539377

Trevino, K. M., Balboni, M., Zollfrank, A., Balboni, T., & Prigerson, H. G. (2014). Negative religious coping as a correlate of suicidal ideation in patients with advanced cancer. *Psycho-Oncology, 23,* 936–945. http://dx.doi.org/10.1002/pon.3505

Trzepacz, P. T., Baker, R. W., & Greenhouse, J. (1988). A symptom rating scale for delirium. *Psychiatry Research, 23,* 89–97.

Trzepacz, P. T., Mittal, D., Torres, R., Kanary, K., Norton, J., & Jimerson, N. (2001). Validation of the Delirium Rating Scale-Revised-98: Comparison with the Delirium Rating Scale and the Cognitive Test for Delirium. *The Journal of Neuropsychiatry and Clinical Neurosciences, 13,* 229–242. http://dx.doi.org/10.1176/jnp.13.2.229

Turan, O., Yemez, B., & Itil, O. (2014). The effects of anxiety and depression symptoms on treatment adherence in COPD patients. *Primary Health Care Research and Development, 15,* 244–251. http://dx.doi.org/10.1017/S1463423613000169

Turk, D. C. (2002). A cognitive-behavioral perspective on treatment of chronic pain patients. In D. C. Turk & R. J. Gatchel (Eds.), *Psychological approaches to pain management: A practitioner's handbook* (2nd ed., pp. 138–158). New York, NY: Guilford Press.

Turk, D. C., & Melzack, R. (2011). *Handbook of pain assessment* (3rd ed.). New York, NY: Guilford Press.

Turk, D. C., Wilson, H. D., & Swanson, K. S. (2012). Psychological and physiological bases of chronic pain. In A. Baum, T. A. Revenson, & J. Singer (Eds.), *Handbook of health psychology* (2nd ed., pp. 149–174). New York, NY: Psychology Press.

Turner, N., Welches, P., & Conti, S. (2013). *Mindfulness-based sobriety: A clinician's treatment guide for addiction recovery using relapse prevention therapy, acceptance and commitment therapy, and motivational interviewing.* Oakland, CA: New Harbinger. Retrieved from http://search.proquest.com.proxy.cc.uic.edu/docview/1539476310?accountid=14552

Unni, E. J., & Farris, K. B. (2011). Unintentional non-adherence and belief in medicines in older adults. *Patient Education and Counseling, 83,* 265–268. http://dx.doi.org/10.1016/j.pec.2010.05.006

Urrutia, I., Aguirre, U., Pascual, S., Esteban, C., Ballaz, A., Arrizubieta, I., & Larrea, I. (2012). Impact of anxiety and depression on disease control and quality of life in asthma patients. *Journal of Asthma, 49,* 201–208. http://dx.doi.org/10.3109/02770903.2011.654022

U.S. Department of Health and Human Services. (2013). *HIPAA administrative simplification, regulation text, 45 CFR parts 160, 162, and 164.* Retrieved from https://www.hhs.gov/sites/default/files/hipaa-simplification-201303.pdf

Vale, A. (2008). Alcohol withdrawal syndrome. *The Foundation Years, 4,* 55–58. http://dx.doi.org/10.1016/j.mpfou.2008.02.010

Vellinga, A., Smit, J. H., Van Leeuwen, E., Van Tilburg, W., & Jonker, C. (2004). Competence to consent to treatment of geriatric patients: Judgements of physicians, family members and the vignette method. *International Journal of Geriatric Psychiatry, 19,* 645–654. http://dx.doi.org/10.1002/gps.1139

Vieira, A. A., Santoro, I. L., Dracoulakis, S., Caetano, L. B., & Fernandes, A. L. (2011). Anxiety and depression in asthma patients: Impact on asthma control. *Jornal Brasileiro De Pneumologia: Publicacao Oficial Da Sociedade Brasileira De Pneumologia e Tisilogia, 37,* 13–18.

Viner, R., Fiest, K. M., Bulloch, A. G. M., Williams, J. V. A., Lavorato, D. H., Berzins, S., . . . Patten, S. B. (2014). Point prevalence and correlates of depression in a national community sample with multiple sclerosis. *General Hospital Psychiatry, 36,* 352–354. http://dx.doi.org/10.1016/j.genhosppsych.2013.12.011

Voaklander, D. C., Rowe, B. H., Dryden, D. M., Pahal, J., Saar, P., & Kelly, K. D. (2008). Medical illness, medication use and suicide in seniors: A population-based case-control study. *Journal of Epidemiology and Community Health, 62,* 138–146. http://dx.doi.org/10.1136/jech.2006.055533

Vodermaier, A., Linden, W., MacKenzie, R., Greig, D., & Marshall, C. (2011). Disease stage predicts post-diagnosis anxiety and depression only in some types of cancer. *British Journal of Cancer, 105,* 1814–1817. http://dx.doi.org/10.1038/bjc.2011.503

Volkow, N. D., Baler, R. D., Compton, W. M., & Weiss, S. R. B. (2014). Adverse health effects of marijuana use. *The New England Journal of Medicine, 370,* 2219–2227.

Wagner, G. J., Goggin, K., Remien, R. H., Rosen, M. I., Simoni, J., Bangsberg, D. R., & Liu, H. (2011). A closer look at depression and its relationship to HIV antiretroviral adherence. *Annals of Behavioral Medicine, 42,* 352–360. http://dx.doi.org/10.1007/s12160-011-9295-8

Waldroup, W. M., Gifford, E. V., & Kalra, P. (2006). Adherence to smoking cessation treatments. In W. T. O'Donohue & E. R. Levensky (Eds.), *Promoting treatment adherence: A practical handbook for health care providers* (pp. 235–252). Thousand Oaks, CA: Sage. http://dx.doi.org/10.4135/9781452225975.n15

Wang, S. M., Chang, J. C., Weng, S. C., Yeh, M. K., & Lee, C. S. (2018). Risk of suicide within 1 year of cancer diagnosis. *International Journal of Cancer, 142,* 1986–1993.

Washington State Department of Health. (2016). *Washington State Department of Health 2015 Death With Dignity Act report.* Retrieved from http://www.doh.wa.gov/portals/1/Documents/Pubs/422-109-DeathWithDignityAct2015.pdf

Weiss, R. D., Greenfield, S. F., & Mirin, S. M. (1994). Intoxication and withdrawal syndromes. In S. E. Hyman & G. E. Tesar (Eds.), *Manual of psychiatric emergencies* (3rd ed., pp. 279–293). Boston, MA: Little, Brown.

Weiss, R. D., & Iannucci, R. A. (2009). Cocaine-related disorders. In B. J. Sadock, V. A. Sadock, & P. Ruiz (Eds.), *Kaplan & Sadock's comprehensive textbook of psychiatry* (9th ed., pp. 1318–1331). Philadelphia, PA: Wolters Kluwer.

West, S., & Kenedi, C. (2014). Strategies to prevent the neuropsychiatric side-effects of corticosteroids: A case report and review of the literature. *Current Opinion in Organ Transplantation, 19,* 201–208. http://dx.doi.org/10.1097/MOT.0000000000000065

Wheeler, K. J., Roberts, M. E., & Neiheisel, M. B. (2014). Medication adherence, part two: Predictors of nonadherence and adherence. *Journal of the American Association of Nurse Practitioners, 26,* 225–232. http://dx.doi.org/10.1002/2327-6924.12105

Wilbourne, P. L., & Miller, W. R. (2002). Treatment for alcoholism: Older and wiser? *Alcoholism Treatment Quarterly, 20,* 41–59.

Wilkinson, A., Gavine, A., & Black, K. (2009). Lithium toxicity presenting as delirium in an older patient. *The Practitioner, 253,* 28–30.

Williamson, G. M. (1998). The central role of restricted normal activities in adjustment to illness and disability: A model of depressed affect. *Rehabilitation Psychology, 43,* 327–347. http://dx.doi.org/10.1037/0090-5550.43.4.327

Williamson, G. M. (2000). Extending the activity restriction model of depressed affect: Evidence from a sample of breast cancer patients. *Health Psychology, 19,* 339–347. http://dx.doi.org/10.1037/0278-6133.19.4.339

Winter, L., & Parks, S. M. (2008). Family discord and proxy decision makers' end-of-life treatment decisions. *Journal of Palliative Medicine, 11,* 1109–1113. http://dx.doi.org/10.1089/jpm.2008.0039

Wise, M. G., Hilty, D. M., Cerda, G. M., & Trzepacz, P. T. (2002). Delirium (confusional states). In M. G. Wise & J. R. Rundell (Eds.), *The American Psychiatric Publishing textbook of consultation-liaison psychiatry: Psychiatry in the medically ill* (2nd ed., pp. 257–272). Washington, DC: American Psychiatric Association.

Witkiewitz, K., & Marlatt, G. A. (2004). Relapse prevention for alcohol and drug problems: That was zen, this is tao. *American Psychologist, 59,* 224–235. http://dx.doi.org/10.1037/0003-066X.59.4.224

Witkiewitz, K., & Marlatt, G. A. (2009). Relapse prevention for alcohol and drug problems. In G. A. Marlatt & K. Witkiewitz (Eds.), *Addictive behaviors* (pp. 403–427). Washington, DC: American Psychological Association.

Wolf, E. J., & Mori, D. L. (2009). Avoidant coping as a predictor of mortality in veterans with end-stage renal disease. *Health Psychology, 28,* 330–337. http://dx.doi.org/10.1037/a0013583

Wong, C. L., Holroyd-Leduc, J., Simel, D. L., & Straus, S. E. (2010). Does this patient have delirium? Value of bedside instruments. *JAMA, 304,* 779–786. http://dx.doi.org/10.1001/jama.2010.1182

World Health Organization. (2002). *Prevention of hospital-acquired infections: A practical guide* (2nd ed.). Retrieved from http://www.who.int/csr/resources/publications/whocdscsreph200212.pdf

World Health Organization. (n.d.). *Health care-associated infections fact sheet.* Retrieved from http://www.who.int/gpsc/country_work/gpsc_ccisc_fact_sheet_en.pdf

Wroe, A. L. (2002). Intentional and unintentional nonadherence: A study of decision making. *Journal of Behavioral Medicine, 25,* 355–372. http://dx.doi.org/10.1023/A:1015866415552

Yohannes, A. M. (2013). Is it quality or quantity of social support needed for patients with chronic medical illness? *Journal of Psychosomatic Research, 74,* 87–88. http://dx.doi.org/10.1016/j.jpsychores.2012.11.009

Young, R. F., & Kahana, E. (1989). Age, medical advice about cardiac risk reduction, and patient compliance. *Journal of Aging and Health, 1,* 121–134. http://dx.doi.org/10.1177/089826438900100108

Zaal, I. J., & Slooter, A. J. (2012). Delirium in critically ill patients: Epidemiology, pathophysiology, diagnosis and management. *Drugs, 72,* 1457–1471. http://dx.doi.org/10.2165/11635520-000000000-00000

Index

B

T

About the Author

Susan M. Labott, PhD, ABPP, received her doctorate in clinical psychology from Northern Illinois University and completed a postdoctoral fellowship at Henry Ford Hospital. She is a professor of clinical psychology in psychiatry at the University of Illinois Hospital and Health Sciences System; in this setting she developed and directed an inpatient health psychology consultation service as well as outpatient health psychology services for 18 years. She is board-certified in clinical health psychology by the American Board of Professional Psychology. She also has interests in ethics and chairs the Social/Behavioral Institutional Review Board at the University of Illinois at Chicago.